Alain Topor

Managing The Contradictions

D1740476

Alain Topor

Managing The Contradictions

Recovery from severe mental illness

LAP LAMBERT Academic Publishing

Impressum / Imprint
Bibliografische Information der Deutschen Nationalbibliothek: Die Deutsche Nationalbibliothek verzeichnet diese Publikation in der Deutschen Nationalbibliografie; detaillierte bibliografische Daten sind im Internet über http://dnb.d-nb.de abrufbar.
Alle in diesem Buch genannten Marken und Produktnamen unterliegen warenzeichen-, marken- oder patentrechtlichem Schutz bzw. sind Warenzeichen oder eingetragene Warenzeichen der jeweiligen Inhaber. Die Wiedergabe von Marken, Produktnamen, Gebrauchsnamen, Handelsnamen, Warenbezeichnungen u.s.w. in diesem Werk berechtigt auch ohne besondere Kennzeichnung nicht zu der Annahme, dass solche Namen im Sinne der Warenzeichen- und Markenschutzgesetzgebung als frei zu betrachten wären und daher von jedermann benutzt werden dürften.

Bibliographic information published by the Deutsche Nationalbibliothek: The Deutsche Nationalbibliothek lists this publication in the Deutsche Nationalbibliografie; detailed bibliographic data are available in the Internet at http://dnb.d-nb.de.
Any brand names and product names mentioned in this book are subject to trademark, brand or patent protection and are trademarks or registered trademarks of their respective holders. The use of brand names, product names, common names, trade names, product descriptions etc. even without a particular marking in this works is in no way to be construed to mean that such names may be regarded as unrestricted in respect of trademark and brand protection legislation and could thus be used by anyone.

Coverbild / Cover image: www.ingimage.com

Verlag / Publisher:
LAP LAMBERT Academic Publishing
ist ein Imprint der / is a trademark of
AV Akademikerverlag GmbH & Co. KG
Heinrich-Böcking-Str. 6-8, 66121 Saarbrücken, Deutschland / Germany
Email: info@lap-publishing.com

Herstellung: siehe letzte Seite /
Printed at: see last page
ISBN: 978-3-8484-4545-5

Zugl. / Approved by: Stockholm, Stockholm University, 2001

Contents

Part I

Part II

Foreword

A doctoral dissertation is a collective effort. Never have I been so dependent on the help and support of so many people as in this endeavour. Those who contributed most, of course, were the study's interview subjects who spoke so openly about their lives – the persons who are subjects of this dissertation. They remain anonymous, although several of them were so proud of what they had experienced that they wished to speak out in their own names.

The one person who has patiently guided me through all the phases of the dissertation is my intrepid supervisor, Professor Anders Bergmark, Department of Social Work at Stockholm University. His confidence in my ideas, his criticisms, encouragement and support are what have sustained me throughout.

Next on the long list of persons who made this work possible are Marit Borg, Elin Kufås, Carsten Bjerke and Johan Svensson, my colleagues in the Nordic Recovery Research Group. The work we did together has extended the bands of our friendship beyond the limits of the project.

Then there are my colleagues at the Department of Social Work at Stockholm University who, throughout the whole of my work to finalise this text, graciously allowed me to use them to test possible formulations and interpretations, offering me constructive criticism to help me on my way. I am grateful to them and to my colleagues who acted as opponents of the various sections of the dissertation: Eva Jeppsson Grassman, Jan Blomqvist, Tommy Lundström and Jan-Håkan Hansson.

Many others at the Department have also encouraged and supported me during my work on this dissertation, among them the members of the seminar group that meets every month under the leadership of Anna-Lena Lindquist the Dean of the Department to discuss social work and research in connection with mental disorders and disability.

A special thanks also my colleagues at the R&D unit of the Western Stockholm Psychiatric Sector, my employer during most of the time I was engaged in writing the dissertation: in particular, Anne Denhov, Irene Karebo Larsén, Christina von Rosen and Dag Tidemalm. They caught many of the weaknesses in how I was handling the material and offered valuable suggestions for remedying them. Special thanks also to Rolf Stackenland, the sector's Head of the Division of Psychiatry and Senior Psychiatrist.

Weddig Runquist and Noella Bickham also have my heartfelt gratitude, for their invaluable linguistic comments and for so much more: Weddig Runquist for his mastodont job in finding and collating all the references, and Noella Bickham for her Homeric effort in preparing the English translation.

Leaving the academic world for a moment, I need only look back at how it all began, on why the dissertation took the direction it took, to be reminded of how much I am indebted to the users and personnel I met at EMMA and Balder, two of the first day centres opened by the social services in Stockholm for "lonely people". The gatherings I witnessed there taught me that change was indeed possible.

My thanks also to the staff and patients with whom I worked, first on ward 53 at Långbro hospital in Stockholm, and afterwards when we moved out of the psychiatric hospital and into Skarpa, an outpatient programme within Southern Stockholm's Enskede-Skarpnäck Psychiatric Sector, under the innovative leadership of Filipe Costa, Head of the Division of Psychiatry and Senior Psychiatrist. It was here that I first got an inkling that chronicity was not inevitable; this conviction has subsequently been a guiding light throughout my professional life.

Johan Cullberg and Sonja Levander in Stockholm, Sandra Escher and Marius Romme in Maastricht, Loren Mosher in San Diego, and Anna Scoppio, Fabio Pittuco, Franco Rotelli, Guiseppe Dell' Acqua in Trieste showed me that psychiatry can indeed think along new channels and find "new ways" to work with persons with severe mental suffering.

To all my friends who let me use them so shamelessly, as friends can be used, my deepest gratitude. They have supported me in my darkest times of dismay and wildest flights into euphoria, in particular Magnus Sundgren, Birgitta Sandström and Leif Öjesjö.

My family, Agneta Guterstam and Sanna Topor have had to undergo so many trials and tribulations during these past years, with endless discussions, and interminable rounds of proof-reading, and with having to put up with my shifts of mood. Dare I hope that there were some moments of joy, as well?

The final stages of this work were financed in part by the Joseph Guinchards Stipendium. This support gave me the leeway I needed to collect my thoughts and bring the work to completion.

But whatever its merits and shortcomings, the ultimate responsibility for this piece of work is mine alone. It has been a great adventure and I would not have missed it for anything.

Alain Topor

In examining their actions and lives one cannot see that they owed anything to fortune beyond opportunity, which brought them the material to mould into the form which seemed best to them. Without that opportunity their powers of mind would have been extinguished, and without those powers the opportunity would have come in vain.

From *Machiavelli*, "The Prince"

1

Introduction:
Background, aims, methods

Chronic mental disorders?

Many people suffer from mental disorders. One of the concerns of psychiatric research is to find out what causes these disorders and how to cure them or make them more manageable. It is clinical psychiatry's task to administer the actual treatment. Throughout the history of psychiatry the definitions of mental illness and the apportioning of madness among the disorders have constantly shifted. There is no consensus on what causes the disorders or diagnoses, nor on what are the most appropriate ways to successfully treat them.

Whenever research has been able to determine the causes of a particular mental disorder and developed a successful treatment for it, the disorder ceases to be classified as belonging to the domain of psychiatry. A case in point is a condition that eventually proved to be the terminal stage of syphilis (*paralysie generale*). It was treated as a mental condition until its cause was determined and it could be treated as a somatic illness (Collé & Quétel 1987). This may explain why the concept "cure" occurs so seldom in psychiatric literature and why there is widespread pessimism about the possibility for patients to recover once they have been diagnosed as severely mentally disturbed. They are by definition chronically ill.

Nevertheless, research results indicate that a significant number of patients diagnosed as severely mentally disturbed eventually improve and some even recover completely. However, there is little documentation on the relationship between particular treatment interventions and recovery and what in the treatment has brought about the recovery.

1

The main question of this study

Despite the lack of successful treatments for people with severe mental disorders, a large number of patients nevertheless recover. What is known today about recovery from severe mental disorders? To what can the improvement in these patients' condition be attributed? And how do these factors impact on the recovery process?

Aims

The aims of the dissertation are twofold:

1. to present what is known today about recovery from severe mental disorders
2. to present the findings of a study on recovery from severe mental disorders from the perspective of those who have recovered, with respect to:

- the course of the recovery process
- which factors according to the interview subjects influenced their recovery
- the interview subjects' descriptions of how these factors have influenced their recovery

It is not the purpose of the dissertation to investigate the effectiveness of specific forms of treatment. On the contrary, the study focuses on finding the common elements in the recovery accounts of persons who have been exposed to various interventions, regardless of whether these interventions can be characterised as treatment or as factors having to do with the person's social life.

Because of its dual aim, the dissertation is divided into two separate but interrelated parts, with different methodological approaches and requirements.

What is known today about recovery

Part I of the dissertation is primarily a literature study where the pertinent works were selected using a number of databases (Medline,

EMBASE Psychiatry, EMBASE Social Work Abstracts. SPRI-line). The search words consisted of a combination of concepts for recovery (recovery and cure) and concepts for chronic illnesses (schizophrenia, psychosis, mental illness and mental disorder). Rather less emphasis has been given to the wealth of literature on rehabilitation and none at all to nursing research. In addition to the literature obtained through the database search, the study also comprises articles listed in the bibliographies in the literature or obtained by contacting researchers in the relevant fields of inquiry.

The literature study is divided into six sections:

1. definitions of the concepts of chronicity and recovery
2. treatment interventions and recovery
3. other factors of relevance for recovery
4. the process of recovery
5. the consequences of research on recovery for the state of the art in psychiatry
6. current research questions

The literature study is a prerequisite for the empirical study in that it:

- provides a background to the empirical study and puts its results in context
- has led to definitions of the central concepts of the empirical study
- has influenced the choice and treatment of the research questions and methods
-

However, the relationship between the literature study and the empirical study is rather more complex than this. The central concepts used at the beginning of the empirical study were obtained from Warner's division of recovery into social and total recovery (1985). The reason for choosing a qualitative method for the study is the generally acknowledged need for qualitative studies of the factors contributing to recovery that are taken up in the literature (Strauss &

Estroff 1989, Strauss & Hafez 1981). The decision to collect concrete in-depth descriptions of what Bertaux calls "*recits de pratiques en situation*" (stories of practice in context[1], Bertaux 1997, p. 8) was motivated by earlier research results and by psychiatry's use of abstract descriptions of both treatment forms and patients (Topor 1996a, b).

The method used in the empirical part of the study is described below. During certain phases, the compilation and analysis of both the literature and the interview material were carried out simultaneously.

In-depth study of recovery practice

The second aim of the dissertation necessitated an empirical study of recovery from problems that have been diagnosed as severe mental disorders. In the field of medicine, including psychiatry, qualitative methods are met with some scepticism. Studies based on small populations, which thereby preclude statistical analysis, and where there are no control groups, are required to justify themselves, unlike research in the humanities and social sciences where qualitative methods are more readily accepted. In the present study, the choice of a qualitative method for conducting an in-depth investigation of data obtained from a small population is a logical consequence of the study's aims. Breier (1988) points out that the advantage of studies of this type is that they offer:

> ... the opportunity for intensive examination of complex interactive phenomena that influence the course of each individual patient. (p. 589)

The empirical study is designed to generate new knowledge. The questions it attempts to answer concern the course of the recovery process and the nature of the contributing factors in the recovery that recur in the life stories of people diagnosed as having severe mental disorders. Sixteen individuals who were earlier treated for severe mental disorders and fulfil specific criteria for recovery were interviewed about their experiences (see Chapter 2 on the definition of recovery).

4

An improbable blend of ideas

In the study certain methodological approaches are used that seem contradictory:

- Bertaux and Bourdieu: Bertaux's field of study is life stories (1981, 1986, 1997); Bourdieu is renown not only for his critique of "the biographical illusion" (1994), but also for a work he did with biographies that has attracted a good deal of attention (1997, in English translation 1999).

- Glaser & Strauss and Bourdieu: In their work on the grounded theory method, Glaser and Strauss (1967, Glaser 1978, Strauss & Corbin 1990) emphasised the importance of the researcher's unfamiliarity with and receptivity to the field of inquiry under study. Bourdieu (1993) has called this stance sociological naivety and rejects the idea of trying to approach an object of study without a preliminary analysis of the field under study.

However, on closer inspection, the apparent contradictions between these authors' work seem to refer more to shades of emphasis than to irreconcilable positions. As this study will try to show, the various perspectives inherent in their work can profitably be combined with one another.

In general, Bertaux's and Glaser & Strauss' work are points of reference in the data collection phase of this study. The tools of grounded theory are used for analysing the data. From Bourdieu the study incorporates some of the ideas and lines of reasoning that he developed in connection with his work with biographical accounts. Thus, Bourdieu's work both complements and is a critical point of reference throughout both parts of the study.

Grounded theory

The research method upon which the study is based is grounded theory. This method was chosen for the following reasons:

5

1. Glaser and Strauss' description of how their method originated corresponds to the aims of this study: to proceed from a "naïve" position in the search for knowledge in a meagrely researched field of inquiry.
2. Glaser and Strauss' presentation of how they developed grounded theory has certain parallels with the leading ideas of this study: it is not a matter of confirming an already existing theory or developing a method of treatment, but of investigating and analysing what people do when faced with a problem that goes beyond their normal terms of reference.
3. The procedures that are a part of grounded theory provide structure to the flexibility that is needed in the data collection phase when investigating a relatively unknown field of inquiry where special receptivity is needed when compiling and analysing the data. Within the framework of grounded theory, the analysis of the material collected should have a bearing on both the preparation of the question guide for subsequent interviews and the selection of interview subjects.
4. The method's requirement that the theory or, in this case, the hypotheses that are formulated during the course of the research be grounded in the data corresponds to a conscious intention in my own approach. This intention is to ensure, as far as possible, that the collection and analysis of what the interview subjects have to relate have not been screened in advance to comply with a preconceived pattern (Strauss & Corbin 1990).

Psychiatry has been characterised as reason's monologue on madness (Foucault 1972). Usually when patients' voices are listened to, they have already been interpreted in terms that confirm the authors' own preconceptions. I am aware, of course, that a wholly naïve perspective is an impossibility; nevertheless, I have endeavoured to let the interview material itself guide me – to be open to being astonished. This means resisting the lure of clever formulations and stories that seem to confirm my expectations and instead, by applying the craftsmanship upon which grounded theory rests, to use to best advantage what the interview subjects have to offer.

The above standpoint is problematic in several respects, two of which will be elaborated here: the feasibility of a naive approach and the quality of the results.

Why a naive approach?

In their book *The discovery of grounded theory: Strategies for qualitative research*, published in 1967, Glaser and Strauss stated that when designing a study, "the initial decisions are not based on a preconceived theoretical framework". (p. 45) Many scholars have pointed out the impossibility of this standpoint. No researcher is a *tabula rasa*. At the same time, however, there have been few studies on recovery from severe mental disorders. Furthermore, when I began my own research on recovery, I was familiar with only a minor and rather special line of inquiry that had to do with the occurrence of recovery. In psychiatry, on the other hand, there are a number of theories purported to be concerned with the causes and treatment of mental disorders. The research on recovery indicated, however, that there was little connection between care and treatment based on these theories and actual recovery (Warner 1985). Thus a naïve approach was not only desirable, it was practically unavoidable.

In recommending that the approach to the object of study be free from a preconceived theoretical filter, Glaser and Strauss (1967) also emphasised that the researcher should be "sufficiently *theoretically sensitive*" (italic in the original, p. 46) when doing the research. Theoretical sensitivity, which develops first after many years experience of doing research, has to do with the researcher's personality, competence in arriving at theoretical insights and knowledge of existing categories, hypotheses and theories within the appropriate fields of inquiry (Glaser 1978). In addition to theoretical sensitivity, the researcher must make a conscious effort to "scrutinize the literature" (Strauss & Corbin 1990, p. 280) for theoretical elements that may be relevant for the emerging theory.

Unlike theoretical sensitivity, which is needed throughout the whole of the research process, the researcher's naivety comes into play primarily when meeting the subjects of the inquiry for the first time and when constructing the initial categories to be used in the data analysis.

Naivety has two functions: it puts the researcher in an open frame of mind with respect to the data, and it discourages any attempt to force reality to fit a preconceived pattern.

Thus, theoretical naivety in relation to the field under study need not result in research becoming "tape-recorder sociology" (*sociologie au magnétophone*) as Bourdieu (1997) feared.

Glaser and Strauss' idea of theoretical sensitivity might even be regarded as a critique of tape-recorder sociology; that is, as being contrary to the wholly naïve approach. In reference to researchers who apply grounded theory, Strauss and Corbin (1990) write:

> They accept responsibility for their interpretative roles. They do not believe it is sufficient merely to report or give voice to the viewpoints of the people, groups or organizations studied. (p. 274)

There is nothing in grounded theory that necessarily contradicts Bourdieu's description of the ideal position of researchers in relation to their data. On the other hand, compared with Bourdieu, Glaser and Strauss' approach clearly implies greater respect for, if not acceptance of, the utterances of the persons under study. Sometimes Bourdieu seems to be saying that he knows better than the respondents what they really mean by what they say, or what they should say and why they do not say it, as posited by the researcher's analysis of the structural conditions of the situation under study:

> Social agents do not innately possess a science of what they are and what they do. More precisely, they do not necessarily have access to the core principles of their discontent or their malaise, and without aiming to mislead, their most spontaneous declarations may express something quite different from what they seem to say. (p. 620)

Here, the researcher not only interprets his/her material, but also assumes the right to over-interpret it. The respondents do not mean what they say. This approach gives the researcher the right to reformulate the subject's utterances to suit the researcher's own "correct" analysis.

This problem has special import in the case of people who have been hospitalised for psychiatric care. The persons we interviewed in this study have experiences from "total institutions" (Goffman 1961). Such institutions have the power not only to redefine the patients but to ensure that they redefine themselves and are redefined by others. Psychiatry's power to redefine the identities of its patients is not restricted to the locked hospital ward. Even though psychoanalysis, for example, frequently asserts the importance of listening to the patient/client, it does so with the aim of hearing something other than what the person actually says. By applying an interpretative filter, the analyst extracts an idea or truth about a person that goes beyond what that person means or is even aware of (Gauchet & Swain 1980, see also Freud 1905/2000).

People who have undergone psychiatric care tend, therefore, to internalise the institutional discourse about themselves; they view their lives in terms of the discourse and reproduce that discourse in their utterances as research subjects (see Hydén 1995). This appears to actualise Bourdieu's position again, when in fact his position reproduces the traditionally dominant discourse where psychiatric patients are presented as being unable to comprehend themselves, to know their own good, to realise the causes of their suffering and to accept the treatment that might neutralise or alleviate their condition.

Even if Bourdieu is correct in his criticism of researchers whose methods call to mind the superficiality of the opinion poll or impressionistic journalism, it is no argument for distrusting experience or the possible emergence of theories grounded in experience. The grounded theory approach is not undertaken primarily for moral considerations – such as giving a voice to those who lack a forum – but to develop knowledge, to introduce new perspectives to the field of psychiatry and thus shed light on its inherent contradictions or, as Bourdieu (1999) himself writes:

> We hope that this structure will have two effects. It should become clear that so-called "difficult" spots ("housing projects" or schools today) [or in our case madness and psychiatry] are, first of all, *difficult to describe and think about*, and that simplistic and one-sided images (notably those found

in the press) must be replaced by a complex and multi-layered representation capable of expressing the same realities but in terms that are different and, sometimes, irreconcilable. Secondly, following the lead of novelists such as Faulkner, Joyce or Woolf, we must relinquish the single, central, dominant, in a word, quasi-divine, point of view that is all too easily adopted by observers – and by readers too, at least to the extent they do not feel personally involved. We must work instead with the multiple perspectives that correspond to the multiplicity of coexisting, and sometimes directly competing, points of view. (p. 3)

That there is a "behind the scenes" analysis in this study becomes apparent in, for example, the use of the concept "total institution" and in the decision to present certain unsaturated results in addition to the main results. However, in the endeavour to generate a new theory, it is not the researcher's task to lay a prefabricated filter over the data, but rather to problematise the relationship between the filtering system and the empirical foundation (including the method for compiling the data). Data collected according to an unconscious, taken-for-granted filter are inaccessible for problematisation. The answer is implied in the question.

Common sense

Another risk implicit in an experience-based approach such as grounded theory is that the results never rise above the level of "common sense" (Alvesson & Sköldberg 1994). There are two different ways of understanding what this risk implies. The first is that the results are self-evident. In countering this criticism, one may well ask whose common sense are we talking about. In the course of the work on this dissertation, I have combed many basic texts in psychiatry to find the origins of the ideas that predominate in psychiatry today. My search has uncovered several contradictory ways of reasoning in psychiatry about, for example, chronicity in connection with mental illnesses, what it means, what causes it and how it is expressed. This means that the results of my study will probably be regarded by some as merely common sense and by others as completely "non sense", not to mention all the possible intermediate positions.

The second is that the results reported remain at the same level of abstraction as the empirical material itself. Strauss has clearly taken this second implication seriously. In an article written together with Corbin (1990), he states that this is not only a risk, but often a reality in much of the research based on grounded theory. Glaser and Strauss (1967) emphasised from the beginning that theory construction is a central aspect of the grounded theory approach.

In this study the aim is to produce what Bertaux describes as:

> … a collection of credible hypotheses, a model based on observation, rich in descriptions of "social mechanisms" and in interpretations (rather than explanations) of the observed phenomena. (Bertaux 1997, p. 19)

The effort to uncover relationships among the hypotheses and categories that have emerged in the present study can be regarded as a first attempt to formulate a substantive theory, but one that is by no means a formal theory.

After many years of collaboration, Strauss, in the later years of his life, no longer agreed with Glaser on what constituted grounded theory. That the two originators of the model could be in basic disagreement about the essence of grounded theory gives special import to Starrin's words (1996):

> Through the years GT has met with increasing acceptance within the academic community. But the theory can be understood in different ways. My view is that the robustness (vitality) of GT lies more in the spirit than the letter. As long as the ambition of its supporters is not to *prescribe* a methodology but *rather* to give *inspiration* to engage in a "process of creation", then GT fills an important role. If GT becomes a mechanically applied rule book, then it has lost its vitality. (Italics in the original, p. 119.)

Life stories

Another point of reference for the present study is the life story method developed by Bertaux (1986, 1997), among others. Bertaux distinguishes between his use of life stories and methods based on life histories. Both Bourdieu and Bertaux point out the risks implicit in the "biographical illusion", risks with which Bertaux has long struggled to manage with the help of his "ethnosociology" and which Bourdieu has tackled in his work *The Weight of the World: Social Suffering in Contemporary Society* (1999; original title in French *La misère du monde* [1993]).

Bertaux collected his life stories by means of interviews and thus they are not strictly autobiographical. Rather, Bertaux points at the dialogical element of the collection as a quality criterion. In his adaptation of the method, life stories are not isolated accounts given by single individuals. They are not concerned with an inner truth; they are not stories about the whole of a person's life. Rather, they are "stories of practice in context" (Bertaux 1997, p. 8) and focus on specific aspects of the person's life.

Bertaux (1997) advocates adopting an ethnosociological perspective within the framework of the life-story method. He regards as possible areas of inquiry what he calls "social worlds" (*monde sociaux*, p. 13) that are constructed around specific activities – first and foremost situational categories (*categories de situations*, p. 15) such as single mothers or unemployed university graduates – and social trajectories (*trajectoires sociales*, p. 15).

Regarding the latter category, Bertaux sees certain problems in that the plurality of life trajectories and the role played by chance make it more difficult to use life stories when making sociological studies of social trajectories. If life stories are used in this context the trajectories being studied must be strictly delineated. The recovery process of severely mentally disordered persons may constitute such a limited social trajectory.

The credibility of life stories?

A crucial question throughout the whole of the study is what is the credibility of the material we have collected and analysed (Bertaux 1997, Hydén 1995, 1997, Kaufmann 1996, Slavney & McHugh 1984)? We discuss, in the following, four aspects of this question:

- The credibility of people suffering from mental disorders. The question is whether we can regard as plausible the life stories told by people who are now, or have been, severely mentally disturbed. This question has received a good deal of attention in recent years in connection with patient satisfaction questionnaires and life quality studies in psychiatry. The one extreme is to question whether people with severe mental disorders are able to express themselves rationally. In an American standard work, for example, the authors write:

> It is not possible to do consumer research on psychiatric hospitals. Although patients often have their own standpoints, these are often determined by their illness and their own subjective experiences. (Mayer & Rosenblatt 1974, p. 433; see also Tatossian 1994)

Expecting people who have been diagnosed as severely mentally disturbed (and therefore, as some would assert, are by definition still afflicted, whether or not their condition is immediately apparent) to comment on their disorder and what may have helped them toward recovery is a logical impossibility. They had, and thus still have, lost their reason.

The other extreme is to assume that, by the very fact of their experiences and life stories, former patients have greater veracity than professionals in psychiatry. This is a tempting position to take considering that the patient perspective is seldom if ever valued, or is valued only to the extent that it confirms the hypotheses of one or the other professional group (Gerhardt 1989). Nevertheless, although such an approach could throw new light on familiar territory, I have chosen to attribute no greater veracity to the patients' accounts than I do to the accounts of the other actors concerned. I have purposely made no attempt to verify or invalidate the life stories collected in this study.

- *Pseudo questions.* To what extent is the response determined by the question? Recovery presupposes that there is something to recover from; it presupposes that the person in question has experienced a period of great difficulty which he or she has been able to some extent to overcome; to have gone from "worse" to "better".

13

- *The past viewed in the light of the present.* The interview material consists of the subjects' reflections about a period in life that is behind them. Which factors determine what events they choose to talk about in the interview and how do they talk about them? To what extent has the "past" been reconstructed in the light of the present?
- *The reality content of life stories.* This aspect concerns the relationship between responses and the actual unfolding of events – "reality". Are the interview responses a story linked to an actual course of events or a narrative that follows the general rules governing stories of this kind, or are they both?
- *The reality content of life stories.* The fourth aspect concerns the relationship between responses and the actual unfolding of events – "reality". Are the interview responses a story about an actual course of events or a narrative that follows the general rules governing stories of this kind, or are they both?

In essence, the last three aspects are concerned with the relationship between texts and real life. Are the collected life stories merely constructions, their content wholly determined by the interviewer, the aims of the interview, the conventions on how to respond to questions and how to tell a story, by the research question and by the interview subjects' aims and position taken at the actual time of the interview; or do these stories have a point of reference outside themselves and other texts, to an actual course of events.

The realist perspective asserts that there is an unmediated relationship between the story/text and reality; the words we use are a direct reflection of reality. In a constructivist perspective, on the other hand, life is the story. "The story does not represent reality, the story creates reality" (Öberg 1997, p. 69).

In presenting the results of the study, I discuss in greater detail the relationship between narrative conventions and reality and how they are intermixed in the interviews. On a principle level, I refer to Öberg's concept "retrospective reflexion" as a fruitful position. On the one hand, it is difficult to defend a purely realist perspective, which its advocates have also acknowledged (Bertaux 1997). On the other hand, from a purely constructivist perspective texts would seem to be the only thing we can talk about. We can produce new texts that refer to other texts which in turn refer to still other texts. From an extreme constructivist perspective it would be difficult to explain how narrative conventions originate at all. By concentrating the search for them in the texts themselves and asserting that texts refer only to other texts, we risk forgetting that narrative conventions must in some sense have a source that, for lack of a better word, could be called reality. That some conventions continue to be used indicates that they bear some relation to real life. Texts reflect something outside the text. And even if the reflection is not a perfect match, the text can be a good enough reflection of that something. If there were no such correspondence, life stories would be like a madman's speech in and about an insane world. But it is also likely that we cannot live in accordance with just any story. This is a question that the Swedish social psychologist, Johan Asplund (1970), was discussing when he wrote:

> But [Ludvig von Bertanffy] seems to mean that this relativity entails a kind of bankruptcy of the truth concept. Yet there has to be some kind of correspondence, an isomorphy, between reality and our perception of it, between reality and our "categories" and "laws". If for no other reason than that the absence of isomorphy would be a disaster in the struggle for life. (p. 78)

Retrospective reflection asserts that there is a relationship between a life story and reality: "The narrator strives for a true and factual representation of his/her life. He/she never puts post-modern question marks around 'fact' or 'truth'". (Öberg 1997, p. 78) According to Öberg, life stories open a window, albeit an opaque one, to history, culture and the mind. Life stories have to do with the tellers' reflective meditation about themselves. The teller and the main character in the story are not the same person. And yet, in a sense, they are:

> Retrospective reflection generates tension because it involves a relationship which (a) the subject in an interview situation has to (b) the life story's subject and to (c) the subject "outside the story" to which the life

story refers. This tension can be studied by analysing the life story's structuring principle – its "plot" or "intrigue". (Öberg 1997, p. 80)

Bertaux (1976, quoted in Heinritz & Rammstedt [1991]), was one of the first to question "the biographical ideology"; he wrote about "the monumental error of the biographical ideology" that left its imprint on much of the earlier research using biographical material (Sartre 1971, Sève 1972, Thomas & Znaniecki 1927). A biographical ideology:

> … was to consist of the mixing together of life stories with life itself and presupposing that each individual life is coherent and has meaning simply because a life is lived from beginning to end by one and the same subject. (p. 350)

This critique is the basis upon which Bertaux developed his way of working with stories of practice in context.

Few have taken Bertaux's criticism to heart.[2] Bourdieu, for example, does not refer to it when, nearly a decade later, he discussed the same question in his article "L'illusion biographique" (The biographical illusion) (Bourdieu 1994). He too regards life stories as artefacts that emanate from and support the notion that a life is coherent and unambiguous. Instead of life stories, he introduces his own concept, *trajectoire*, track or trajectory, which he defines as

> … a series of positions that are assumed successively by one and the same agent (or group) in a room that is in the process of becoming and is constantly changing. (p. 71)

Working with biographical material in practice

Many scholars who use interviews in their research seem to assume that there is a correspondence between the material they have compiled and reported on and a reality beyond the text. This premise gives rise to the question of how to collect the research data so that it lies as close as possible to the reality one is attempting to describe. In connection with his comprhensive interview study, Bourdieu (1999) writes that "… all kinds of distortions are embedded in the very structure of the research situation." (p. 608)

The risk of distorting something implies that there is something to distort, something about which we can acquire knowledge that could also be more or less distorted, something outside the text and outside the interview situation. Kaufmann (1995) criticises this way of looking at distortion and argues that it cannot possibly be about distortions of what we presume to know about a reality that exists beyond all distortions, but rather about variations of one and the same reality:

> It is not so much a question of a distortion of reality as when constructing categories of meaning. Ordinary people do not distort, they form, they produce meaning, truth (their truth). (p. 63)

Distortion or variation; in the last analysis these writers seem to agree that purposeful choices have to be made, both when conducting the interview and when analysing the material.

Bourdieu (1999) argues, for example, for a reflex reflextivity (*réflexivité reflexe*) in order to:

> ... perceive and monitor *on the spot*, as the interview is actually taking place, the effects of the social structure within which it is occurring (p. 608, italic in the original)

In practice, this means to make oneself aware that the study intrudes on a person's life and that this intrusion has consequences. One way to become aware of the consequences is to clarify how the subject of the inquiry understands the situation and the difference between this understanding and the investigator's. The inequality or imbalance between the subject and the investigator has to be dealt with. There are two main sources of the inequality. First of all, it is the investigator who initiates the encounter and dictates the rules. Secondly, it is the investigator who most often possesses greater cultural capital in the form of, for example, linguistic and symbolic goods. To counteract as far as possible the symbolic violence that may be implied in the interview situation, Bourdieu argues that the relationship has to be one of "active and methodical listening" (p. 609). This way of listening differs from the spontaneous actions of even a good interviewer because it affects the very structure of the relationship. In the study *The Weight of the World: Social Suffering in Contemporary Society* (1999) the investigators came into contact with the interview subjects partly through the subjects' friends and acquaintances: "Social proximity and familiarity provide two of the conditions of 'nonviolent' communication." (p. 610) Throughout the investigation, Bourdieu continues, it is important that the person who agrees to participate feel "...that they may legitimately be themselves...". (p. 612)

Bertaux (1997) acknowledges the relevance of these objections, but asserts that the ethnosociological perspective provides tools for dealing with them. The basis for this perspective is the idea that:

> ... existence precedes consciousness, which does not prevent us from thinking that the latter can have repercussions for existence through our actions. (p. 8)

In obtaining a number of "stories of practice in context" that were compiled by means of theoretical sampling:

> ... we have at our disposal a series of testimonies about one and the same social object. Compiling these testimonies enables us to cast off the retrospective colouring and isolate what is the common core of the collected experiences corresponding to their *social* dimension, which is precisely what we are trying to describe. This core should be sought in actions and practices rather than in the representations. (Bertaux 1997, p. 37, italic in the original)

What Bertaux is stressing here is variation (*"l'exigence de variation"*, p. 25) when its comes to the data collection and a concentration on compiling stories of practice; that is, stories whose focus is not on the subject's inner life, value judgements and conceptions but on his/her actions and the context in which they occur: "... the social context about which they have acquired practical knowledge through their experiences". (p. 17)

The striving for plurality can also be said to be at the heart of theoretical sampling as it is used in grounded theory. Glaser and Strauss (1967) stressed the importance of forming the group under study during the actual investigation, as the initial categories emerge.

A central procedure in theoretical sampling is to include new informants in the group under study who differ in a crucial way from the earlier informants. Theoretical sampling can be said to have two concurrent and contradictory aims:

1. to critically examine the emerging categories and create new ones by purposely looking for persons and situations bearing characteristics that contrast with the characteristics of the persons and situations already collected and analysed
2. to achieve saturation in the emerging categories whereby the researcher concentrates on obtaining material that, besides confirming the existing categories, also opens up new dimensions

But where theoretical sampling seeks to validate the central categories in the emerging theory, Bourdieu (1999) stresses the importance of not trying to resolve the contradictions and tension between different world views by rationalising them:

> … it is not enough to explain and present each view on its own. We should also confront them with one another, just as they are confronted in reality, not in order to relativise them by letting their views play against one another ad infinitum, but, on the contrary, just by putting them side by side, to bring to light what results from the clash of different or antagonistic world views; that is, what is, in some cases, the *tragedy* that is created from the clash, where concessions and compromises between viewpoints are impossible because they are all grounded in a social rationale. (p. 17, italic in the original)

Various viewpoints have emerged during the course of the interview study and are discussed in relation to viewpoints in psychiatry. This has sometimes necessitated going back to the historical sources of contemporary psychiatry, which are then confronted with excerpts from the interviews.

Plurality as a methodological principle

Because of various difficulties, we have had to devise special strategies for coming into contact with individuals in the target group of the study and determining who should be included on the basis of specific criteria. By incorporating these strategies into the study, we have endeavoured to satisfy the requirements for theoretical sampling. We have aimed at plurality when it comes to:

- *The interview subjects.* The persons to be interviewed were recruited in accordance with the following variables: sex, age, country (Norway and Sweden), place where they were treated (urban or rural environment), recovery status, family situation, employment situation and housing conditions. We also varied the recruitment procedure so that it included both persons who have recovered by their own assessment and those whom others have assessed as recovered.
- *The forms of psychiatric interventions* to which the interview subjects have been exposed. Variation in the extent and form of treatment intervention, which includes medication, various forms of psychotherapy, social support and social interventions. Two forms of intervention were shared by all the interview subjects: periods of hospitalisation (with one exception) and medication prescribed at some time. During the final phase of the data collection we enlarged the criteria for selecting the interview subjects by including in the study a person who had never been hospitalised.
- *The interviewers.* A group of five persons was responsible for collecting and discussing the material. In forming the group we purposely sought to diversify the group in terms of gender and professional background. Two of the group's members are women and three men. They represent five different professions (occupational therapy, psychiatry, social work, sociology and clinical psychology).

We also sought to obtain diversity among the respondents, but within the range of the predetermined variables, with the one exception from the hospitalisation criterion. Apart from these inclusion criteria, the interview subjects are a relatively heterogeneous group.

Multiplicity as a recruitment goal could have an impact on the generalisability of the collected data. By varying not only the persons who were recruited for the study, but also how they were recruited, we attempted to establish a broad base for our material. The interview group does not consist only of people who were prepared to talk about their experiences and who contacted us on their own initiative. With such a group, no matter how valuable it might be for certain purposes, a special problem arises that has perhaps been best formulated by William James: "Stories happen to people who know how to tell them." (Quoted in Öberg 1997, p. 99) Some of the respondents were recruited by others and were uncertain whether they had anything to say, which is evident in the wide variation in the length of the interviews.

Nordic Recovery Research Group

The main part of the material was collected by a project group, Nordic Recovery Research Group (NRRG). The group devised a joint interview guide and conducted 14 of the 16 interviews. I personally conducted five of the 14 as well as the remaining two. Because their professional backgrounds were varied, the members could throw light on different points of interest during the preparatory, interview and analysis phases. Consensus was reached on all questions that arose during the course of the work and everyone in the group felt enriched by the discussions. The absence of contention in the group can perhaps be explained in that no one in NRRG is affiliated with a specific school of psychiatry. No one felt obliged to defend specific theoretical perspectives and so we could avoid contentious discussions on theory.

A second reason for there being so little contention in the group could be that everyone was clear about the prerequisites for the study. The purpose of the work was not to confirm a specific theory; on the contrary, it was to search for the common elements in our material. What we may have lost through this tendency for eclecticism is difficult to determine. An aspect that we missed in the analysis and which we became aware of through our discussions was the gender perspective.

To ensure that the project group worked from a common conceptual platform two seminars were arranged prior to the start of the data collection phase. The seminars dealt with grounded theory and were led by Bengt Starrin, who has used grounded theory in a number of studies and written a number of books on the theme.

NGGR's work has so far resulted in two reports (Borg & Topor 2001 and Topor, Svensson, Bjerke, Borg & Kufås 1998), one licenciate dissertation (Borg 1999) and two published articles (Borg, Bjerke, Kufås, Topor & Svensson 1998, Topor 1998). An introductory review of the literature on recovery was written by Topor (1997).

For the purposes of this study I have revised the previously published literature review; I have also independently coded all the interviews that were part of the NRRG-study as well as the two interviews I later conducted on my own. Thus, I hope that I have both made good use of the diversity of perspectives in the project group and produced a work of my own.

Procedure and ethical considerations

Contacting people who have suffered from severe mental disorders involves many practical problems and ethical considerations. In our society mental problems are often associated with feelings of shame and guilt, which are intensified through stigmatisation and discrimination. People with a past history of hospitalisation who are now able to manage a life outside of hospital, and even outside psychiatry, tend to erect a barrier between that period in their lives and their current life, an exception being those who become involved in user organisations. There are no special grassroots movements for safeguarding the interests and experiences of people who have recovered, and which we could approach in connection with a study of this kind. Another practical problem is that people who have totally recovered are, by definition, no longer in contact with psychiatry.

To contact in writing people who had been hospitalised in the past for mental problems is generally considered to be unethical. We rejected this approach to avoid the risk that some of the prospective respondents might interpret such a letter as indicating that they still "belonged to" psychiatry. There was also the risk that the letter might be opened by someone other than the addressee and perhaps cause problems in the person's present life. An advertisement in the mass media was a method we considered but rejected because it would be difficult to manage a likely flood of phone calls in an ethically defensible manner.

The study has been reviewed and approved by the Norwegian Regional Committee for Medical Research Ethics (Regionale Komité for Medisinsk Forskningsetikk. Helseregion II). We discussed in the NRRG the suitability of submitting the study for review by an ethical committee. The argument against doing so was that several of the participants were no longer in contact with psychiatry and had been recruited without any assistance from psychiatry. To ask a medical ethical committee to rule on these persons' involvement in the investigation might be an ethical problem in itself. The argument for requesting an ethical review, on the other hand, was that it would provide a good test of the study's design.

We used different ways to come into contact with the interview subjects. We took contact with people who were regarded, and who regarded themselves, as being "socially recovered"[3], several of whom were still receiving outpatient care and/or social service support in connection with their mental problems. These contacts were established mainly through user organisations and through colleagues who were acquainted with the prospective participants and could give them introductory information about the aims and terms of the study.

We also contacted people who were regarded as totally recovered and who were no longer receiving social support or psychiatric care of any kind. These contacts were made through user organisations, through personal contacts and in connection with public lectures on the recovery theme. We recruited one interview subject after hearing him tell about his life in a radio programme.

All of the prospective participants were informed orally about the aims and design of the study. They were also told that they could leave the study at any time during the interview process but not after they had approved the interview transcription. Those persons who were still in contact with psychiatry or the social services were given a guarantee that the interviewers were not connected in any way with the interview subject's activities in these arenas. We informed these persons specifically that should they decide to discontinue their participation, their decision would not affect in any way the support they were receiving from psychiatry and the social services.

We explained to the participants that we would have certain problems to guarantee their anonymity. Although we changed the names of persons and places and the times when various events occurred, because of the research method's concentration on detailed descriptions of concrete situations, there was a possibility that the interview subject would be recognised. We discussed this risk carefully with the respondents. Several wished to appear with their real name. But as this conflicted with our initial ethical considerations and as not all the respondents had the same wish, we did not grant the wish; all names are fictitious.

Everyone whom we contacted or who took contact with the project group were interviewed. One person left the project after reading the interview transcription. Three persons whom we contacted and who were interviewed were subsequently excluded from the study when it became apparent that they did not fill all the selection criteria. In two cases the interview subjects had never received psychiatric care although they had had severe mental problems. In the third case it was revealed during the interview that the person in question had been hospitalised on one occasion during the two-year period immediately preceding the study. In all three cases the interviews were completed to the end but not used in the study. [4]

I chose to accept the diagnoses for which the interview subjects stated they had been treated. This choice is open to criticism on two accounts:

1. The diagnosis for which the patient was treated may be unreliable and thus unsuitable for research purposes. This position relies on the idea that diagnoses reflect an objective condition in the person's mind. However, it is my judgement, based on the research reported in Chapter 2 in connection with the chronicity and recovery concepts, that the diagnoses lack objectivity. Severe mental disorders do not seem to be clearly defined illnesses with specific etiologies and courses of development. Nevertheless, the assumption that an individual probably has the

diagnosis for which he or she has had long-term treatment is defensible if we also make the further assumption that psychiatric diagnoses do not constitute objective frames of reality, but are based on various traditional ways in psychiatry of combining various behaviours to form diagnostic entities.

2. Patients are unreliable when it comes to what they know about the diagnosis or diagnoses they have been given. Some research findings indicate, however, that the self-reported diagnoses of current and former mental patients are fairly reliable. (Cutting & Dunne 1989, Distefano, Pryer & Garrison 1991)

With a single exception, all the respondents could name one or more psychiatric diagnoses for which they had been treated. In the one exception the person was unsure of the exact wording of the diagnosis. This person was critical of psychiatric diagnostics in general and therefore did not attribute any special weight to the diagnosis.[5]

The interviews

Polanyi (1985) distinguishes between life stories and reports. Reports are like simple presentations or compilations, whereas life stories convey actions in context. Polanyi's distinction corresponds to Bertaux's division between life stories and chronicals. (1997, p. 32)

In the present study, the aim of the interviews was to obtain life stories. Our intention was to collect the experiences of a group of individuals and their reflections on their experiences. We were not interested in abstract commentaries that bore little or no relation to concrete experiences. Chase (1995) stresses the importance of the manner in which the questions are posed: sociological questions tend to elicit sociological responses. In her survey of feminist research, she writes:

But the abstraction of such talk – its disconnectedness from their actual lives – made it hollow. (…) the idea of putting sociological questions on the table is naïve – even when done in a collective, feminist spirit – because such questions produce answers that have little to do with how people live their lives. (p. 4)

Chase argues that human beings are bearers of stories of their own lives and experiences which they want to share. Thus in the interview situation the responsibility for the discourse should be left to the person being interviewed:

> Our task as interviewers is to provide the interactional and discursive conditions that will arouse her desire to embrace that responsibility. (p. 12)

Also Bourdieu (1999) embraces the idea that people are bearers of stories; he writes about the joy of expressing oneself (p. 615), and elaborates further:

> By offering the respondent an absolutely exceptional situation for communication, freed from the usual constraints (particularly of time) that weigh on most everyday interchanges, and opening up alternatives which prompt or authorize the articulation of worries, needs or wishes discovered through this very articulation, the researcher helps create the conditions for an extra-ordinary discourse, which might never have been spoken, but which was already there, merely awaiting the conditions for its actualization. (p. 614)

But despite the stress Bourdieu puts on the shadow cast by structural conditions over what is said in an interview and the need for lucid analyses of the situations illuminated in the interview in order to comprehend what the interview subject is saying (even beyond what he/she says), Bourdieu tends to make a fetish of the interview situation. In *The Weight of the World: Social Suffering in Contemporary Society* (1999), which consists mainly of interviews, life stories, that he compiled with the help of colleagues, Bourdieu and his associates describe the interview as:

> ... a sort of *spiritual exercise* that, through *forgetfulness of self*, aims at a true *conversion of the way we look at* other people in the ordinary circumstances of life. (Italics in the original, p. 614)

Furthermore, he recommends that the interviewer's attitude should be one of "a sort of *intellectual love*". (p. 615)

Admittedly, the interview situation can become highly emotional at times, but in Bourdieu's approach there is a gap between the spiritual experience of the interview itself and the subsequent cool-headed analysis. We have attempted to reduce that gap by using a semi-structured interview guide that was developed during the course of the interviews (see Appendix 1). The purpose of the interview guide was to ensure that certain obligatory areas would be included. The manner and order in which these areas were discussed were left to the dynamics of each interview. Besides tracing the respondents' life course and ensuring that most of the preselected areas were commented upon, the interviewers' primary task was to obtain as concrete and detailed descriptions as possible of the situations and events being presented by the respondents. (See Strauss & Corbin 1990, Strauss & Hafez 1981)

The series of interviews had gotten underway before the literature review was completed. Our knowledge of recovery was limited at the initial phase to the findings of several epidemiological studies and to Jerome Franks' (1963) study of the non-specific factors in psycho-therapy. However, that study was concerned only with neuroses. So, our point of departure was truly one of "genuine" naivety with respect to the possible responses we could expect in the interviews.

As mentioned earlier, everyone in the project group had professional experience of psychiatric care, either as a clinician, a researcher or both. Taken together, the group represented an intricate combination of theoretical and practical sensitivities. The project group met on five occasions to discuss the interview material and to develop the inter-view guide.

Before beginning the interview, we presented its aims and purpose in everyday language: we wanted the persons' help to learn what had had an impact on the their recovery; or using Bertaux's terms: "How did it happen?", or "How did it come about?" (*Comment ca marche?*, 1997, p. 17). Each interview began with the question: "How did it all begin?" without specifying what was meant by "it all". In all of the interviews the recovery process itself was discussed, but the process that led to the person's being placed under psychiatric care was also raised by the respondents. This theme seemed to constitute a necessary component in recovery stories. From this initial question a series of life stories unfolded.

The interviews focused on detailed descriptions of concrete situations that had relevance for the recovery process and on the covariance between the actors and other prerequisite factors in each situation. The condition that Bertaux (1997) posited for ensuring that an interview will lead to practical knowledge is that it is "...oriented toward the description of personal experiences and the contexts in which they occurred." (p. 17)

All aspects that had significance for the recovery process were followed up with questions like What? Who? When? Where? How? Can you tell me more about that? and What happened after that? We used the same questions whenever contradictions, interruptions and gaps occurred in the stories. We were careful not to try at all cost to resolve any contradictions occurring in the stories, but rather to concentrate on illuminating their various components.

Tension tended to rise as the interviews progressed. Judging by the respondents' comments, there were primarily two reasons for the heightened tension. The first was, of course, that the interview revived situations where the respondents had experienced themselves as vulnerable with little or no control over their own lives. The second reason was that the revival of the past and the concrete questions we asked resulted in their asking themselves new questions about what they had experienced. There were several occasions when respondents remarked: "No one ever asked me that before". And we cannot eliminate the possibility that they had never asked themselves those questions before either. What has emerged in these interviews is something new, something other than the ready-made question-answer sequences with which many people under psychiatric care have become so familiar.

Particularly the professional clinicians among the interviewers reacted to the emotionally charged atmosphere of the interviews. They commented on the unconventionality of the interview situation where they asked questions of people who had a history of being a mental patient without being in a position to offer them advice, recommend treatment or make decisions. In this interview situation the questions were not intended to bring about a change in the respondent, and this was a radical departure from the kind of clinician-patient relationship to which several of the interviewers were accustomed.

The interviews were carried out at the venue chosen by the respondent: in one's own home, at a café, a day centre or at the administration office of a psychiatric facility. All of the interviews were tape-recorded. In three cases, the interview extended over two or more occasions. The length of the interviews varied between 45 minutes and some 10 hours.

Transcription

The whole of each interview was transcribed. All forms of transcription from speech to written language entail decontextualising.

> The interview is an evolving conversation between two people. The transcriptions are frozen in time and abstracted from their base in a social interaction. (Kvale 1996, p. 166.)

There are different schools regarding transcriptions. At one extreme there is the school that advocates transcribing "everything" just as it was recorded, including pauses, sighs, laughter and so forth; at the other extreme it is considered enough to merely summarise the interview and to include only a few of the actual words spoken at the time. In the first instance, the aim is to capture the whole of the communication occurring during the interview. The problem with this approach is that, no matter how hard we try to write down "everything" that appears on the tape, we will nevertheless miss all of the non-verbal communication (body movements, facial expressions and gestures) as well as certain aspects of the verbal communication, such as intonation, which give the spoken word a particular value. The attempt to capture "everything", in the extreme case, risks becoming a grotesque elaboration of the language at the expense of other aspects of the interchange. Such an endeavour also implies an attempt to resolve the contradiction between the separate rhetorical forms of speech and written language. In the hope of rendering all aspects of the conversation, it is easy to forget that:

> Transcripts are not copies or representations of some original reality, they are interpretative constructions that are useful tools for given purposes. (Kvale 1996, p. 165)

Still another problem with this method of transcription is that the resulting text is difficult to read and cannot easily be handed over to the interview subject for final approval.

The other extreme implies a large measure of arbitrariness in that so little of the actual taped material is transcribed. A highly condensed text leaves a great deal to the researcher's own discretion and little room for surprises. This method of transcription conflicts with the explorative aim of the study, which is to capture the respondents' own words and ways of formulating their experiences.

Deciding which transcription method to use depends at what level the material is to be analysed (Kvale 1996). Kvale discusses three grounds for determining the choice of transcription level: For whom is the transcription intended? For what purpose? and lastly, What are the ethical considerations? These include confidentiality and the possibility for respondents to recognise themselves in what they have said.

We have tried to achieve a balance between reproducing the interview verbatim (spoken language as written language) and interpreting the interview (from spoken language to written language). The aim has been to retain as much as possible of the spoken language, the expressions used, the process which the respondent has gone through to find the right words for formulating his/her experiences (which means testing and rejecting alternative formulations) and the dialogue between the respondent and interviewer that is implicit in spoken language. No words have been changed or added.[6] However, repetitions and profane language that had no significance for the content and structure of the life story were deleted.

The choice of transcription level has also influenced how interview excerpts are used in the presentation of the results. Often they are quite long to give a better idea of the respondent's reasoning. In such manner we hope to dispel any illusion that the analysis and hypotheses presented are the only possible ones (Bertaux 1997).

A transcription was sent to each respondent for final approval. In about half of the cases this resulted in suggestions for changing certain details, which we also did. These changes mostly concerned clarifying a particular course of events and the correct spelling of the person's name. In no instance was it necessary to delete parts of the interview or change the story content (with the exception of the person who left the study at this stage).

The analysis

The aim of the study is to find common components of recovery practice over and above the individual variations. But the study also concerns real-life people, their lives, experiences of suffering and occasions for rejoicing. To preserve traces of the individuals and their specific histories, each person was assigned a new name and the stories of practice have on occasion been reproduced in their context.

The material was analysed in two steps, the first by the project group and the second by myself. The transcriptions were read through several times whereby a number of analytical categories successively emerged.

The quotations that belong to each of these categories were grouped together and read in their new constellations. The risk with this procedure is that quotations are taken out of context and some of the context is lost. To reduce this risk the excerpts were often coded to include more than the specific "point" being made. Consequently, the amount of coded material became fairly extensive, but we considered the advantages of this procedure to outweigh the disadvantages.

Repeated readings of the text pertaining to the different categories brought to light a number of characteristics or features of each category. A central concept in grounded theory is "saturation", which means that the data compiled under a specific category occur often enough in different interviews to make new interviews unnecessary; consequently, the category and its characteristics can be assumed to be grounded in experience. Saturation in the context of research is determined on a subjective, not a statistical, basis.

31

The question of saturation is crucial because it reduces the risk that the researcher will extract from the material only what he/she expects to find. In much of the psychiatric literature clinical observations are reduced to anecdotes having little scientific value (Strauss & Hafez 1981) or to clinical renditions whose only function is to illustrate a particular line of reasoning. They thus acquire an expressive function, says Bertaux (1986, 1997), which jeopardises the results:

> The most common mistake is to put forward an hypothesis, for example one regarding a social mechanism, and then presenting an excerpt from a life story that "illustrates perfectly" this mechanism. Separate incidences may thus be assigned the status of having confirmed a generally applicable hypothesis; furthermore, it is quite likely that the order of the discovery has been reversed artificially. If the quoted excerpt illustrates the hypothesis especially well, a likely reason is that the excerpt provides the basis for developing the hypothesis during the course of the research; is it an *indicium* which one now wishes to give the status of *proof*? Insofar as this is a normal procedure among writers of essays, it is scientifically unacceptable. (1997, p. 113; italics in the original, teanslated form the French)

Saturation does not concern quantity alone; all aspects of a particular category must be elaborated. Deciding whether saturation has been reached always involves some uncertainty. That some of the categories can be found in the work of other researchers is a likely indication that saturation has indeed been reached. In other cases further research is needed to enrich, supplement, confirm or invalidate the resulting hypotheses and analyses.

In reporting on the results of the study, a number of categories and characteristics are presented where saturation was not reached, but which could nevertheless be important for contradicting the content of saturated categories and thereby counteract the invention of a one-dimensional meta-narrative on recovery and its components.

Burke's pentad

Burke (1945) has devised a pentad (five associated aspects) which I found useful for presenting the results of my own study. As Asplund (1980, p. 129) has suggested, Burke could very well be regarded as the co-founder of social psychology along with George Herbert Mead. But in the Swedish literature Burke's work is seldom mentioned[7]. Asplund introduced Burke in 1980 and refers to him again in an essay on the sociology of sports (1987a) where he expresses his regret at not having properly introduced Burke in Sweden the first time.

Burke, who wrote for the most part about fiction, found in his literature analyses that a pentad always appeared in stories about what people do and why they do it.

The pentad consists of:

- Act, what was done?
- Scene, when and where it was done?
- Agent, who did it?
- Agency, how did he/she do it? and
- Purpose, why? (p. XV)

Later in the book Burke subdivides the third category into agent, friends ("co-agents") and enemies ("counter agents") (p. XIX-XX).

The questions that Burke associated with his pentad correspond to the questions we used to elucidate further the "stories of practice in context" we obtained through the interviews. Thus it is not surprising, but is nevertheless interesting, that the analysis and the application of theoretical sensitivity revealed a connection between the outcomes of this study and Burke's own work.[8]

In reporting the results, I use both Burke's pentad and an aspect of the pentad emphasised by Asplund (1980, 1987a), namely that a social event can be understood only by referring to the whole of the pentad, not just one or a few of its key terms. Burke expressed it this way:

We have also likened the terms to the fingers, which in their extremities are distinct from one another, but merge in the palm of the hand. (1945, p. xxii)

No one aspect of the pentad is sufficient in itself; all are necessary if we are to comprehend what people say about what they do.

Burke's pentad serves as a point of departure in presenting the results of the study. However, we depart from the pentad's culturally determined formal structure and Burke's way of formulating the key terms in order to get a better view through the "opaque window" to reality opened up by the stories of practice. In the report on the results of the study, the aspects of the pentad are reviewed in light of the stories of recovery practice in context.

---

[1] Translations of the excerpts in French are my own unless otherwise indicated.

[2] Roos (1992) is one of the exceptions.

[3] This concept is defined in connection with the literature study.

[4] We hope to be able to use the material from the two persons who had not had contact with psychiatry in a later study.

[5] The interview subjects are presented in greater detail in Part II and in Appendix 2.

[6] Translating the interview excerpts into English involved special problems. Spoken language contains many colloquial expressions which of course cannot be translated word for word into another language. The English translator has endeavoured to match the tone and style of the interview subjects' utterances and to use whenever possible corresponding colloquial expressions in English that would be recognisable to both British and American readers.

[7] In Sweden Blomkvist (1996, 1999) and Hydén (1992) have referred to Burke in their own work.

[8] Other scholars quoted in this study who refer to Burke's work are Barrett (1996), Bruner (1987) and Mattingly (1994).

Part I

2

Chronic disorders
and recovery

The point of departure for this study is a paradox: the implied contradiction between the existence of chronic disorders and of recovery from these disorders. It is thus of central importance to explore how these concepts are defined and implemented in practice. To do so we need to answer certain questions. With respect to the first concept, chronicity, we need to know: How is chronic illness defined within psychiatry? and What criteria are used when determining whether a particular state of ill health is chronic?

And with respect to the second concept, recovery, we need to know: How is recovery defined? and How can a patient's recovery be measured?

Both these concepts, chronicity and recovery, must be problematised for the purposes of this study.

The terms chronicity and recovery occur in other scientific disciplines besides psychiatry. Recovery is discussed in connection with drug abuse treatment and research (Blomqvist 1996, 1999; Greenberg 1994) and chronicity occurs in connection with somatic illnesses (Strauss et al. 1984). In the following presentation the use of these terms is limited to the field of psychiatry.

Chronicity

Although frequent reference is made to chronicity in psychiatric research as well as clinical practice, the term has seldom been defined (Bachrach 1988, Belliveau Krausse & Tomaino Slavinsky 1982). The

37

book by Sander, Smith and Weinman (1967) entitled *Chronic psychoses and recovery* is a case in point. Despite the book's promising title, the authors offer no definition of chronicity and in the book's index we find only one pertinent reference: "Chronic, see Length of illness". (p. 336) The Swedish Academy's word list (1985) offers a definition that also takes the duration factor into account but makes an important distinction: "Chronic" in the sense of "constant, persistent", but also "progressively deteriorating, incurable". Two aspects of chronicity stand out in this definition: duration, which is life-long; and progression, by which is meant the tendency toward an inevitable progressive deterioration.

According to Lanteri-Laura (1997) references to chronicity in connection with psychiatric illnesses date back to the latter part of the nineteenth century. Before that time, psychiatry textbooks conveyed an air of optimism about the possibility for mental patients to recover. Lanteri-Laura mentions three decisive factors in the introduction of chronicity as a concept within psychiatry:

- *The establishment of large asylums* whose daily operation depended on having a staff of patients who could work the fields and perform simple maintenance tasks. This prolonged the patients' stay and made their adaptation to life outside the hospital more difficult.
- *The emergence of the degeneration theory.* Degeneration was thought to be an immutable and predestined process that proceeded along two axes; the first was between generations and the second was the illness course within a single generation. Degeneration means:

  > an irreversible chronicity which of necessity progresses from an initial phase of anxiety to beginning paranoia to a third phase marked by meglomania and leading finally, to intellectual deterioration. (p. 38)

- *A renewed interest in dementia* in connection with the rapid rise in longevity. Because of improved living conditions people live longer and thus dementia has become more common. Dementia's course of development served as a model for ways of conceputalising chronicity.

The idea of a natural course of development

Behind the chronic illness concept lies the notion that there is a natural course of development inherent in the untreated illness. Certain illnesses have a short life span; chronic illnesses have a long life span, usually extending over the patient's lifetime. This aspect of chronicity emerges clearly in associated notions of persistent illness, long-term care, incurability, therapy-resistance, severe mental disturbances and mental handicap.

The idea of a natural course of development presupposes that the illness is of organic origin, conforms to a given pattern and follows a given course: "... an inflexible natural history of the disorder." (Harding, Zubin & Strauss 1992, p. 27) The illness is thought to develop through a series of phases, and the progressive deterioration of the individual's mental state is usually taken for granted. New symptoms appear, earlier symptoms become worse, even though there may be periods in which the patient seems free from symptoms. But unlike the episodic illnesses that are of short duration, in chronic illnesses a new episode is called a relapse, a "falling back" into illness. The implication is that the person has never truly recovered from the illness, even though he/she no longer exhibits any symptoms. Pathological processes have continued to operate under the surface.

Chronicity as identity

Ever since the 1930s a distinction has been made between infectious illnesses and chronic illnesses. Through proper treatment, medical science could effectively intervene in the developmental course of infectious illnesses. The treatments cured the patients, they were no longer chronically ill (Burish & Bradley 1983, Strauss et al. 1984). In the case of illnesses defined as chronic, treatment is not directed toward a cure, but toward symptom reduction where the patient's co-operation plays a key role. In the place of a cure, a new concept has appeared in connection with chronic illness – "quality of life" (Terra 1994). Another common term is "palliative care" (Strauss et al. 1984). This has led in recent years to the illumination of a new aspect of chronicity – chronicity as identity.

In research on somatic diseases, attention is given to the social and psychological consequences of chronicity. A chronic illness does not constitute a limited episode in a person's life; rather, it tends to pervade all facets of daily life and makes deep inroads into the individual's self-identity. "Chronic diseases are disproportionately intrusive on the life of the patients", write Strauss et al. (1984, p. 13). Often persons so afflicted have to adapt their lives to fit strict routines and may have to give up many of the activities that interested them before the onset of the illness. The treatment may have serious side-effects, and this also reduces the person's chances to live a normal life. The fluctuating character of a chronic illness makes it difficult to plan for the day, never mind the future. Financial problems usually follow in the wake of a chronic illness. A chronically ill person may have to take extended sick leaves or even exit from the job market altogether. And a chronically ill person may feel driven to experiment with forms of treatment that have not been approved by the medical community and are therefore not covered by the national insurance system.

Because of the tremendous impact chronic illnesses have on a person's life over such a long period of time, they tend to play a dominant role in how chronically ill persons are regarded, both by themselves and by the people in their surroundings. Very little attention has been paid in psychiatry to the social and psychological aspects of chronicity. This may be because the disorders that come under psychiatric care are, by definition, an assault on the person's whole identity and social life. An altered sense of identity is regarded in most cases as a symptom of the illness and not as an expression or reflection of the person's altered social situation and the psychological dilemma with which he/she must now contend.

Chronicity in psychiatry

In psychiatry the various aspects of chronicity have been summarised in four criteria that are applied singly or in various combinations (Bachrach 1988): diagnosis, duration, hospitalisation and functional disability.

Diagnosis

There is still some uncertainty in psychiatry about which diagnoses to associate with chronicity. Nevertheless, in Minkoff's (1978) view: "The population of chronic mentally ill is best defined according to diagnosis". (p. 12) The diagnoses he refers to are schizophrenia, manic-depression, alcoholism, organic brain damage associated with senility and syphilis, developmental disabilities and certain forms of drug dependency and personality disorders.

Bachrach (1988), on the other hand, writes that although there is general agreement among psychiatrists about diagnosing schizophrenia and other forms of psychosis, "there is less certainty" (p. 383) when it comes to the other diagnoses.

Schizophrenia as a chronic illness

The discussion in the following is based mainly on the literature pertaining to schizophrenia. My purpose here is to take a closer look at which theories and hypotheses about chronicity and recovery dominate within the field of psychiatry.

Schizophrenia can be said to be the prototype for a psychiatric chronic illness diagnosis, psychiatry's chronic mental illness *par excellence*. This is partly because the criteria for schizophrenia listed in diagnostic manuals correspond well with the characteristics ascribed to this condition; and partly because, in terms both of number and consumption of care and treatment, schizophrenic patients predominate in psychiatric inpatient care.

An official inquiry of the Psychiatry Commission (Official Reports of the Swedish Government 1992:73) found that at the end of the 1980s 2% of the adult population in Sweden, or some 171,800 individuals, suffered from psychosis in some form. A fourth of these, some

41

43,000 persons or 0.5% of the adult population, displayed symptoms that fulfilled the criteria for the diagnosis schizophrenia.

The duration of the illness and its course of development and organic etiology are central aspects of the definition of schizophrenia: "... it represents an organic mental disorder characterised by progressive irreversible intellectual and emotional deterioration" (Ludwig 1971, p. 7). Because its organic basis has not been localised, schizophrenia is classified among the so-called "functional psychoses" (as opposed to the organic psychoses).

The Swiss psychiatrist Eugen Bleuler (1950) first used the term schizophrenia as a refinement of Kraepelin's diagnosis dementia praecox (Boyle 1993, Fredén 1991, Garrabé 1992, Kraepelin 1971). The various symptoms exhibited by patients were classified as a single diagnosis because they were considered to be manifestations of a single illness having a common origin (etiology) and a similar course of development progressing toward the same terminal stage. The course of the illness was characterised by early onset and progressive deterioration toward dementia and idiocy.

By definition, schizophrenia, like other severe forms of psychosis, pervades the whole of the person's identity. Bleuler distinguished for example between primary and secondary symptoms. Primary symptoms had an etiologic status, whereas secondary symptoms were regarded as stemming from the primary ones. The main primary symptoms are sometimes referred to as the Four A's: Autism, Associative disturbances, Ambivalence and Affect disorder. Bleuler regarded hallucinations and delusions as secondary symptoms. Obviously these symptoms have a crucial impact on the patient's ego functions and ability to relate to the social environment.

The same notion of schizophrenia can be found in the current literature. A paper published by the Swedish Psychiatry Association (1996) lists the most common symptoms for the diagnosis of schizophrenia as:

> (...) delusions, disruption of thought patterns, self-absorption, emotional disturbances, hallucinations and cognitive disorders; that is, disruptions in the ability to take in, conceptualize, and impart information. Besides pro-

ducing a disturbed sense of reality, the illness also has an adverse effect on the individual's relationships with family and friends, work capacity and possibility to lead a normal social life. (p. 11)

Henry Ey, a leading French professor of psychiatry, has summarised the various definitions of schizophrenia:

The loss of the entity that constitutes the individual, regression into delusions, detachment from reality, disturbance in communication are all various aspects of the emergence of a person without person and of a world without world, which is the very essence of the disorder schizophrenia. (1977, p. 64)

The schizophrenic – from the perspective of psychiatry, the person is indistinguishable from the illness – becomes *incomprehensible*. Jaspers, who has greatly influenced how European psychiatrists regard schizophrenia, asserts that the impossibility to understand the schizophrenic is an insurmountable barrier to being able to feel empathy for such a person:

If we try to get some closer understanding of these primary experiences of delusion, we soon find we cannot really appreciate these quite alien modes of experience. They remain largely incomprehensible, unreal and beyond understanding. (Jasper, quoted in Barrett 1996, p. 222)

The image of the schizophrenic as someone other than, as someone qualitatively different from, other people occurs in diverse psychiatric traditions and underscores the notion that the total breakdown of the ego is the foremost reason for chronicity:

But the "burned-out" schizophrenic is an empty shell – (s/he) cannot think, feel or act... She or he has lost the capacity both to suffer and to hope – and at present, medicine has no good remedy to offer for this loss. (Quoted in Davidson & Stayner 1997, p. 5)

Should the chronicity ever be reversed, there is no way in which human intervention could bring about such a reversal. The person is an empty shell, a creature so incomprehensible to others, so alien, that it is impossible to feel empathy for the person, a creature detached from social contexts and human relationships, one that can be affected only by chemical and surgical procedures. It is this quality of chronicity that is of key importance when establishing a schizophrenia diagnosis:

> If a patient who had all the symptoms of dementia praecox improved, Kraepelin routinely considered the patient to have been originally misdiagnosed. (Harding, Zubin & Strauss 1987)

Problems

In defining chronic illness psychiatry faces two major problems: one is the difficulty to establish reliable diagnostic categories; the other is the indistinct boundary between organic and socio-psychological aspects of the etiology of the diagnosis and of the chronic course of the illness. Despite the seemingly precise data on the diagnostic criteria, as discussed earlier, and despite the large number of people who exhibit different kinds of mental disorders and the copious consumption of medical treatment, the criteria for different diagnoses vary widely with respect to the main symptoms, onset of the illness, the course of the illness and the terminal phase. These variations occur not only over time, but also concurrently between different traditions in the same country and between different cultures. This leads, in turn, to widely varying estimates of the actual number of persons with schizophrenia, despite repeated attempts from psychiatrists to find universal and indisputable criteria.

There have been periods, for example, when North American psychiatrists were much more likely to diagnose patients as schizophrenic than were psychiatrists schooled in Western Europe. In a study by Kramer (1969), a patient was diagnosed as schizophrenic by 14 of 42 American psychiatrists but by only one of 42 English psychiatrists. Conversely, a further 14 of the 42 American psychiatrists diagnosed one and the same patient as having a "personality disturbance" compared with 30 of the English psychiatrists. (See also Brockington & Nalpas 1993 and Leff 1977) This study clearly shows that psychiatrists who come from the same cultural world but from different scholastic traditions often arrive at different diagnoses. But Kramer's study also shows that even psychiatrists within the same cultural world and who use the same diagnostic instruments may arrive at quite different diagnoses. Warner (1985) concludes:

> ...which patients are labelled schizophrenic varies from country to country, from time to time and from one psychiatrist to another. (p. 60)

A great effort has been made in recent years to bring into alignment the different definitions of the diagnoses listed in the two leading diagnostic handbooks – the ICD of the World Health Organization and the DSM of the American Psychiatry Association. To achieve greater reliability, modern diagnostic handbooks now use elementary descriptions of specific sets of behaviour for each diagnosis. Patients exhibiting a certain number of the listed behaviours automatically fill the criteria for the diagnosis. But the effort to improve reliability has been at the expense of validity (di Paola 2000a, b, Kirk & Kutchins 1992). As a result, American psychiatrists are now much more restrictive in diagnosing schizophrenia, which has led to assigning new diagnoses to some patients who had been treated for years for schizophrenia.

The effort to formulate more precise psychiatric diagnoses has also led to a substantial increase in the number of diagnoses. In 1840 American diagnosticians assigned a single diagnosis for all known mental disorders; 40 years later the number of diagnoses had increased to seven. In 1952 DSM-I listed 106 diagnostic categories. In 1968 DSM-II listed 182, increasing to 265 in the DSM-III from 1980, and to 292 in the revised edition from 1987 (Berner 1992). The question, however, is whether this increase in the number of diagnoses addresses the basic problem of diagnostics in psychiatry; i.e., the discrepancy between, on the one hand, discrete categories that are intended to reflect specific illnesses and, on the other, the complex personalities of patients. Strauss et al. (1979), in their study of the relationship between patients and diagnoses, found only limited correspondence between patients and the constellations of symptoms of which different diagnoses were considered to consist:

> The implications of these findings for clinical practice and research are considerable. The diagnostician dealing with real patients is apparently forced to place patients into discrete diagnostic categories based on rela-

tively severe levels of symptomatology, even though a great number of patients actually fall between the categories or exhibit low symptom levels where the categories themselves have relatively little meaning. (p. 111)

The diagnostic procedure fails to take into account patients' subjective experience, the meaning they extract from their symptoms and experiences, although both research and clinical practice show that the same symptom may have a different meaning and function for different patients. (See among others Corin & Lauzon 1992.)

To obtain greater reliability, the authors of later editions of the DSM have concentrated on symptoms, ignoring both etiologic considerations and theoretical concepts like "neurosis". Consequently, psychiatry's diagnostic procedure is still at a primitive level: "The conceptualization of schizophrenia is still at an early stage of development". (Weiss 1989, p. 325)

With respect to the etiology of the illness, Eugen Bleuler's son, Manfred Bleuler (1963) concluded:

Today we can look back to the great work of two or three generations of psychiatrists all over the world, who wished to discover the specific cause of schizophrenia and did not find it. This failure has been called the scandal of psychiatry. It is rather the tragedy of psychiatry of the first half of the twentieth century. (p. 25)

The uncertainty about etiology has led a number of writers to once again question the existence of schizophrenia as a uniform diagnosis. Several researchers and clinicians (e.g. Alanen 1997 and Cullberg 1993) have suggested that schizophrenia is not a single disorder but several, each of which has different causes. Boyle (1990, 1993) argues convincingly that the cases of schizophrenia studied by Kraepelin and others actually concerned an entirely different illness that was first diagnosed some years later. She remarks that the kinds of patients described by Kraepelin and Bleuler "are almost never seen today". (Boyle 1990, p. 14) With the exception of delusions and hallucinations, none of the symptoms described by Kraepelin and Bleuler occurs in the classifications used today. Their descriptions of schizophrenic patients correspond, however, to symptoms found in *encephalitis letargica*, an infectious disease that was common at the time. *Encephalitis letargica* results from Parkinson's disease and was first described by von Economo in 1917.

So, diagnoses of psychiatric patients seem to be an uncertain basis for determining chronicity, whether it concerns the individual patient or whole groups of patients. We can therefore conclude: "Diagnosis and prognosis should be treated as different dimensions of psychosis". (Harding & Strauss 1984, p. 1599)

Duration

The duration of the illness is described in the literature as being closely connected to the diagnosis in that different diagnoses are defined as having different natural courses and thus are of varying duration. Chronic diagnoses connote a lifelong illness course. But because the grounds for establishing a diagnosis are uncertain, it is not possible to connect a given duration to a particular diagnosis. In many cases this has led to replacing the term "the chronically ill" with "the long-term ill" and "the long-stay patient". However, there is no consensus on just how long is long. The tendency is to equate the duration of the illness with the length of the person's stay in hospital:

> I have used the traditional criterion of two years' continuous stay in the mental hospital as the defining characteristic of being a long-stay patient – that is of being chronically hospitalized. (Bott 1976, p. 108)

It is thought that certain diagnoses may become episodic, which makes it even more difficult to ascertain the actual duration. Determining duration and the prognosis for the terminal phase becomes even more complicated, however, because it is uncertain whether a patient who was cured from a chronic illness has really been cured or whether recovery is a temporary or permanent stage in the chronic course of development. Kraepelin describes, for example, a case in which 39 years had elapsed between two occasions where an person showed distinct symptoms of schizophrenia; he defined these two occasions as two phases of one and the same illness. (Kraepelin 1971)

In the case of schizophrenia, it has been shown that, contrary to Kraepelin's view that lifelong duration was decisive for establishing the diagnosis, the life course of patients diagnosed as schizophrenic varies greatly. (See among others Bleuler 1978, Carpenter & Kirkpatrick 1988, Huber 1997.) We will return to the question of duration in the section in this chapter on recovery.

Hospitalisation

For some years a simple criterion for chronicity was admission to hospital for psychiatric care. Persons who were or had been hospitalised as a psychiatric patient were regarded as chronic, even if they had since been discharged.

In 1989 in Sweden there were 12,509 occasions on which patients diagnosed as schizophrenic were hospitalised. Patients diagnosed as schizophrenic are generally hospitalised for fairly long periods of time. The average time patients spent in care in 1989 was 165 days. These patients often have recurrent hospitalisations during a succession of years, in total some 2,068,543 days of institutional care. Jonsson (1993) estimated that these patients constituted between 30 and 40% of all patients hospitalised for psychiatric care and were responsible for about half of all treatment days.

Problems

But even such a clear-cut criterion as hospitalisation or consumption of inpatient psychiatric care causes problems. It is difficult, for example, to fine suitable ways of measuring the effects of treatment interventions or the length of time that the treatment is actually necessary. Possible units of measurement are the number of admissions and/or number of days spent in care. The form of the admission – voluntary or coercive – and the time elapsed since the latest admission could also be of interest. But for none of these units of measurement is there consensus among professionals.

The situation becomes even more paradoxical when factors external to the individual and the illness play a role in determining whether a particular individual is to be considered chronically ill. Often such factors as access to hospital beds, local conditions affecting psychiatry and the provision of social services, and labour market policies play a major role in determining the length of hospital stays and thus also in determining chronicity.

Lastly, in recent years a network of activities and programmes have been developed to enable people with mental disorders to live in the community. These intermediate forms of care are in many cases comparable to hospitalisation with respect to the amount of care they provide. But because they lie outside the administrative framework of the health and medical care system, these forms of care are not included in the "hospitalisation" criterion. (Topor & Karebo Larsén 2000) Nevertheless, because of the simplicity of this criterion, it is still used in the USA to determine the chronicity diagnosis of individual patients and thereby their right to be the recipients of a variety of social support measures. (Bachrach 1988, p. 385)

Functional disability

Bachrach (1988) refers to the occurrence of functional disability as a criterion of chronicity:

> There appears to be a growing consensus that disability should be given consideration at least equal to that of diagnosis, and probably more. Diagnosis is, in short, a necessary but not sufficient condition for defining chronic mental illness. (p. 384)

The interest in functional disability for persons with mental disorders arose in connection with the wave of hospital shut-downs that swept across psychiatry after the end of the second world war. It soon became apparent that many patients discharged from psychiatric hospitals had difficulty coping with life outside the institution, even many of those who no longer displayed clinical symptoms. Moreover, new problems arose when it became possible to discharge patients who earlier were judged to be chronic and were expected to spend the rest of their lives in an institution. How was this to be interpreted in relation to the body of knowledge in psychiatry? To what extent was this knowledge actually about institutionalised human beings rather than about "real illnesses"?

In step with the closing down of the psychiatric hospitals, a range of activities and programmes have been devised to support discharged patients who have difficulty living outside the institution. This difficulty has sometimes been interpreted as indicating the continued progression of the illness (as a symptom), sometimes as indicating residual functional disabilities and sometimes as indicating the social consequences of the treatment itself, foremost that of institutionalisation (psychological damage caused by long-term hospitalisation).

Much of the interest in functional disability concerns the need to administrate various interventions for persons discharged from the psychiatric hospital. It is one thing to provide medical treatment for an illness, but on what basis are support and help in daily life to be arranged for people who lack visible signs of physical or biological injury? The relation between chronic mental illness, functional disability and administrative routines is made clear in the following excerpt from the Arizona Checklist for Chronic Mental Illness Determination:

> The chronically mentally ill are defined as those persons whose emotional or behavioral functioning is so impaired as to interfere grossly with their capacity to remain in the community without supportive treatment or services of a long-term or indefinite duration. The mental disability is severe and persistent, resulting in a long-term limitation of their functional capacities for primary activities of daily living such as interpersonal relationships, homemaking and self-care, employment or recreation. (Quoted in Bachrach 1988, p. 384)

When hospitalisation, symptoms and diagnosis lost their earlier presumed clarity as criteria for a chronic illness, functional disability – experienced difficulties in daily life presumably caused by a biological condition – became a new criterion. Deinstitutionalisation has resulted in a shift of focus from the disorder itself to the social consequences of the disorder; i.e., to the person's ability to live a normal life and the obstacles connected with this endeavour.

In Sweden the concepts of handicap and functional disability were applied to persons with mental disorders in connection with the National Mental Health Survey and the so-called Mental Health Reform[1] (Official Reports of the Swedish Government 1992:73). The reasoning here is that mental illness leads to brain damage which leads to certain residual symptoms or functional disabilities (hypersensitivity, withdrawal, shortcomings in personal care and hygiene). These in turn can constitute a handicap when it comes to communication, physical mobility, holding down a job and participation in social interaction. The handicap arises as a result of shortcomings in the community's support of persons with functional disabilities.[2] (Grunewald 1997, 1999)

So it is possible for a person to overcome a handicap, but the underlying brain damage and resultant functional disability remains unchanged. The illness and the functional disability are biological phenomena. The handicap arises when the disability related to these biological phenomena are improperly managed and the person is given too little support.

Problems

The line between illness and functional disability is hard to draw and functional disability is sometimes referred to as a "residual illness". Functional disabilities are considered to be as chronic as the underlying illness was once thought to be. Thus the concept functional disability faces the same problems of definition as the chronicity concept discussed earlier. How long is a long time? How extensive must a person's difficulties be to rank as a functional disability? Where does one draw the line between a functional disability and normal variations in how people live their lives?

Another problem with the functional disability concept has to do with an alternative perspective that has come to the fore in conjunction with psychiatric research findings on the damaging effects of institutionalisation. Research on what effects institutions have on the patients residing within their walls has problematised psychiatry's view of diagnoses and the symptoms that are thought to characterise them.

51

Barton (1959) regarded the harmful effects of institutionalisation as an illness in itself, brought about by life within the institution ("institutional neurosis") and closely resembling known mental disorders:

> ... a disease characterized by apathy, lack of initiative, loss of interest more marked in things and events not immediately personal or present, submissiveness, and sometimes no expression of feelings of resentment at harsh or unfair orders. There is also a lack of interest in the future and an apparent inability to make practical plans for it, a deterioration in personal habits, toilet, and standards generally, a loss of individuality, and a resigned acceptance that things will go on as they are – unchangingly, inevitably and indefinitely. (p. 14)

Also Gentis (1969) regarded chronicity as a consequence of the interplay between mentally ill persons and their environment:

> What creates chronicity is, so to say, a kind of interplay between the ill person and his environment. It is a matter of complicity between the schizophrenic and the hospital in order to secure a special kind of life for the ill person (...) (p. 39)

The relationship between, on the one hand, the observations of clinicians and the theoretical discourses based on these observations and, on the other hand, the institutional conditions where the observations were made is particularly revealing in Kraepelin's case. The institution where he worked in Heidelberg became a meeting-place for "chronic" patients in the area. Patients who were helped by the treatment interventions practised at that time were never referred to his institution and he himself lacked the possibility to arrange the referral to other institutions of patients who were not helped by his own brand of treatment. (Barrett 1996) What is remarkable here is how the clinics were able to disregard these institutional conditions and project onto the individual the whole responsibility for the observed course of events.

Research on the iatrogenic consequences of institutionalisation has shown that symptoms regarded as being of key importance when establishing a diagnosis are not inherent in the "illness" itself, nor in the "functional disability", but have to do with how the person is received in the community; that is, the symptoms in fact reflect a particular social order.[3]

In this perspective, the cause of chronicity, which has long been sought within the individual (biological or psychological characteristics), is not inherent in the illness itself, a part of the natural order, but rather is clearly connected with the person's life in the society. In extension, the negative effects of institutionalisation are carried over into the discharged patient's life outside the institution through the process of stigmatisation. (Belliveau Krauss & Tomaino Slavinsky 1982, Goffman 1961) Stigmatisation makes it impossible for patients leaving hospital to return to their former life. Both their own self-image and the way others perceive them have been shaped by the culture's predominant notions of insanity and chronicity. Persons whom psychiatry defines as chronic assume psychiatry's definition of themselves. They learn what behaviour is expected of them as people who are chronically mentally ill (disregarding the important role played by the side-effects of medication and the negative effects of institutionalisation) and are treated according to these expectations, both within and outside the domain of psychiatry.

In several cases it has been possible to show that certain symptoms that had been regarded (and sometimes still are) as indications of severe mental disturbance were in fact a result of hospitalisation. Punell (1970) determined therefore that "Delineating chronic schizophrenia in a hospital population can (...) be very difficult..." (p. 3562)

Bettelheim (1986), in relating his experiences as a prisoner in a German concentration camp during World War Two, described how his fellow inmates developed such symptoms as reduced reality orientation, perception of the world as a confrontation of good and evil forces, loss of temporal orientation and a mounting inability to plan for the future. Bettelheim's point is that even normal individuals, and not only persons with mental disorders, may exhibit signs of chronic illness when subjected to certain environments. What we know about a mental illness cannot be separated from the situation in which it occurs and is studied, nor from the person himself/herself who is seeking to learn more about the illness. (See also Vail 1966)

Nor should these symptoms be treated as functional disabilities, as residual signs of an illness. They could just as well occur in "healthy" people if they were forced to live under certain adverse conditions. Thus the division between illness (biological), functional disability (consequence of, or rest of, the illness) and handicap (which is what results from treating a functional disability with inadequate forms of social support) is a problematic one; this division lies at the core of the handicap discourse in psychiatry.

Such a perspective also calls into question the notion that mental problems are chronic; how such problems are expressed and how they develop depend on social interactions and not on an inherent "natural course" of the illness itself.

Seen from this perspective, the chronic course of development, which we have been told is characteristic of the severely mentally disturbed patient's condition, is not inherent in the disorder itself nor in any natural course of development, but clearly has to do with the kind of life the designated patients are forced to live.

Recovery

A number of terms have been developed in psychiatry for describing a benign course of development: cure, remission, readjustment, rehabilitation, improvement and recovery. I have chosen the term recovery as my point of departure in the discussion that follows. To talk about a "cure" implies a one-sided concentration on the individual's symptoms and symptom reduction. Rehabilitation focuses on the individual's functional capacities and their course of development. Both of these concepts are connected to forms of intervention where professional groups do something with, to and for the individual. The recovery concept, on the other hand, embraces all three aspects (symptom, function and handicap) of the individual's situation and places the person in a broader life perspective that also includes the individual's own efforts and contributions and those of his/her social network. (See McGorry 1992)

In the Swedish edition of the *English-Swedish Dictionary* from 1969 (Läromedelsförlagen Språkförlagen 1969), the verb "to recover" is associated with the notions of recovering – for example, one's kingdom, health or voice; with recovering one's balance; and with getting well and "being on the mend". The connotations of "recovering" are regaining, getting back, reinstating and getting well. To avoid the medical connotations of "getting well", I have chosen the Swedish term *återhämtning* when talking about recovery. The recovery concept also has the advantage in Swedish of implying that the person who has recovered (*återhämta sig* is a reflexive verb in Swedish) plays an active role in this process.

It is interesting to note how seldom the recovery concept is defined in the extensive psychiatry literature in which it occurs. One reason might be that to have recovered has long meant to have become as one was before the onset of the illness; so nothing more need be said about it. The concept requires no definition. All that need be done is to ascertain through tests that the person has truly become normal again. In the work of Kraepelin, as in that of many current researchers and clinicians, the need for definition was replaced by the use of various tests and other clinical methods of investigation to trace remaining signs of the illness or its residual effects. Taken together, these instruments are intended to assess two aspects of the individual's current life: the first is the presence of symptoms or residual sign of symptoms, and the second is the social effects resulting from the illness. Following upon these two, and as a logical consequence, is a third aspect: whether the person is currently undergoing treatment of any kind. In the literature on psychodynamics, whether or not the person shows "insight" is still another factor in determining recovery.

The first three measures can constitute the elements of a definition of recovery. A radical definition of recovery has to do with the total absence of symptoms, treatment and resulting social effects. From this radical position, some researchers have devised a system for grading the extent of recovery. A person may be cured although his/her social situation has not altered; similarly, a person can be trained and rehabilitated with respect to certain functions although there is no change in the symptoms. (McGorry 1992)

Recovery can imply a return to a former identity or the emergence of a new one. Both positions can be found in the literature. In the last analysis, this way of grading the extent of recovery is itself a radical definition – if a mirror-image of the total recovery definition. In recent years both members of the research community and the patient movement in the USA have broadened the meaning of recovery. At the centre of this expanded definition is the patient's subjective experience of having regained control over his/her life. Anthony (1993) writes for example:

> Recovery is described as a deeply personal, unique process of changing one's attitudes, values, feelings, goals, and/or roles. It is a way of living a satisfying, hopeful, and contributing life even with limitations caused by illness. Recovery involves the development of new meaning and purpose in one's life as one grows beyond the catastrophic effects of mental illness. (p. 15)

As we have ascertained earlier, certain diagnoses are regarded as chronic and therefore irreversible. However, Emil Kraepelin discussed the idea of recovery in his book *Dementia Praecox* (English translation of the 8th edition[4], 1971). The problems he pointed out concern the criteria used for making the original diagnosis, the extent to which the diagnosis can be considered valid, and the criteria for observing the improvement and for ascertaining the duration of the improvement. (p. 185-188)

Diagnostic criteria

Kraepelin found that some contemporary psychiatrists had reported a greater probability for recovery for patients diagnosed as suffering from dementia praecox than he did[5]. He expressed this in a remarkably paradoxical statement: "... in spite of the ease with which the great majority of the cases can be recognized, there is still a great uncertainty."[6] (p. 186)

The implication is that although the diagnosis was simple enough, many psychiatrists still made mistakes and included in the dementia praecox diagnosis even patients with other kinds of problems; it was these patients who later recovered. Despite the claim that the condition was easily diagnosed, Kraepelin's work has led to the emergence of two schools of thought when it comes to defining chronic illness in psychiatry, particularly in connection with schizophrenia. The one maintains a narrow definition whereby recovered patients who fulfil certain specified criteria are eliminated from the diagnosis group altogether. The other proceeds from a broader definition which makes it possible to report a higher number of patients as recovered. Traditionally, European psychiatrists have favoured the narrow definition, although recent negotiations between WHO and APA have led to a tightening up of the American diagnostics.

As severe mental disorders (illnesses), first and foremost schizophrenia, are described as chronic illnesses, finding a high percentage of patients who have recovered would constitute a contradiction in terms. Bleuler (1911[7], English translation 1950), who coined the term schizophrenia, wrote:

> As yet I have never released a schizophrenic in whom I could not still see distinct signs of the disease; indeed there are very few in whom one could have to search for such signs." (p. 256, italic in the original)

The choice of diagnostic criteria is one way to limit in advance the proportion of verified recoveries. However, this strategy proved to be inadequate due to the unreliability of the prognosis variables under discussion. Consequently, although diagnosis variables were chosen for their power to predict a chronic course of development, there were patients even in this group who recovered.

Warner (1985) has shown that in Scandinavia, where a strict diagnosis has long been used, the share of patients diagnosed with schizophrenia who have recovered is as high as in countries like the USA, with the same pattern of variation over time. For this reason, some clinicians and researchers have introduced *a posteriori* verification whereby recovery of schizophrenic patients is explained as cases of mistaken diagnosis.

This argument was used in Sweden, for example, to explain the recovery of Elgard Jonsson, a patient diagnosed as schizophrenic who had been treated for many years at various institutions. Eventually he received psychotherapy by Barbro Sandin and has since then been pronounced completely cured. But in the debate his recovery set off, there have been statements to the effect that since he has undeniably recovered, he must have been incorrectly diagnosed from the start.

The Danish psychiatrist Langfeldt (1937) devised a separate diagnosis for patients who exhibited symptoms of schizophrenia – "typical schizophrenia" – but who also exhibited a positive development. The diagnosis "schizophreniform disorder" was given to patients who exhibited several of Langfeldt's criteria for a positive outcome; for example, sudden onset of the illness and adequate functioning of the personality prior to onset.

The tradition of establishing exclusion criteria in order to retain schizophrenia as a chronic diagnosis is clearly expressed in the widely used diagnostic handbook (DSM) of the American Psychiatry Association (APA). In the third edition (APA 1980), one of the criteria for a schizophrenia diagnosis was the presence of symptoms for at least six months (p. 184), which axiomatically excluded all patients who had had a rapid recovery. The DSMs conclusion was:

> A complete return to premorbid functioning is unusual – so rare, in fact, that some clinicians would question the diagnosis. However, there is always the *possibility* of full remission or recovery, although its frequency is unknown. (p. 185, italic in the original).

The latest edition (APA 1994, 4th edition) has retained the six months or more criterion. A difference compared with the preceding edition is that the duration of the active symptoms has been reduced to one month "or less than one month if symptoms are successfully treated." (p. 278)

As for the probability that patients may recover, the writers of the DSM-IV say that it depends on how the disorder is defined. (p. 282) And yet, the consequences they describe apply only to a narrow definition: "Complete remission (i.e., a return to full premorbid functioning) is probably not common in this disorder." (p. 282) The criteria for "schizophreniform disorder" and schizophrenia are the same except for the duration of the disorder.[8]

The time dimension

Closely related to diagnostic reliability is the question of how long patients should show an improvement before they can be pronounced recovered. Kraepelin writes:

> An improvement, which resembles recovery, may certainly persist far longer than a decade. We shall be able to pronounce a final judgement about the issue of an apparently cured case only after a very long time, and must even after ten or twenty years make up our minds to having few cases verified. (p. 187)

The question is how long must an individual show signs of recovery before the onset of a new illness episode is regarded either as a relapse or as a whole new bout of illness.

In actuality the follow-up of patients is limited in most cases by financial considerations and the difficulty of getting in touch with people after a long time has elapsed. Most follow-up studies found in the professional literature cover periods between one and two years. A few have followed patients for between five and ten years. (Vaillant 1978, WHO 1979) None of these studies corresponds to the temporal criteria established by Kraepelin. Only a few cover longer periods of time (Bleuler 1978, Harding et al. 1987a, b), but these studies are concerned only with the period of recovery.

Harding (1986) has found still another problem with follow-up studies of this kind. Normally they use two points of measurement, the first at a base line and the second at the time of follow-up, which is termed "outcome" and even "end state". However, what is regarded as outcome or end state becomes "course" if and when a new follow-up is made at a later time. Usually we have little knowledge about the time between the two points of measurement. Harding summarises her conclusion in an aphorism: "Two cross-sectionals do not a longitudinal make". (p. 200)

Extent of recovery

After having pointed out that the same patient can be diagnosed differently by different experts, or even by the same diagnostician on different occasions, Kraepelin (1971) asserted that even if agreement could be reached on a diagnosis, it would still be necessary to agree on what was meant by "recovered". Here too, experts disagree. There are different degrees of recovery. Kraepelin made a distinction between "cure" and "recovery with defect" (p. 186). A "cure" means the total absence of all signs of mental disorder. "Recovery with defect" means that even if the most disturbing symptoms have disappeared, the knowledgeable observer can still find traces of personality alterations that can be linked to the illness. Although Kraepelin's division was based on the clinical symptoms, it recurs in later literature both as "best outcome" and "second best outcome" (WHO 1979), and as "total recovery" and "social recovery". (Warner 1985)

Total recovery

Several writers, among them Bleuler (1950), include a return to the functional level and lifestyle prior to the onset of the illness – *"resitutio ad integrum* or at least *status quo ante"* (p. 255, italics in the original) – as a criterion for total recovery. But Bleuler also points to some of the problems this approach raises. First of all, because the illness often has an insidious beginning, it is difficult to determine an actual point in time for its onset and thus to know anything about the individual's life prior to onset. Another problem has to do with the early onset of the illness, often occurring during puberty or even earlier, which makes it difficult to ascertain "What is a peculiarity of character and what is a schizophrenic symptom?" (Bleuler 1950, p. 256) A return to the level of functioning of an adolescent or even younger child is hardly an adequate sign of a good recovery. A complete return to a condition prior to the onset of illness is a problematic measure of recovery.

Despite the difficulty in defining the criteria for total recovery, this type of recovery is considered very rare. According to Bleuler, psychiatrists who claim that a former patient has totally recovered are either lacking in psychological skills or have had insufficient time to carry out their examination of the patient. (p. 256)

Manfred Bleuler's son, Manfred Bleuler (1978), conducted one of the most thorough follow-up studies of patients diagnosed as schizophrenic and their families. In this work he also questioned the criteria raised by his father and Kraepelin for determining total recovery. His first objection is that, upon close examination, it is possible to find psychotic symptoms in every human being. If we were to follow the approach of the meticulous studies mentioned earlier, no one could be classified as recovered:

> ... there is also a danger (...) of applying excessively refined methods in determining recovery. As Uchtenhagen shows, in the framework of these studies, often test results reveal a normal, healthy person as schizophrenic. As soon as the possibility is taken seriously that in every normal person's being there lies concealed some schizophrenic form of life, considerably more care will be applied before considering every schizophrenic manifestation in life as an indication of psychosis. (p. 187)

Nor can recovery from schizophrenia, Manfred Bleuler asserted further, be compared with recovery from other illnesses and injuries because schizophrenia attacks the personality itself. This leads Bleuler to draw two conclusions. The first is that schizophrenia may be a way certain individuals have of managing their lives; in its milder forms, it may actually be a way of life rather than a pathologic condition.

> Possibly his schizophrenic life is an inner necessity for him. The deeper we learn to feel our way into the schizophrenic, the less certain becomes our judgement as to what his recovery might mean, and whether a social readaptation would be the patient's own well-being – his own greatest personal achievement". (p. 188)

If milder forms of schizophrenia can in some cases be regarded as a relatively adequate way of living one's life and if all people display some signs of schizophrenia, then determining total recovery becomes a problem.

Bleuler's second conclusion is that psychosis is such an overwhelming experience for the individual that a return to what is ordinarily considered normality might be impossible. Psychosis is an experience that must leave its mark on any normal person:

> It is difficult to determine what would constitute the completely healthy processing of the outrageous experience of a schizophrenic psychosis. It often seems to me that it is more nearly pathological when a patient can discuss his former psychosis with unconcerned objectivity, and acts as if he had not been the victim of it (...). (p. 192)

Manfred Bleuler concludes that determining the extent of recovery is and will always be a subjective exercise.

Insight

A special criterion for determining the degree of recovery has been launched primarily within psychodynamic psychiatry. McGlashan (1987) suggested that patients be classified as recovered according to how well the illness episode has been integrated into the ego. He distinguishes between persons regarded as recovered who minimise the importance of their illness episode and the impact of their experience of psychiatric treatment. The individual looks upon his illness episode as a clearly limited event that is alien to himself and his life. McGlashan calls this way of relating to the illness as "sealing over" and argues that the underlying problem behind the patient's becoming ill has not been solved.

The second way of relating to the illness according to McGlashan is "integration": the person looks upon his/her experiences during the period of illness as part of his/her life history. Through integration, individuals gain greater insight into their way of functioning and can benefit by these experiences in their present and future life.

Problems

Greenfield, Strauss, Bowers and Mandelkern (1989) pointed out, however, that insight is an ambiguous concept which in many studies has been reduced to mean the patient's concurring with the caregivers' view of his/her problems. In several studies a criterion for insight is the patient's acceptance of the justification for his/her admission to in-patient psychiatric care. In the study of 21 patients diagnosed as functionally psychotic, Greenfield and his colleagues found that nearly all the patients had a complex way of relating to their symptoms and to the kinds of treatment they received and tended to mix together aspects of "insight" and "denial". They concluded that:

> ... traditional descriptive and psychoanalytical concepts of insight into psychotic illness – judging whether the patient is capable of acknowledging he has an illness or the 'integration versus sealing over' conceptual model of recovery style – are incomplete and inadequate. (p. 250)

Mild relapse or social recovery?

Although Kraepelin, Bleuler and their successors concluded that there was very little likelihood of total recovery for schizophrenia patients, they could nevertheless describe a number of cases where patients were able to engage in social relationships outside the institution:

> Therefore we do not speak of *cure but of far-reaching improvements* and differentiate them from the severe deteriorations (in which the patient is wholly incapable of social relations) and from the mild deteriorations which include all the rest of the cases between the two extremes. (Bleuler 1950, p. 256, italics in the original)

The areas of life that are usually referred to when determining the degree of "far-raching improvement" include work capacity, the ability to live outside psychiatric institutions, and the ability to establish and maintain social relationships with marriage as one of the more advanced forms.

In his study Manfred Bleuler used the following criteria as indicative of a "mild" relapse stage: the person is able to carry on balanced conversations, at least about matters that do not directly concern his/her hallucinations. Furthermore, the person does not act in a bizarre manner in face-to-face interaction, although his/her behaviour might be regarded as eccentric; the person lives outside the psychiatric institution or on a calm unlocked ward and participates in some form of work or recreational activity. This means in effect that the psychotic symptoms may still occur "beneath the surface". Furthermore, continued treatment and support may still be required.

There are certain problems connected with establishing the criteria for social recovery. A common problem is that most of the above criteria refer to matters that have little to do with the patient's condition, abilities or motivation. The possibility to participate in working life depends to a great extent on the job market situation and on what kinds of support are available to persons with functional disabilities to help them re-enter the job market. What kind of housing is available to someone who has been hospitalised for psychiatric care depends, of course, on the overall housing situation – the availability of adequate housing – but also on whether there are supportive measures to facilitate the individual's transition from institutional life to a life lived outside the institution. Participation in "occupational activities", in a social network, in family life, is also dependent on how the social life of the community is organised. The conditions for social life are quite different in an agrarian society, for example, compared with life in an urban society.

Contact with outpatient care

One aspect that must be taken into account when determining recovery is whether the patients continue to be under psychiatric care. This includes continued medication, psychotherapy and special measures to facilitate employment and recreation. It is difficult to apply common criteria when different countries have different laws governing which public authorities are responsible for which forms of intervention. Supportive measures defined as being community based may occur within both the social services and psychiatry, but also through voluntary organisations. Rehabilitation can be provided by the social services, psychiatry or the regional social insurance office. Most writers of psychiatric literature today accept the idea that persons can be regarded as socially recovered even though they still receive treatment and support. The problem is to determine the highest level of such interventions at which a person can still be regarded as socially recovered.

Warner (1985) has concluded that it is very difficult to standardise the criteria and measuring instruments for the kinds of social variables being discussed here. In their follow-up study of several hundred patients discharged from hospital in the middle of the 1950s, Harding et al. (1987a, b) used a variety of measuring instruments: Global Assessment Scale (GAS), Level of Function Scale (LOF), Brief Psychiatric Rating Scale (BPRS), Community Adjustment Scale (CAS) and 12 additional scales measuring in all 21 different areas of functioning. The subjects of the study were also assessed using interviews. In two of the follow-up groups, the measurements yielded straightforward results. The subjects scored consistently high or low on all scales. But in 45% of the cases, the subjects' scores were mixed, with high results on certain variables and low scores on others. Determining whether or not patients had recovered and what characterised their recovery remained a matter of subjective assessment on the part of the investigators. (Harding 1986)

Contact with inpatient care

In much of the research it has been practically impossible for the investigators to make follow-up assessments of patients who had been discharged. It is difficult to keep in contact with discharged patients. Furthermore, to make high quality clinical assessments of a large group of current and former patients is a very time-consuming and costly undertaking. To surmount this problem, the course of the illness and recovery are defined operationally, the criterion being that the patient was not hospitalised at the time of the study or at a specific time period prior to the study (see Warner 1985). In the section in this chapter on chronicity, we saw how hospitalisation could serve as a criterion for determining if a patient was chronically ill. The advantage of this measure, says Warner, is that it is unambiguous. But in fact even this measuring variable has certain complications. One of the problems of using admission to hospital as a criterion for determining whether or not a person has recovered is that it thereby excludes all other criteria pertaining to the individual's life. The measuring instrument becomes the criterion. The researchers search under the nearest lamppost for a key they dropped in a dark alleyway.

The number of available hospital beds varies greatly between districts and within the same district over time. Therefore the probability that a person will be hospitalised does not depend solely on how the person feels. A crucial factor in measuring consumption of inpatient care is access to hospital beds and outpatient facilities. (Stein & Test 1978)

Another consideration concerns legislation, which changes over time and varies from country to country. This affects in turn the boundary between psychiatry and correctional care or drug abuse treatment. Shifts in the areas of responsibility between psychiatry and other care and support providers affect access to treatment and housing alternatives outside the domain of inpatient care. This is occurring in Sweden as resources are being transferred from psychiatric wards and nursing homes to community services in connection with the psychiatric dehospitalisation reform. For the persons concerned, the reform meant the end of their stay in the psychiatric hospital. These changes took place above the heads of the persons concerned; and they took with no regard to whether the person's life situation had changed in the least.

Recovery as a process

The definitions of and criteria for recovery that we have discussed so far have proven to be problematic. They all represent attempts to establish dividing lines in the complex and varied lives of individual persons according to what are supposed to be unambiguous objective criteria. But judgements of the mental states of patients are based mainly on a single instrument consisting of the psychiatrist and his subjectivity in relation to the patient, the criteria set out in the diagnostic manual and his/her own past experience. The judgements of the ability of patients to return to civil society depend on economic and social factors outside the individual patient's control. Strauss & Carpenter (1981) wrote:

> Real patients do not have 'an' outcome. One patient with continuous hallucinations may be fully employed, while another patient, unable to function outside of the home, may take extensive responsibility in family

affairs. (…) In the past, the use of a global outcome judgement may have provided the clinician with an opportunity to synthesize the broad range of information concerning outcome functioning into one variable, but it had also the unfortunate effect of suggesting that such a conceptualization is a fully adequate representation of reality. (p. 60-61)

In contrast to the dichotomy recovered/not recovered is the idea of recovery as a process that touches upon the individual's whole life. This view has been launched by a number of researchers, several of whom have personal experience of mental disorder (Deegan 1988, Chadwick 1997, Harding 1986). The patient's situation and mental state should be judged on the basis of a broader knowledge of the patient's life:

> Let us suppose that some of the so-called loners have always been loners and preferred their own company to others? Was their behavior prodromal and now considered to be residual or are there not substantial numbers of people outside of, or working for, the mental health system who live alone and who are quite happily functioning at work and caring for themselves who do not maintain relationships? (Harding 1986)

Just as Manfred Bleuler found symptoms of schizophrenia in "normal" people, aspects of "normality" can be found in persons exhibiting symptoms of severe mental disorder. Psychosis is seldom a condition that envelops the individual's whole personality all of the time. Deegan (1988) regards it more as a process than a condition, a long-term process of creating a new self-image (Rakfeldt & Strauss 1989, Strauss 1989b); an ego that is not completely subjected to the illness; an ego that means that the patient is not entirely helpless in relation to the illness. (Strauss, Harding, Hafez & Lieberman 1987)

For Deegan, it is important to understand that patients are not simply *restored*, like a car is repaired. Rather it is a question of actively (re)establishing a new way of conceptualising the self, not as the self that existed prior to the illness, nor as a passive acceptance of the illness and its accompanying limitations. Patients "recover themselves" (in Swedish, they *återhämtar sig*).

From a similar perspective McGorry (1992) distinguishes between recovery and rehabilitation. To recover means that the patient assumes an active role in the recovery process in contrast to rehabilitation programmes where the patient is seen primarily as a recipient of various supportive measures. Moreover, recovery focuses more on the illness whereas rehabilitation focuses more on the consequences of the illness: handicap and functional disability.

Against this background recovery can be regarded as a development process in which the individual regains (reclaims) his/her self and his/her power over his/her own life (Leete 1989). The goal is not normalisation but "… to embrace our human vocation of becoming more deeply, more fully human". (Deegan 1997a)

The passage from Anthony (1993) quoted earlier runs along the same lines:

> … recovery is a deeply personal, unique process of changing one's attitudes, values, feelings, goals, skills, and/or roles. It is a way of living a satisfying hopeful and contributing life even with the limitations caused by the illness.

A consequence of such a perspective is that the ones who are best able to judge the extent of recovery are the persons (patients) themselves (Tooth, Kalyanansundaram & Glover 1997).

The danger of adopting such a perspective is that it might replace the subjectivity of the psychiatrist with the subjectivity of the patient. In cases where no one could possibly characterise certain persons as having recovered, they themselves, despite considerable suffering and disability, might consider themselves fully recovered.

If recovery from severe mental disorders is conceptualised only in terms of process, then there is the risk of the process being endless, which opens the backdoor to chronicity. Even persons who fulfil high level criteria for recovery risk, like the sober alcoholics in the AA movement, being defined for all time in terms of their earlier diagnosis.

[1] The term "mental handicap" already appeared in the Socialtjänstlagen (Government Bill 1979/80, p. 299) but had few consequences in practice or in the professional and public discourse. See also Cullberg and Grunewald (1988).

[2] The National Board of Health and Welfare (1997:8) distinguishes between functional impairment (loss of function – biological) and functional disability (loss of ability – psychological/social).

[3] See Wing & Brown's (1970) classic study of the effects of change on patients' symptomatology at three mental hospitals in England.

[4] Kraepelin made extensive revisions of his book between the different editions. The book has been published in nine editions in all between 1883 and 1919. (see Garrabé 1992.)

[5] Kraepelin reported finding nine terminal stages for dementia praecox: cure, "cure with defect", "simple deterioration", "imbecility", "hallucinatory deterioration", "hallucinatory insanity", "dementia paranoides", "flighty silly deterioration", and "dull apathetic deterioration".

[6] Kraepelin's words have a modern echo in Ey, who writes sixty years later: "Even if a poor prognosis is a necessary element (clinically, historically and logically) in the schizophrenia concept, it is far from being an indisputable necessity for all clinical work". (Ey, 1977, p. 134)

[7] Bleuler's text is based on the 7th edition from 1899 of Kraepelin's book but also on the 1886 edition. Thus his view of recovery for patients with schizophrenia is more pessimistic here than in other editions. (See Garrabé 1992.)

[8] See, however, the French criticism against putting schizophrenia on par with schizophrenic-type psychosis (or its French variants *bouffée délirante* and *schizophrénie aigues*) which is regarded as being of long-term duration.

3

The probability of recovery

Longitudinal studies

The probability that a person will recover from a severe mental disorder depends, as we have seen, to some extent on what diagnostic and recovery criteria are being applied, in what time period, in what part of the world and grounded in what theoretical school. Follow-up studies of patients treated for schizophrenia show that the disorder can develop in different ways and that in many cases the course of development is positive.

Ciompi

Ciompi and Muller (Ciompi 1980) conducted a study on 228 patients with the diagnosis schizophrenia, all of whom were born in the last quarter of the 1800s. The length of time between the patients' first hospital admission and the time of the study averaged 36.9 years. So, in terms of the length of the follow-up, this study is certainly one of the most comprehensive.

The results show a wide variation in the course of development of the illness. Ciompi distinguished eight basic types of development that varied as to onset, development and terminal stage (see Fig. 1, p. 72). The most common course consists of the sudden onset of the illness followed first by a period of intermittent recovery and relapse and then by an end state where the person has recovered. Even cases where the onset of the illness occurs slowly can eventually result in a recovery. Ciompi (1980) wrote:

The global outcome of schizophrenia, measured at the final state, was favourable in 49% of the cases, of which 27% had totally recovered and 22% had only minor relapses, compared with 27% with unfavourable outcomes of medium and serious degree. In comparison with the situation at first hospital admission, their mental health had totally or partly improved in about two-thirds of the cases. (p. 26)

A fourth of the patients had been hospitalised for 20 years or more, but as many as 47% had been hospitalised for short periods amounting to less than a year. Although the average age of the patients was 74 years at the time of the study, over half of them performed work of some kind, a third of them on a full-time basis and the rest part-time. Ciompi concluded that the probability that patients with a schizophrenia diagnosis would improve had been grossly underestimated:

> Just as in the normal life process, what we call illness can represent the complex and varied reaction of a person, with all his sensitivity, ideosyncrasies, personality structure, behaviour and patterns of communication and earlier and current experiences, to a similarly complex and global situation. (p. 32)

With such a broad spectrum of possible courses of development for the illness, the schizophrenia diagnosis can no longer be distinguished as a chronic illness in that only a minority of patients actually develop along the course predicted by the diagnosis. Ciompi's 1980 study also shows that it is possible for patients to recover regardless of whether the symptoms appeared suddenly or after a slow progression.

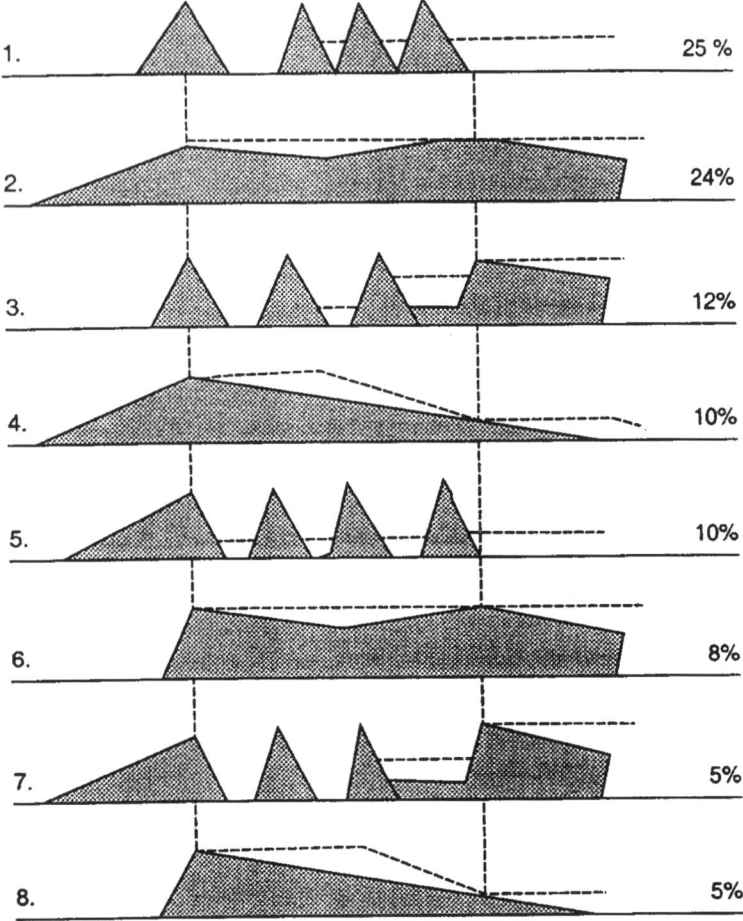

Figure 1. Long-term development of schizophrenia (the dotted lines represent variations in the same course of events).
Source: Ciompi 1980.

Bleuler

The variation found in the possible outcome for patients diagnosed with schizophrenia calls into question the occurrence of the disorder as initially defined. Manfred Bleuler, the son of Eugen Bleuler, the clinician who first introduced the term schizophrenia, published a study at the end of the 1970s in which he followed the evolution of the disorder for 208 patients at Burgholzli hospital in Zurich, the same place where his father had worked (Bleuler 1978). Bleuler found the same range of variation in the patients' life histories as did Ciompi. Bleuler, using a stringent definition of schizophrenia, found that after an average of five years, the disorder usually stagnated and that, contrary to expectations, the majority of the patients diagnosed with schizophrenia recovered totally or socially. Moreover, the patients' condition was still amenable to change long after they had been certified as chronically ill, in some cases decades later. In most cases, these changes represented an improvement. Bleuler concluded therefore that:

> The following general rule applies: Some two-thirds to three-fourths of schizophrenias are benign, and only about one-third or less are malignant. In addition, the frequency of the two opposing types of "end states" should be mentioned. About one-third of the "end states" are long-term recoveries, and about one-tenth to one-fifth are the severe chronic psychoses. (p. 414)

Harding and associates

Harding and her colleagues conducted a follow-up study of a group of patients who had been discharged from a psychiatric hospital in Vermont between 1955 and 1965 (Harding, Brooks, Ashikaga, Strauss & Breier 1987a, b). The patients, who constituted the hospital's residual population of severely disturbed chronics, had participated in a comprehensive rehabilitation programme prior to their discharge. For the purposes of the study the patients were re-diagnosed in accordance with DSM III criteria; 82 were judged as fitting the criteria for a schizophrenia diagnosis. Harding and her associates found that between a half and two-thirds of this group of patients showed no signs of deterioration after discharge, but rather "an evolution into various degrees of productivity, social involvement, wellness, and competent functioning." (Harding et al. 1987b, p. 730)

A total of 82% of the patients who matched the criteria for schizophrenia had not been hospitalised during the year immediately preceding the follow-up. Forty per cent had held a job during this period; 68% exhibited only minor or no symptoms at all; 68% had formed close or relatively close friendships.

An interesting aspect of this study is that when comparing the 213 patients who matched the DSM-II's broader criteria for schizophrenia with the 82 patients who, when re-diagnosed, matched the more stringent criteria of DSM-III, these diagnoses were of no value for predicting patient outcome.

Harding et al.'s study is especially noteworthy in that it shows that even patients who had been categorised as belonging to the residual group of a chronic population were able to break the yoke of chronicity. The study problematises the ability of professional judgements to predict individual development. Lastly, the Harding study points at the importance of social interventions for recovery.

McGlashan

McGlashan's study (1984) of patients at Chestnut Lodge, a psychiatric institution closely affiliated with the pyschoanalytic school, is usually cited to lend support to the pessimism regarding the probability of recovery of patients diagnosed with schizophrenia. However, this study has serious limitations in that what it has evaluated is a specific method of treatment applied at a particular psychiatric institution,; it has not measured the outcome for people with a schizophrenia diagnosis. Furthermore, the study is strongly biased in that inmates at Chestnut Lodge are usually recruited from among those patients who showed no progress while hospitalised in other institutions. So, the patients who were the target group in McGlashan's study had spent long periods of time in hospital and others had finally given up on them. They did not constitute a normal population but a group that excluded those who had already recovered.

WHO

That schizophrenia occurs in different cultures has been taken as proof that the illness is universal, that it has a biological basis and that socio-cultural factors have only secondary importance. In a follow-up study conducted by WHO, a comparison was made between the illness course of patients with a schizophrenia diagnosis in industrialised countries and those from developing countries. The patients were monitored for a two-year period. The results showed that 28% of the patients from the industrialised countries and only 13% of the patients in the developing countries belonged to the "worse outcome" category. In the category of patients who had the best outcome, 15% were from the industrialised countries and 35% from the developing countries (WHO 1979).

A five-year follow-up of the same patients (Leff, Sartorius, Jablensky, Korten & Ernberg 1992) confirmed these results. In this later study, 27% of the patients from the developing countries had experienced only one psychotic episode during the five years they were monitored. The corresponding figure for patients from the industrialised countries was 8%. Half of the patients from the developing countries had recovered (in terms of occupational activity, human relationships and sexuality) in the periods between psychotic relapses compared with 15% of the patients from the industrialised countries.

Richard Warner (1985) concluded in a commentary to the two-year follow-up:

> The general conclusion is unavoidable. Schizophrenia in the Third World has a course and prognosis quite unlike the condition as we recognize it in the West. The progressive deterioration, which Kraepelin considered central to his definition of the disease, is a rare event in non-industrial societies, except perhaps under the dehumanizing restrictions of a traditional asylum. The majority of Third World schizophrenics achieve a favorable outcome. The more urbanized and industrialized the setting, the more malignant becomes the illness. (p. 156)

Contemporary studies – a summary

Harding (1988) reviewed the data from a number of studies (Table 1) and found that:

> Together these studies found that one-half to two-thirds of more than 1,300 subjects studied for longer than 20 years achieved recovery or significant improvement. (p. 479)

Table 1. Results from five follow-up studies of patients with a schizophrenia diagnosis.

	No. of patients	% totally recovered	% socially recovered	% recovered
Bleuler 1972	208	23	43	66
Harding et al. 1986	269	34	34	68
Huber et al. 1975	502	26	31	57
Tsuang et al. 1972	186	20	26	46
Ciompi & Muller 1976	289	29	24	53

Source: Harding (1988).

Manfred Bleuler (1991) has perhaps best summarised how these results have affected what we know about the course of schizophrenia when he wrote:

> *There is no specific course for the disorder.* Instead, the outcomes of schizophrenic psychoses are extremely diverse, varying among prolonged recovery, intermittent course, and prolonged psychosis of severe or mild degrees. For a long time, many psychiatrists believed that a precise definition of the diagnosis indicated a specific prognosis. Experience has shown that no matter how we formulate the diagnosis, it never insures predictable course and outcome. (p. 5, italic in the original; see also Huber, Gross, Schuttler & Linz 1980)

Meta-studies

Longitudinal studies have been conducted on patients diagnosed as schizophrenic for as long as the diagnosis has been in use. One of the most comprehensive meta-study of the recovery of patients with a schizophrenia diagnosis was made by Warner (1985). Warner compiled 87 studies conducted between 1919 and 1979 of patients hos-pitalised between the 1880s and the 1970s (see Fig. 2, p. 79). In the analysis, he divided the data from these studies into five distinct time periods:

- *1881-1900.* The end of the 19th century could be characterised as a time of pessimism about the effects of treatment at the same time as there was a deep economic recession. It was also during this period that Kraepelin introduced the concept dementia praecox. The overview includes four studies from this period. The percentage of recovered patients varied between 0 and 13%; only one study referred to social recovery and placed 15% of the patients in this category. Because there were so few studies, Warner subsequently excluded this time period from his overview.
- *1901-1920.* During this period, which includes World War I, unemployment declined and there was a nascent optimism about the new treatment methods that were being introduced. Twelve studies from this period are included in the overview. The aver-age percentage of totally recovered patients was 20%, with a range of 2 to 30% for all twelve studies. The average percentage of socially recovered patients was 40%, with a range of 19 to 60%.
- *1921-1940.* During this period unemployment rose dramatically and new treatment methods such as electric shock therapy (ECT) and lobotomy were introduced. Twenty-five studies are included from this period. The average percentage of totally recovered patients was just over 10%, with a range of 0 to 23%, and of socially recovered patients 30%, with a range of 8 to 45% for all 25 studies.
- *1941-1955.* The post-war years were a time of economic growth and full employment in many countries. These factors were coupled with renewed optimism in connection with advances in social psychiatry (therapeutic communities and day care facili-ties). Seventeen studies are included. The average percentage of totally recovered patients was just over 20%, with a range of 12

and 41%, and of socially recovered patients just over 40%, with a range of 26 to 59%.

- *1956-1980.* During this period the growth rate in many industrialised countries declined and unemployment rose. Beginning in the second half of the 1950s, modern psychopharmaceuticals like chlorpromazine and lithium came into widespread use. Twenty-nine studies are included. The average percentage of totally recovered patients was 20%, with a range of 7 to 52%, and of socially recovered patients just over 40%, with a range of 21 to 81%.

A similar pattern was found concerning the respective percentages of admissions and discharges from psychiatric hospitals. An average percentage of just over 55% of the patients were discharged during the first two decades of the 20th century. This figure first declines by 5% for the next 20-year period, and then rises by just over 20% to an average of 70% for the period between 1941 and 1955, when the number of hospital beds was being reduced in several European countries and the USA. Thereafter, the effects of a deliberate policy of deinstitutionalisation that was introduced in several countries in the 1960s and 1970s began to be felt. The average for the period 1955-1980 was more than 80%.

Regarding the probability of patients diagnosed with schizophrenia to recover, Warner's study throws light on an interesting phenomenon. The average percentage of socially recovered patients during the time periods reported varies between 30 and 40% and of totally recovered patients between 10 and 20%. These figures should be somewhat unexpected in that they apply to what has generally been regarded as a chronic disorder.

In still another meta-review, comprising in this case 320 studies (Hegarty, Baldessarini, Tohen, Waternaux & Oepen 1994), the authors found similar high percentages of recovered patients. The conclusion that Hegarty and his associates drew, however, was that the variations between the different time periods depended largely on what definitions of schizophrenia were being used at the time.

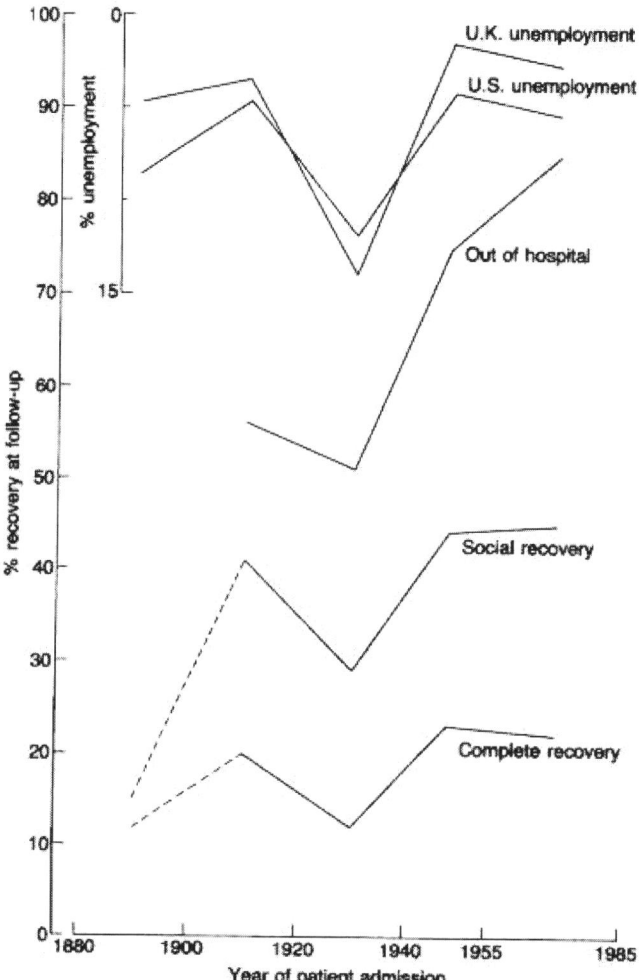

Figure 2. the outcome for schizophrenia in Europe and North America based on 85 studies (Warner 1985), and the inverted data on unemployment for USA and Great Britain during the same period.

How a diagnosis is defined and which criteria are deduced from these definitions of course play a significant part in determining the outcome of an illness. But even if Warner (1985) and Hegerty et al. (1994) disagree about the background to the varying percentages of recovered patients found in their respective overviews, their studies show that patients do recover – regardless of socio-economic aspects and set of diagnostic criteria.

So why the pessimism?

The research results reported here give rise to two questions: Why is the view of schizophrenia as a chronic incurable disorder still so strongly maintained among clinical staff in psychiatry? and How can the recovery of patients diagnosed as schizophrenic be explained?

Reasons for pessimism among clinical staff

We can discern a number of factors that explain the continued pessimism surrounding many diagnoses in psychiatry. Manfred Bleuler, whose research results contrast strongly with those of his father Eugen Bleuler, offered this anecdote (1978) to explain his father's growing pessimism about the possibility for schizophrenia patients to recover:

> From 1886 to 1898, E. Bleuler dedicated himself completely to his community of schizophrenics as director of the remote psychiatric clinic of Rheinau, which was then in a isolated rural sector of Switzerland. Two decades later during and after the first world war, he went back to Rheinau to visit about once a year, usually when the weather was fine during the summer. His former schizophrenic patients always greeted him warmly and enthusiastically. Much as these greetings pleased him, he usually made the painful observation, "Most of them did seem to have deteriorated". Then, depressed, he would ask, "Is there really nothing that can stop this disease?" If he spent all his life wrestling with the question of whether there was an "organic process" at the basis of schizophrenia, it was mainly because of experiences like the above. But E. Bleuler did not know how many improved patients were out for their Sunday walk during his visits, and certainly not how many had been released and were living at home, recovered. Had he known, and if he had not continued to meet

only the most severe cases among his old problem children, his assessment of the schizophrenia would have been strongly influenced. A number of generations of clinical psychiatrists had experiences similar to this. (p. 413)

Bleuler's anecdote takes on an even more general meaning in a study of the grounds upon which researchers and clinicians base their knowledge of a variety of problems and illnesses (Cohen & Cohen 1984; see also Harding, Zubin & Strauss 1992). Clinicians base their knowledge of psychiatric problems and illnesses on the patients they meet in the course of their practice and who either have sought their help voluntarily or under coercion. Thus, treatment staff meet a select group of patients who have in common the fact that they are ill; patients who feel well are not part of the staff's world of experience. In cases where the problems and illnesses extend over different time periods and where treatment is not expected to result in a cure, clinical staff are more likely to meet patients ("chronics") who have spent a longer time in care than patients with shorter periods of time in care, even though the latter group is the larger one.

The same can be said about longitudinal studies where patients with the longest time spent in care have a much greater chance to be part of the research population than patients with shorter times in care. Cohen and Cohen (1984) call this phenomenon "the clinician's illusion" arising as a "consequence of using a prevalence sample as a substitute for an incidence sample" (p. 1180).

Still another bias in support of pessimism about the schizophrenia diagnosis is the attempt by certain groups in psychiatry to introduce incurability as a diagnostic criteria. A case in point was the attempt to formulate special diagnoses for patients who exhibited sufficient criteria for a schizophrenia diagnosis but who had nevertheless recovered. (See Chapter 2 in the present study).

The greatest difference between the clinicians' observations and the actual status of the population occurs, according to Cohen & Cohen (1984), when the following five factors are present:

- large variations in illness duration
- a fluctuating illness course which means that different organisations become responsible for patient care at different times
- unclear definitions of illness and onset
- reduction of symptoms through treatment but without achieving a cure
- treatment provided by specialists who later lose contact with the patients who have recovered

Cohen & Cohen concluded by referring to two other sources of bias which distort clinicians' and researchers' understanding of the course of different long-term illnesses. Clinicians and researchers seldom, if ever, come into contact with people who display symptoms of the illnesses but who nevertheless manage on their own and even recover without ever coming into contact with the mental health system. In a prevalence study, those patients who have not already recovered make up an inordinate share in relation to their actual number. The patients who became ill and recovered prior to the time of the study do not become part of the research population, which makes patients with chronic characteristics the dominant group in the study.

A final factor behind the pessimism is the difficulty to either give a tenable explanation of severe mental disorders (see Barrett 1996) or establish a significant correlation between treatment interventions and patients' social and total recovery (McGlashan 1988). In the face of psychiatry's demonstrated pessimism, few clinicians and researchers have the inclination to study recovery from severe mental disorders.

Treatments and their results

Ambitious attempts have been made to relate the reduction of hospital beds, the probability of readmission to psychiatric care and the frequency of recovery among severely disturbed patients to the development of modern psycho-pharmaceuticals and/or to the introduction of psycho-social interventions into psychiatry. An important point of departure for this field of research, and which is seldom taken into account, is Hasting's observation that:

...any treatment under test must exceed by a significant difference these spontaneous outcomes if it is to be of value. (1958, p. 1065)

The results obtained through the prescribed treatment must be better than the outcome for patients who have never treated. Treatment research continually yields new results. New techniques, new medicines, individually and in combination, have been tested and evaluated. While the following presentation makes no claim to giving a complete overview of the research field, it should be a sufficiently useful for the purposes of this study.

Psycho-pharmaceutical interventions

There are numerous studies showing that neuroleptic medicines are superior to placebos for reducing the symptomology of psychotic patients. But should incontestable proof that psychoactive drugs reduce symptoms ever be forthcoming, this finding must still be put in relation to the patients' recovery. There are also a number of studies (among them Anthony & Liberman 1986, Carr & Katsikitis 1987, Hogarty 1984, Hogarty et al. 1986 and Talbott 1981) showing that treatment with psychoactive drugs reduces the probability that patients will be readmitted to hospital.

Some 60% of the patients with a schizophrenia diagnosis who were released from hospital and who were administered psychoactive drug treatment through the outpatient clinic had no relapse within a year after discharge. The remaining 40% had suffered a relapse. The findings from these studies must be viewed in the light of the studies that show that also between 10 and 20% of the patients who were administered a placebo remained out of hospital (see also Guelfi 1994, Kleinman 1988, Zarifan 1988).

One of the problems with follow-up studies of psychoactive drug treatment is that many patients stop using the drugs, usually because of their severe side-effects. Thus, the real relapse frequency among patients being treated with these drugs is often higher than the 40% mentioned above, a figure that is based on a sample of patients who continued with the prescribed treatment.

The vast majority of patients who suffer from psychosis and are under psychiatric treatment are prescribed some form of neuroleptic medication. But this is a complex issue, as a number of studies show. For example American (Cole, Goldberg & Klerman 1964) and British (Leff & Wing 1971) studies show that between 5 and 7% of patients with a schizophrenia diagnosis do not "respond" to psychoactive drugs, neither with respect to symptom reduction nor relapse frequency. After these studies were conducted, new psychoactive drugs have been introduced which may have an effect on the percentage of patients who are helped by medication.

Rosen, Engelhardt, Freedman and Margolis (1968) and Rosen et al. (1971) investigated the effect of psychoactive drugs on the relapse frequency of 400 patients with a schizophrenia diagnosis. They divided the patients into two groups using a prognostic instrument that included such variables as the patient's previous level of social competency, previous history of treatment and results on psychological tests. Upon their release, the patients in both groups were divided again into two groups, one that was given traditional neuroleptic medicines and the other a placebo. For the patient group who had a poor prognosis, treatment with psychoactive drugs clearly had an effect. Only some 30% of the patients in this group had to be readmitted compared with some 60% of the patients who received a placebo. On average, the patients who were prescribed neuroleptic medicines stayed out of hospital for a longer period of time than those who were given a placebo. The former were readmitted on average first a year after discharge, the latter after six months.

For the patients who had a good prognosis, however, the picture was the reverse. Between 12 and 28% of the patients who were given psychoactive drugs (depending on which medication was administered) had to be hospitalised compared with just over 7% of those who were given a placebo. Also with respect to the length of time before the patients were readmitted, the picture was the reverse of that of the group with a poor prognosis. The patients who were given neuroleptic medicines were readmitted to hospital on average between six months and just over a year (depending on what medication was administered). Patients who had received a placebo remained outside of hospital for an average of 30 months before being readmitted. This study implies that there is no simple cause-effect connection between treatment with neuroleptic medicines and length of the period between hospital stays. Rather, the relationship is complex, where social and psychological factors also play a significant role.

There is widespread belief among professionals and laypersons alike that the reduction in the number of hospital beds in psychiatric care, which was carried out in most of the industrialised countries after the second world war, is related to the introduction of a growing variety of medicines at the beginning of the 1950s. But this is not entirely true. Studies of the number of hospital beds in psychiatric care in various European countries show instead that this reduction began several years before, even several decades before, modern psychoactive drugs came into general use. In Sweden it took more than ten years after these medicines came into use before the first reductions were made in the number of hospital beds; instead, these facilities were expanded during this ten-year period. In France, Belgium, Austria, Spain and West Germany, there were more hospital beds in the 1970s than in the first half of the 1950s before psycho-pharmaceuticals came into widespread use (Pilgrim & Rogers 1993, Sedgwick 1982).

In the USA there was a noticeable reduction in the number of hospital beds in 1956, which led Pollack & Taube (1975, quoted in Gronfein 1985), to conclude:

There appears to be no question that the sudden decrease in the state mental hospital population in 1956 (...) was due to the widespread introduction of psychoactive drugs into the mental hospitals. (p. 438)

Gronfein's (1985) and Sculls' (1984) statistical studies indicate that the picture is much more complex. In the USA, the number of beds in psychiatric hospitals began to decline in 17 of the states even before 1946. Statistics on discharges from American psychiatric hospitals showed a rising trend between 1946 and 1954; that is, after the introduction of psychoactive drugs. But even if the discharge rate increased after 1954, Gronfein's study shows that:

... while a majority of the states did experience a greater increase in discharge rates after drug introduction than before, fully 40 percent of the states showed the reverse pattern. (p. 448)

Warner's overview (1985) shows also that the percentage of discharged patients in follow-up studies decreased in the period between 1900 and 1040, but increased sharply between 1941 and 1955. The increase continues after 1956, if at a slower rate. (See Figure 2.)

When it comes to the consequences of treatment with neuroleptic medicines for patients' social or total recovery and for their consumption of hospital services, it is difficult to establish any clear correlation.

The data in Warner's metastudy (1985) show that the widespread use of clorpromazine did not result in any statistically measurable changes in the percentage of patients with a schizophrenia diagnosis who recovered either socially or totally.

After reviewing a number of studies, Bental (1990) concluded that:

Only a small proportion of patients benefit from these drugs and that minimal differences in outcome are observed between patients given these medications and those on low dosages or no medication at all. (p. 31)

In an experts' report presented to a consensus conference on schizophrenia (Garrabé & Winkelmuller 1994), it was concluded that:

Even if many studies have been devoted to this subject (whether psychoactive drugs affect the duration of schizophrenia, my note), few of them were able to draw any clear conclusions because of methodological problems, which most of the authors themselves acknowledge in their articles. (p. 81, my transl.)

Treatment with psychoactive drugs can reduce symptoms in many cases. They may even help to prolong the time before a relapse, defined in terms of readmission to hospital. However, help of this kind remains at the symptom level and does not affect the causes that lie behind the symptoms, whether these are situated in the individual's genetic constitution, brain functioning, childhood or current general social situation.

The social consequences of neuroleptic medicines vary sharply; the reduction of symptoms can be an opportunity to help the person manage aspects of life than may have been a contributing cause of the disorder, but it can also be used to as an excuse to terminate other forms of treatment when the patient no longer constitutes a danger to his/her environment. The belief that severely mentally disturbed patients could be cured by means of neuroleptic medicines has had the effect that accounts of social and psychological treatment strategies introduced before the mid-1950s and reflected in the discharge policy practised at that time have been overlooked in the history books. The replacement of psycho-social treatment interventions with medical treatments might explain the contradictory numbers found in the statistics over the percentage of recovered patients during the period after the second world war.

Psychotherapeutic interventions

By psychotherapy is meant, in the context of this study, talk therapies that are based on psychodynamic theory. Freud was quick to adopt a negative view of the possibility of using psychoanalysis to treat patients with severe mental disorders. In his *Orientering i psychoanalysis* [Orientation in psychoanalysis] (1980), a collection of his early lectures between 1915 and 1917, Freud wrote:

> In the meantime there are now other types of illnesses where we, despite the similarities in the condition, have never succeeded with our treatment. (…) These patients, paranoids, melancholics and sufferers of dementia praecox, are generally unaffected by and inaccessible to psychoanalytic therapy. Why is this so? Not the lack of intelligence; our patients must of course have a certain measure of intellectual ability. (p. 361) (…)
>
> Our observations have taught us that patients with narcissistic neuroses are incapable of transference or only have a residual capacity. They reject the doctor, not through hostility but through indifference. For this reason they are inaccessible to influence; what he says never touches them; consequently, the healing process that we can initiate in others – by which we mean the reawakening of the pathogenic conflict and overcoming the repression mechanism – never gets started with them. They remain what they are. Often these patients have tried to find a cure on their own,

attempts that have a pathological outcome. Here nothing can be done. (…) They do not invite transference and therefore are inaccessible for our treatment; we cannot cure them. (p. 368)

These words of Freud have not gone unchallenged in the psychoanalytic movement. In an encyclopaedic work entitled *The Psychoanalytic Theory of Neurosis*, Fenichel (1971) wrote:

An analytic effect on schizophrenics is possible because the regression to narcissism (which was thought to undermine the basis for a transference relationship, my notation) is never a complete one. (p. 447)

Fenichel pointed out, however, that if psychoanalysis was to be used with these patients, it would have to modify some its techniques:

Still, the therapeutic successes that are reported are not yet sufficiently due to a systematic, scientific consciousness of the necessary modifications, but rather to the intuitive therapeutic skill of the respective analyst. (p. 448)

In this passage Fenichel has introduced several themes that still have weight in the analytic discussion of therapies with this category of patients: the insufficient scientific rigour of studies of psychoanalytic therapies and their outcome, and the relationship between the therapist's technique and personality.

Sjöström (1985), in researching the effects of psychotherapy on patients with a schizophrenic diagnosis, discussed a review of earlier studies on the same topic in which were reported:

… rather negative findings from a small number of controlled studies, while more optimistic views are derived from uncontrolled and casuistic reports. (p. 513)

Measuring the part played by psychotherapy in the recovery from severe mental disorders entails far-reaching problems (see among others the National Board of Health and Welfare 1989). One of the problems is to decide which kinds of encounters are to be regarded as "psychotherapeutic". The question touches upon the therapist's qualifications and the "setting" for the therapy. Does psychotherapy merely mean frequent and organised one-on-one sessions with a psychoanalyst who is affiliated with a particular theoretical school? Another problem is that proponents of the psychotherapeutic school have questioned the measurement criteria used in psychiatry. These criteria are primarily concerned with symptomology and social adaptation and seldom attempt to measure "insight". They regard these criteria as superficial and that fail to take into account psychodynamic aspects.

Still another problem is that psychotherapeutic techniques were introduced unevenly into psychiatry's treatment arsenal. This makes it difficult to measure a "before" and an "after" in studies that extend over a particular geographic area or a larger patient population. Generally, however, it can be said that psychodynamic methods and theories began to gain ground in psychiatry after the second world war. Their introduction in Sweden dates from the beginning of the 1970s when projects were initiated in various psychiatric sectors, such as Nacka and Hasselby-Vällingby in the vicinity of Stockholm and Luleå in northern Sweden. This innovation coincided with the national accreditation of psychotherapists.

Keeping these reservations in mind, we nevertheless maintain that the absence of change, (as the studies by Warner [1985] and Hegarty and associates [1994] show), has the same consequences for evaluating the treatment effects of psychotherapy as it does for evaluating the results of psycho-pharmaceutical interventions. In a research overview of the effects of psychotherapy on psychosis, the Swedish National Board of Health and Welfare (1989) concluded that:

> ... the research literature – possibly with two exceptions (May and McGlashan) – shows that psychotic patients can be helped by different psychotherapies. It is, however, very difficult to say anything about the extent of their improvement and what improvement means for the patients themselves. The prognosis is considerably better for psychotic patients with affect disorders or borderline personalities than it is for schizophrenic patients. (p. 47)

It is uncertain, however, if the authors of the National Board of Health and Welfare's review of the research literature paid attention in their evaluation to the incidence of "spontaneous improvement" noted in the follow-up studies that were conducted in the 1900s.

Table 2. A model for summarising the effects of various forms of treatment as presented in the literature.

	Symptom reduction	**Social function**	**Personality change**
Psychosocial treatment	Yes	Yes	Unclear
Insight therapy	No at acute phase Yes at later phase	Yes, at later phase	Unclear

Source: Swedish National Board of Health and Welfare 1989.

Stanton et al. (1984) conducted a comprehensive investigation in Boston to test the hypothesis that insight therapy had a positive outcome for patients with a schizophrenia diagnosis. The patients were divided into two groups. One group received supportive therapy, at most one a week, and the other group insight therapy two to three times a week. The therapies were to continue for two years and all the patients were treated by experienced therapists. The drop-out rate at the end of the two years was high: only 31% of the original 164 patients were still in the project.

The patients who stayed in the project showed marked improvements as measured by a number of variables (fewer thought disturbances, greater ability to form stable interpersonal relationships, less need of medication, etc.). Only small differences between patients in the two groups could be noted. The patients who had received supportive therapy had fewer days of hospitalisation and functioned better in such areas as social adaptation and work. The patients who had received insight therapy showed greater improvements in their ego functioning and cognition. A disconcerting finding, however, was that the patients who had dropped out of the project had significantly fewer days spent in hospital and took less medication than the patients who remained in the project to the end.

In Sweden Cullberg and Levander (1991) conducted an investigation of patients with a schizophrenia diagnosis who were treated successfully with psychotherapy. In the study they elected to use stringent diagnostic criteria both for schizophrenia (all the patients selected for the follow-up group were re-diagnosed according to DSM-III-R criteria) and for recovery. To be included in the study, former patients must not have shown any sign of schizophrenia or psychosis for the two years immediately preceding the follow-up. Nor were they to have been treated on a daily basis with neuroleptic medicines or any other psychoactive drug.

Cullberg and Levander contacted a long list of accredited psychotherapists and supervisors in Sweden. Fifty-five therapists reported immediately on a total of 183 persons whom they regarded has having been successfully treated for schizophrenia by means of psychotherapy. But after the inclusion criteria had been applied to these patients, only eight remained in the group of recovered. Six of the successful cases had been treated by Barbro Sandin, a seventh had a therapist who was under Barbro Sandin's supervision. Cullberg and Levander concluded that:

> … the number of cured schizophrenics is small, supporting the view that compete cure is a rare phenomenon. (p. 260)

The problem with this conclusion is that it does not take into account the conditions for the study; namely, the use of DSM-III-R criteria for schizophrenia tend to exclude cases that have a favourable prognosis.

Psychotherapeutic interventions can play an important role for people with diagnoses of severe mental disorders. For some individuals it can even be crucial. There remains, however, a need to be more precise about what in the treatment itself can have brought about the good effects. Seen in relation to Hasting's (1958) requirement that treatment results must be better than the outcome for patients who receive no treatment at all, the psychotherapeutic research to date has had only marginal success when it comes to recovery.

Psycho-pedagogical interventions

Bleuler (1963) came to the conclusion that:

> We are forced to conclude that no single, specific cause for all schizo-phrenic psychoses has been found. I think that it does not exist. (…) Misery and psychosocial stress of the most varied kinds are more frequent in the life history of schizophrenics than in an average family history. (p. 26)

With the advent of the so called "vulnerability" hypothesis, cognitive methods have received increased prominence in the treatment of schizophrenia and other psychosis diagnoses (Borell 1995, Official Reports of the Swedish Government 1992:73, Zubin & Spring 1977, Zubin, Steinhauer & Condray 1992). The vulnerability hypothesis was formulated as early as the 1940s, say Zubin and Spring (1977), but has later been given a modern interpretation, both by these authors and others (see for example Cullberg 1999). A common feature of the various interpretations is the assumption that mental disorders result from the breakdown of the person's ability to cope with the various facets of his/her life ("coping ability"). This ability is primarily innate and implies in effect that different people have different tolerance levels for stressful situations.

Kopelowicz and Liberman (1996) describe the treatment intervention that has emerged from this hypothesis as a combination of anti-psychotic medicines, social training/learning and support (for example in homemaking, work and recreation). Treatment interventions may also involve members of the person' social network. Here the main issue is the family's over-involvement in the patient's situation. In some families, this involvement is expressed as critical comments made about and to the patient (so called "Expressed Emotions" or E.E.). The primary aim of treatment is to create a protective environment that reduces the number of situations that are stressful for the patient and to help patients find a way that works for them in coping with their symptoms. Based on the Expressed Emotions hypothesis, clinicians have developed a series of pedagogical interventions:

Family interventions are organized around the central goal of providing family members with more information about the disorder and strategies for managing common problems. (Penn & Mueser 1996, p. 609)

There are also various means of combining the patients' own ways of managing their symptoms ("coping strategies") with clinical treatment. In the field of psycho-education, learning programmes have been developed to supplement the patients' own arsenal of coping strategies and to replace those that are less successful. The focus in these cases is on how patients cope with particular symptoms and "early signs" of impending psychosis. Follow-up studies of such interventions show an increase in patients' ability to control and reduce the extent of their symptoms, particularly with regard to the occurrence of delusion (Penn & Mueser 1996). The majority of researchers conclude that the best results in terms of symptom reduction, better social adaptation and fewer relapses and readmissions to hospital are achieved by combining these various psycho-educative interventions together with medication (see for example Liberman et al. 1986).

The frequently referred to review by Hogarty and associates (1986) lent support to this spirit of optimism. They found that in several of the studies in the review, four of ten schizophrenic patients suffered a relapse within a year although they took the prescribed medication. This finding led the research team to initiate a two-part support programme encompassing both patients and their families. The patient's family was offered a psycho-educative programme to help reduce emotional tension (E.E.) in the home and help the family to adopt more realistic expectations of the patient's accomplishments. In addition to medication, the patients were offered a programme to train their social functions. The aim here was to:

... develop the social competence of patients by enhancing both verbal and nonverbal social behaviors as well as developing more accurate social perception and judgement. (p. 635)

The patients were divided into four groups; the first received the family training programme together with medication, the second social training and medication, the third a combination of the three, and the fourth only medication. For the first two groups, the programme reduced by half the number of patients who suffered a relapse and were readmitted to hospital during the project's first year; i.e., from 40% to about 20%. For the group who received a combination of all three interventions, the relapse frequency fell to 0%. For the fourth group, the share of patients who suffered a relapse remained at the expected 40% level. Hogarty and associates concluded that the common factor for the patients who did not suffer a relapse was that the level of E.E. in their respective families had decreased. They pointed out, however, that they did not know what had actually brought about the change:

> The results that we obtained might just as well have followed from factors and processes unknown to us at the moment. (p. 640)

The results from the next follow-up (Hogarty et al. 1991) dampened their optimism, however. At the two-year follow-up, it came to light that although the family interventions still had a significant impact, the effects of social training had disappeared. The combined effects of social training, the family programme and medication had also disappeared. After two years, even the positive effects of the family programme had disappeared.

The conclusion of the study, therefore, is that various interventions in combination were effective in delaying relapses in terms of readmission to hospital, but did not prevent them. This conclusion received added support from a review of similar research endeavours: the treatment programme for schizophrenia patients based on social training contributed to reducing the symptoms and increasing the patient's social adaptation. However, they had no appreciable effect on the number of relapses and readmissions to hospital (Penn & Mueser 1996). Hogarty et al. concluded:

> It is not our intent to turn the hopefulness of the past decade, which followed on short-term treatment gains, into an era of pessimism because such gains might be time-limited. Rather, schizophrenia in its more

prevalent form is a chronic illness, to which most families and dispassionate clinicians would attest. (1991, p. 344)

So, once again, we see that when the evaluation of form of treatment in which the researcher believes wholeheartedly does not produce the expected results, the tendency is to conclude that the absence of a positive outcome can be explained by the nature of the disorder itself, that the disorder is intrinsically chronic.

In closing, we can conclude that at present there are no specific treatment interventions for specific mental disorders that bring about the recovery of the majority of the patients. This gives cause for profound pessimism in the clinical world. It is for this reason that schizophrenia is characterised as a chronic disorder; that is, a disorder in which the course of development is predetermined, is not affected by treatment and persists throughout the rest of the person's life.

4

Roads to recovery

Hypotheses on recovery

Psychiatry has been unable to establish a clear and indisputable connection between particular forms of treatment and the recovery of persons with severe mental disorders such as the schizophrenia diagnosis. To come to grips with the occurrence of recovery among this category of patients psychiatry has adopted two main strategies: elimination and naturalisation.

Elimination

This strategy, discussed above in Chapter 2, is used in connection with patients who have already been diagnosed as well as with first-time patients. A common procedure in research contexts is to ask a psychiatrist experienced in diagnostics to make a new diagnosis of the patients under study by re-examining their hospital records. Patients who had been treated for schizophrenia but were now cured could thereby be assigned a new diagnosis. Schizophreniform disorder, for example, is a diagnosis that was devised in the mid-1930s (Langsfeldt 1937) for just such cases.

Another way to eliminate patients from the chronically ill category is to specify a minimum duration criterion for the diagnosis, thereby eliminating patients who recover "too quickly". What remains is a select group of patients whose symptomology shows a tendency from the start to be of long duration (APA 1980, 1994).

Naturalisation

In contrast to the elimination strategy, naturalisation accepts the idea that patients with chronic diagnoses might recover. However, their recovery is never the result of human intervention, except possibly when psychoactive drugs or surgery is used (Ljungberg 1975). These patients are said to be "spontaneously cured". What this generally means is that the improvement in the patients' condition has come about as a result of the inherent dynamics of the illness itself. The explanation for the cure of patients suffering from a chronic illness could then be found in the so-called "natural" course of development that was specific to this particular diagnosis. These patients would have recovered no matter what treatment they received, and even if they had never been treated at all (Wynne 1988). There is a good deal of research whose aim is to find out whether there are specific personality traits that could explain why individual patients diagnosed as chronically ill nevertheless recovered were cured spontaneously.

Factors related to a positive prognosis

Gender, age, civil status, heredity, type of illness, social network, IQ, occupation, age at sexual debut, personality characteristics prior to becoming ill, occurrence of external events that caused the onset of the illness and types of symptoms are all factors that have been said at different times to have an effect on the course of mental illnesses (Beiser & Iacono 1990, Ciompi 1980, Stephens & Astrup 1963, Vaillant 1964). The type of person who is most likely to have a good prognosis, according to many researchers and clinicians, is an older married woman who has previously worked for a living, has an adequately high IQ, a broad and varied social network and no hereditary complications, who became ill suddenly with so-called positive symptoms[1] brought on by a specific external event and whose personality prior to the onset of the illness is considered to have been fairly well structured.

Strauss and Carpenter's (1978) study along this line of inquiry showed, however, that the value of most of these predictor variables was limited. Those that proved to have good predictive value could be divided into three categories: history of prior hospitalisation, social relationships and occupation prior to onset of the illness.

> Evaluating the relationships of the various predictors with each aspect of outcome showed that each of the three variables – hospitalisation, level of social relations, and level of occupational function – was best predicted by its corresponding predictor variable. Thus social relations before admission were the best predictor of social relation at outcome, work function before admission was the best predictor of work function at outcome, and duration of hospitalisation before the initial evaluation was the best predictor of hospitalisation the year before the follow-up. (p. 62-63)

These three categories of variables, Strauss and Carpenter contended, had prediction value not only for patients diagnosed as schizophrenic, but also for patients with other kinds of mental disorder diagnoses. Their findings were confirmed in later studies. (See Ciompi 1980)

It was further thought that determining such predictor variables would make it possible to distinguish "real" schizophrenia, in the sense "incurable", from other disorders like 'schizophreniform psychosis". Another possible consequence of this line of research was to be the identification of various genetic, biological and developmental psychological explanations for why patients diagnosed as schizophrenic could display a similar set of symptoms but respond differently to treatment (see for example Bleuler 1978 and Cullberg 1993).

So far, however, this line of inquiry has not lived up to expectations. It has not been able to establish a simple direct relationship between personal characteristics and the onset of mental illness; on the contrary, what has emerged instead is the realisation that these factors are much more complex than first thought. In effect, this line of research has invalidated schizophrenia as a uniform diagnosis (Cullberg 1993). But in breaking down the schizophrenia diagnosis into a variety of disorders, it has for that very reason made it possible to retain the psychiatric illness model where types of illness are delineated in objective terms, and each illness is assumed to have its own etiology, specific course of development and specific ways of treating it.

Recovery as an object of research

There has been relatively little research on what persons who have recovered believe has aided their recovery. Instead there is an extensive material in the form of autobiographical narratives in which persons who have received psychiatric treatment describe their journey into and out of psychiatric care. Among the more well-known are *Percival's Narrative* (first published in 1840; new edition in 1961 edited by Bateson); Hannah Green's *I Never Promised You a Rose Garden* (1964); Mary Barnes' *Two Accounts of a Journey Through Madness* (1971); Elgard Jonsson's *Tokfursten* (The Mad Prince, in Swedish) (1986); and Ron Coleman's *Recovery – an alien concept* (1999).

The reputable scientific journal *Schizophrenia Bulletin* has since its debut number published autobiographical articles, some of them on recovery from severe mental disorders[2]. Scientific articles have been written by authors who in their research work make use of their own experiences of severe mental problems to describe their own and others' encounters with psychiatric care. Among them are Patricia Deegan (1988, 1997b) and Cheryl Gagne (Kramer & Gagne 1997), to mention just two.

Particularly during the last two decades of the 1900s, research has been concerned with the process of recovery from severe mental disorders. Especially four aspects of the recovery process have been studied:

- structural conditions that aid recovery
- the personality characteristics of persons who have recovered and their own contribution to the recovery process
- how other people have contributed to the recovery process
- the course of the recovery process

In the following sections we present a number of studies in which the experiences of mental health service users have been compiled and investigated under controlled conditions. In a concluding section, the consequences of this knowledge are discussed in terms of how it affects our way of thinking about severe mental disorders and the kinds of help that could be offered to persons so afflicted. From this review emerges new areas of research that need defining and which form the basis for the empirical part of the present study.

Structural factors affecting recovery

Both evaluative research on particular methods of treatment and follow-up studies of patient groups tend to place the human subjects of the study in a social, political, cultural and institutional vacuum. What were institutions like when Kraepelin constructed the dementia prae-cox diagnosis? What factors in "third world" settings are conducive to recovery? What has come in the place of the psychiatric hospitals that were shut down? And what effect has closing down psychiatric hospitals and establishing alternatives to these institutions (or the lack of alternatives) had on the patients themselves?

Cultural notions about the nature of mental suffering and how persons so afflicted are to be regarded and treated have their roots outside the domain of psychiatry, materialising after a time as institutionalised routines and procedures. These institutionalised practices tend to be self-perpetuating when it comes to justifying their existence. This has led to the emergence of professions, bodies of knowledge and ideologies whose interests coincide with the survival interests of their respective institutions (Conrad & Schneider 1992).

A number of studies have shown that structural factors play a role in determining the probability of recovery. Three such groups of factors are discussed here: the institutional policies of psychiatry and the social services; the labour market; and cultural notions of madness.

Institutional factors

Notions about mental illness in Europe and North America are closely related to the existence of psychiatric hospitals and the monopoly doctors have on all that concerns madness. To be cured, it was long thought that the patient must be removed from the home environment and isolated in therapeutic institutions under strict medical supervision (Castel 1976, Scull 1979). The evolution of psychiatric hospitals from an intended place of treatment to a custodial facility changed people's attitude toward mental illness and those afflicted with it. Madness became an inherent condition of the individual, a genetic and/or psychological defect. A chronic illness.

Research on the effects that institutions and life within them have on patients has largely focused on the routines and social relationships that occur within closed institutions and how these affect the inmates' identity. Several research studies show that it is often difficult to distinguish between, on the one hand, the patient's behaviour, cognition and emotions, which psychiatry defines as symptoms of mental disorder, and on the other, the effects of hospitalisation on a person's identity; that is, the harmful effects of institutionalisation. Bettleheim (1943) described the effect of a stay in a total institution on persons who were not mentally disturbed as a deep regression of the ego structure. The inmates' daydreams became increasingly bizarre, their sense of time became distorted, their ability to postpone gratification deteriorated, they came more and more to regard the world as split into good and evil. Barton (1959) found a similar syndrome among hospitalised patients and called the condition "institutional neurosis" (see Chapter 10).

This similarity between the effects of institutionalisation and symptoms of severe mental disorder implies, in other words, that some of the symptoms psychiatry regards as signs of mental disorders could in fact be effects of treatment. The person's suffering is organised within the special framework of the psychiatric institution.

Goffman's study *Asylums* (1961) has done much to change the general public's attitude toward psychiatric hospitals. At the centre of his analysis is a description of the mechanisms that contribute to re-shaping the individual's self-image. Goffman based his analysis on the study of total institutions, not as physical structures, but as social systems where a central authority has total insight into and overall control over the lives of other people. Power is wielded primarily by means of rules and rituals and, in certain situations, even by the direct encroach-ment on the patients' rights. The process whereby the person's sense of identity is undermined begins even before he/she is admitted to the institution:

> The prepatient's career may be seen in terms of an extrusory model; he starts with relationships and rights and ends up at the beginning of his hospital stay with hardly of either. (1961, p. 125)

> The recruit comes into the establishment with a conception of himself made possible by certain stable social arrangements in his home world. Upon entrance, he is immediately stripped of the support provided by these arrangements. (1961, p. 24)

Without the continued support that the self is accustomed to, a person's identity loses the nourishment it needs to sustain it. During their stay in a psychiatric hospital, patients meet a radically different kind of response than they are used to, which alters the basis for their self-image.

> Here one begins to learn about the limited extent to which a conception of oneself can be sustained when the usual setting of supports for it is suddenly removed. (p 137)

The reshaping of the self occurs in three steps. First, patients are separated from their physical and social environment, which up until then had been a main source of identity. Next, their life before becoming patients is described as consisting of a series of events that lay the groundwork for the ultimate failure – admission to a psychiatric hospital. Their identity is seen as a consequence of these past failures. The goal of treatment is to create a new identity. The result is a radical redefinition of the patients' identity wherein they adopt psychiatry's version of their life histories; they strive to live up to expectations as to how their lives will evolve, either as chronic patients or as "new" persons.

The more "medical" and the more progressive a mental hospital is – the more it attempts to be therapeutic and not merely custodial – the more (the patient) may be confronted by high-ranking staff arguing that his past has been a failure, that the cause of this has been within himself, that his attitude to life is wrong and that if he wants to be a person he will have to change his way of dealing with people and his conception of himself. (p. 139)

The negative development that Kraepelin saw as being decisive for the natural course of schizophrenia could just as well have been a consequence of the stringent rules and regulations that were in force in the Prussian institutions where he worked.

Goffman's analysis of the destructive effect of psychiatric hospitals on the inmates' identity became a basis for the critique of these institutions. At the same time, however, it contained the seeds of optimism. If institutions could break down a person's identity, would it not be possible to reconstruct identity again by reversing these mechanisms? Consequently, considerable effort has been devoted through the years to changing the conditions of life in institutions. If a person's identity could be demolished by environmental factors, it should be possible to build it up again under the right conditions became the rallying cry of the new era. Incidentally, it is interesting to note that this same argument was used to justify the establishment of psychiatric hospitals in the first place. Before, it was life outside the institution that was destructive; now, it was life within its walls that caused the damage. In either case, both the process of demolishing identity and of subsequently reconstructing it were attributed to external factors.

The first task of reforming the institutions after World War II was to normalise the conditions of everyday life within their walls. The number of dormitories and beds per room was reduced. Patients were given closets for their personal belongings. They were allowed to wear their street clothes and to make personal phone calls. Various social and cultural activities were arranged. Mixed wards were introduced. Furloughs were granted more often. Rehabilitation programmes designed to get patients more accustomed to life outside the hospital were further developed.

Studies of the rehabilitation practices of psychiatric hospitals have presented contradictory results. Wing and Brown's (1970) study of three mental hospitals in England during the 1960s showed that the patients' social competence developed parallel with the introduction of social activities and the normalisation of daily life within the institutions. However, the study also showed that these gains were lost when the hospitals subsequently reintroduced stringent institutional routines. Warner (1985) has shown that patients who participated in occupational therapy upon admission had fewer re-admissions than other patients. Anthony, Buell, Sharratt and Althoff. (1972), after reviewing the relevant research, concluded that patients could improve considerably in hospital settings, but that these improvements tended to disappear after they were discharged.

Efforts to create a therapeutic setting proved in many cases to be of limited benefit. Considerable improvements could be made in the institutional setting and in the patients' level of functioning and symptomology. But many of the patients who got better and were discharged had difficulty coping with life outside the hospital. Researchers concluded that comprehensive alternatives to hospitalisation were needed (Basaglia 1987, Stein & Test 1980, Mosher & Burti 1988). These alternatives included further developing the social insurance system and initiating local treatment and support programmes.

Changes in the daily life and routines of institutions and the emergence of alternatives to hospitalisation occurred concurrently with the marked reduction of hospital beds in Europe and North America. As a consequence, the living conditions of people hospitalised for long periods of time changed radically. In Sweden, for example, the number of hospital beds for 24-hour care declined from around 36,000 in the mid-1960s to around 10,000 thirty years later[3]. Thus the probability that a person would have a stay in hospital decreased, in relation to the number of times admitted and the total length of stay in hospital.

Thus, an already doubtful measurement for recovery became even more questionable. Earlier, continued hospitalisation was a means for measuring lack of recovery. The problem with using length of stay in hospital to measure chronicity or recovery is that for over a century there was a steady rise in the number of beds and no alternatives to hospitalisation. Now, with the reduction in the total number of hospital beds, the probability that persons will be hospitalised has also decreased.

Following in the wake of these reductions are a variety of specialised networks and forms of intermediate care. Their aim is to help discharged patients cope with daily life in the community, including occupational opportunities, housing, recreational activities and help to reconstruct a personal social network. Some of these intermediate facilities provide short-term rehabilitation whereby the individual is expected to advance to less regulated forms of support and finally to a life without any psychiatric support. Other intermediate facilities offer support that is unlimited in time with the risk that the support becomes a permanent fixture in the person's life.

Both Stein and Test (1978) and Bachrach (1976) have compiled comprehensive reviews of the research literature. They found that shutting down the psychiatric hospitals has resulted in appreciable improvements in the discharged patients' quality of life, and even in their state of mental health. A decisive factor for securing such improvements was a comprehensive and readily available system of community-based programmes designed to provide support during periods of crisis and for coping with daily life. After a 14-month long follow-up study of a group of mentally disturbed patients, Stein and Test (1980) concluded that no time limit should be set on these forms of support, at least for patients with a long history of hospitalisation. Several other studies (see Stein & Test 1978, Test & Stein 1978) have shown that the positive effects of programmes for discharged patients were obtained only so long as these programmes remained in force. Thus it may be a question of life-long support, the nature and extent of which could vary over time.

Another important result of the studies reported here was that interventions provided outside the hospital setting could reduce the risk of readmission. Patients who received support after discharge expressed more satisfaction with their situation than did patients in a control group who remained in hospital. These results suggest that a varied and flexible programme of community-based support provided outside the hospital setting could contribute to social recovery. However, there is no indication that such programmes affect the number of persons who recover totally.

In the study by Harding et al. (1987a, b) conducted in Vermont, social rehabilitation programmes in combination with medication resulted in the total recovery of a relatively large number of persons. A group of patients were followed up thirty years after they had taken part in a comprehensive and long-term rehabilitation programme, initiated while they were still in hospital and continued after their discharge. This group consisted of patients who were left in hospital when all the other patients had been discharged after being treated with new neuroleptic medicines. Harding (1997) described the state of most of the remaining patients at the start of the rehabilitation programme as one of profound regression.

This study is remarkable in that it follows up a group of patients who from the beginning were classified as "treatment resistant". The rehabilitation programme itself was of a traditional kind. But it departed from tradition in two respects: its duration and the nature of the relationship between patient and care-giver. The programme ran for a ten-year period.

Furthermore, it became apparent that during this period some of the patients and staff members of the rehabilitation team had formed inter-personal relationships. The patients were discharged into the communities where many of the staff lived. They belonged to the same parish, shopped in the same stores and participated in the same activities. Thus, the relationships formed in hospital were carried over into community life and evolved from one of professional distance to greater equality and reciprocity. However, the explanatory hypotheses formulated in the study are still unverified.

The expansion of intermediate forms of support poses new challenges when it comes to understanding what helps people with severe mental disorders to recover and what mental disorder and recovery really mean. Intermediate care could become a parallel society filling the same function that the psychiatric hospitals used to fill. Several research scientists (Estroff 1985, Corin 1990) have pointed out that both the social insurance system and intermediate forms of support entail the risk of long-term recipients becoming "support dependent" and that their recovery would then mean living a marginalised existence.

Intermediate care could also be an open network where even its most extreme parts are integrated into the cultural life of the community (Dell'Acqua & Mezzina 1988). In an open network, persons previously regarded as severely disturbed remain officially under psychiatric care but the support they receive has little resemblance to typical psychiatric care. An example comes from Trieste, Italy where the authors are engaged in mental health programmes where former patients run, among other things, a co-op bar, a radio station and a hotel.

Castell (1987) and Rotelli, de Leonardis and Mauri (1987) have made an important distinction for future analyses of the impact of intermediate forms of support on the identity of persons with mental disorders and on how the general public regards mental illness. On the one hand there is deinstitutionalisation where the sole aim is to close the large psychiatric hospitals, and on the other hand, deinstitutionalisation where the closure of the institutions is accompanied by a change in the relation between normality and madness. It is not only patients who must adapt to the society; society's norms must be based on the actual people who constitute its base. Therefore, support programmes for the mentally ill should not constitute a world apart from "the normal people's world".

> The problem has to do with creating a different relationship between madness, the immediate experience of madness and social structures of normality that could be the structures of deinstitutionalisation. ... So, deinstitutionalisation is not the same as the absence of institutions nor the breaking down of institutional structures. Rather, it could mean deinstitutionalising madness; that is to say, we could create a new culture concerning mental illness which could flourish even through institutions. (Castel 1987, p. 20)

There has been very little research to ascertain whether intermediate forms of support actually contribute to recovery from severe mental disorders. But the findings of several Swedish studies (Topor 1983, 1996, Hydén & Karlsson 1994, Karebo Larsén 1996, Tidemalm 1996, Forsberg & Starrin 1996) indicate that intermediate forms of support might very well play a role in social recovery and could help persons who have been hospitalised to reconstruct a self-image that gives a more prominent place to their own resources.

Work

Work has a central function in psychiatry. The inability to work is taken as an indication of a mental disorder. Moreover, work is described as a possible treatment measure. The patient's return to working life is an important variable for measuring the success of treatment. In the absence of work, by which is meant paid employment, successful treatment implies that the person is engaged in occupational activities where work of some kind is performed but that there are fewer demands on performance and extent of participation. The person does not receive a salary and is not eligible for social insurance benefits connected with the labour market.

C. J. Ekströmer, general director of the "Läns-lasaretterne, kurhusen och hospitalen i riket" (a Swedish hospital and sanatorium in operation in the 1800s), gave an early example of work as a tool for treatment and as a pasttime when he wrote:

> *The mentally ill person's involvement in work*, undoubtedly the most suitable and most beneficial way to influence the minds of the majority of those who are mentally ill, has in recent years resulted in appreciable advances in most of the hospitals; however, there remains much to be desired in this respect. ... the monotone repetition of suitable *diversions*, which are implemented according to plan to provide variety and reward, is hardly less important in treating the mentally ill than the work itself. (Ekströmer 1848, p. 64, italic in the original, my transl.)

Hydén (1995, see also Hydén & Karlsson 1994) point out three characteristics underlying the rehabilitative effects of work:

1) It offers a structure with respect to time (work verses recreation) and place (the home verses the work place).
2) By participating in shared production, the individual comes into contact with other people.

3) Through work and the social relationships these bring about, the person has a place in the society.

In other words, in work, as it is described in psychiatric contexts, several partly conflicting functions are combined. Work implies both treatment and rehabilitation, but is also the goal of these interventions. It is a right, but also a moral duty. Lastly, work has political implications. Through work persons whose only possession is their labour participate in a barter relationship with the surrounding world. By contributing their labour they become citizens.

Two interesting aspects of work that are seldom mentioned are the physical hazards of certain kinds of work and the shift from paid employment to unpaid work/labour, a phenomenon that is seldom discussed in psychiatry as a problem. There is considerable research pointing out the hazards of work in the form of physical and mental injuries resulting from undue stress and the trauma caused by exclusion from the labour market (see among others Diderichsen & Janlert 1983, Gardell 1983). Nevertheless, psychiatry has consistently pointed out only the positive aspects of work.

Work has seldom been discussed in terms of earning a wage, as in Warner's study (1985) referred to earlier. Earnings, money, is usually not regarded as a central factor when it comes to the work of people with mental disorders. The meaning of work for "people like them" is thought to be quite different from what it is for "people like us".

Bergh (1998) has questioned how the work concept is used in connection with people who have been in psychiatric care. He distinguishes between gainful employment on the regular labour market, which is what the studies that Warner refers to are concerned with, and the "occupational pastimes" that have developed after the psychiatric hospitals were shut down. In these programmes paying a wage or salary has been replaced by the notion of work as "meaningful in itself". Because the terms of the regular labour market (payment, democracy, productivity, dismissal) and these occupational pastimes are often in opposition to one another, it could later be a hinder for people who have recovered to re-enter the regular labour market.

Estroff (1985) has pointed out that there is a risk that community-based alternatives to hospitalisation will prove to be just as socially excluding as the psychiatric hospitals once were. In addition, they might also keep discharged patients dependent on psychiatry because it would be too risky to try to live without community support.

In his review of the relationship between psychiatry and political economy, Warner (1985) examined the findings from 85 follow-up studies of patients diagnosed as schizophrenic in relation to unemployment statistics in the US and Great Britain (see Chapter 3, Fig. 2).

The parallels between these two variables are remarkable. Periods of high unemployment coincide with periods when there are few discharges from psychiatric hospitals or few cases of social and total recovery. In periods of low unemployment, there is a rise in the occurrence of these three phenomena. This is not to say, however, that there is a definite cause and effect relationship between unemployment and the probability for patients diagnosed as schizophrenic to recover.

It seems that in the industrialised world the labour market, with its constantly fluctuating need of manpower, has an impact not only on the probability that people diagnosed with schizophrenia will be discharged from hospital, but also that they will recover, either socially or totally.

In connection with this line of reasoning Warner (1985) offered a hypothesis to explain the better prognosis that a study by WHO (1979) found among schizophrenia patients in developing countries. An important factor, according to Warner, is that people who deviate from the norm are less stigmatised in countries where there is no regular labour market. The notion of unemployment as a social norm lacks meaning in the developing countries, Warner pointed out. A person who is unable to work for a certain period of time hardly needs to explain his absence from the labour market. Furthermore, in these countries there are fewer demands on work performance, both when it comes to hours of work and productivity.

The possibility to enter the regular labour market seems to be related, not only to the risk that patients will be readmitted to hospital, but also to their possibility to recover socially or totally. However, it is not known what factors in connection with paid employment contribute to the recovery process. Therefore, it is important to distinguish between paid work and the various forms of occupational programmes that have developed after the psychiatric hospitals were shot down. The apparent relationship between reduced consumption of care and the existence of these programmes might instead be a consequence of the availability of fewer hospital beds. A number of studies have found that persons who participate in occupational programmes derive substantial personal benefit from them. For many of the participants it is possible to se signs of social recovery. However, there are no data on the possibility of total recovery.

Cultural factors

One of the points made in connection with WHO's follow-up study of schizophrenia patients in nine industrialised and developing countries (Leff 1977, WHO 1979) was that in each of the nine countries it was possible to find patients who fulfilled the project's criteria for schizophrenia. Kleinman (1988) pointed out, however, that to obtain this group of patients, the research team had to exclude a large number of patients who did not satisfy the stringent selection criteria. But despite the manner in which they were selected, the patients who were included in the study differed greatly in terms of their symptoms and illness course. The marked differences in outcome between schizophrenia patients from industrialised countries and those from developing countries indicate the need for further research.

The WHO study has been criticised for its methodology. Several authors have looked for weaknesses in the study's design to explain the more favourable outcome for the third world countries. As examples of such weaknesses, it was suggested that the third world sample contained more first-time patients with a better prognosis; that the same diagnostic criteria were not used in all nine countries; and that the most severely disturbed patients in third world countries never come into contact with the health care system. Additional studies were undertaken to meet these objections. (See Kleinman 1988, Leff, Sartorius, Jablensky, Korten & Ernberg 1992, Waxler 1979) Other explanations of the observed differences in outcome have focused on the cultural differences between developing and developed countries.

In a five-year follow-up of the WHO study on schizophrenia, Leff and associates (1992) found that clinical values co-vary with the level of clinical development and that primarily social variables predict the patient's later life in the community. However, the most important factor for determining if patients had a good or poor prognosis was if they lived in an industrialised country or in a third world country, regardless of the other predictor variables:

> This indicates that the superior five-year outcome of schizophrenic patients in developing countries is not explained by the set of predictor variables tested in the modelling procedures. These were chosen because their predictive value for the outcome of schizophrenia had been established by many previous studies. It is evident that the explanation for the better outcome in developing countries needs to be sought elsewhere. (p. 141-142)

A number of studies have been undertaken to try to explain the outcome of the WHO study. Two factors in particular have been mentioned: first, that persons from third world countries can count on continued support from their families if they become mentally ill; and second, that they have the possibility to return to their former occupation or find alternative ways of earning a living after discharge from hospital (Shepherd, Watt, Falloon & Smeeton 1989). A related explanation is that patients in developing countries are shown greater tolerance for their symptoms. A possible explanation for this is that in agrarian societies families are often large and consist of several generations, so that the burden of a sick family member is shared by more people. The measure for "greater tolerance" in the WHO study is the family's "Expressed Emotions". This hypothesis was confirmed in some, but not all, of the third world countries participating in the WHO study. (Leff et al. 1987, Leff et al. 1990)

Waxler (1979) conducted an investigation in Sri Lanka with the aim of testing the methodological problems found in the WHO study. Her results are wholly in line with the WHO follow-up. Forty-five per cent of the schizophrenia patients she followed up were completely symptom free five years after their initial contact with psychiatry compared with 8% for Denmark in the WHO study, to give just one example.

The factors Waxler examined as possible explanations of these differences are family structure, local ("native") forms of treatment, notions of madness and the common values and beliefs of the culture.

Family structure in developing countries, according to Waxler, is broad-based, tolerant and strong. It is easier for the multiple generation family than for the nuclear family to "bear the burden" of having a mentally disturbed person in the family. Furthermore, extended families offer their members in crisis a broader range of alternative roles. Thus, there is less risk of social isolation or that the mentally disturbed person will feel abandoned or become a social outcast.

Treatment interventions, including hospitalisation, are provided for shorter periods of time in developing countries than in industrialised countries. Even when the treatment follows the precepts of established medicine, patients and their families have considerable power over the kinds of treatment offered and the length of the patients' hospitalisation. They can even choose forms of treatment that better correspond to the local culture and combine different elements in the range of available forms of treatment.

Belief systems in developing countries regarding mental disorders often emphasise external explanatory factors. Thus the individual is seldom weighted down with the burden of guilt. In developing countries, it is usual to localise the source of the disorder in the person's own personality. In many developing countries individuals can choose for themselves to change their ways of behaving. A fundamental notion within the belief system is that episodes of madness are of short duration and are curable. The prevailing cultures of these countries encourage the idea that severely mentally disturbed persons have a good chance to recover (see also Nathan 1994, 1998).

With respect to studies that contrast developing and industrialised countries, we must take into account the economic advances that have taken place in recent decades in several so-called developing countries. Comparisons between developing and industrialised countries are often made between agrarian or rural cultures on the one hand, and urban or town cultures on the other. An interesting feature of the WHO study and the research that it has spawned is that the findings point away from individual prognostic variables toward more social and culturally based explanatory models. The studies have raised much controversy in the scientific community.

Kleinman (1988) asserts that also psychiatry employs various belief systems and that we must therefore regard psychiatric diagnoses as interpretations of the other person's experiences, experiences which from the beginning were conveyed to the psychiatrist through that person's own belief system:

> Because language, illness beliefs, personal significance of pain and suffering and socially learned ways of behaving when ill are part of that process of mediation, the experience of illness (or distress) is always culturally shaped phenomenon (like style of dress, table etiquette, idioms of expressing emotion and aesthetic judgements). The interpretations of patients and family become part of the experience. Furthermore, professional and lay interpretations of experience are communicated and negotiated in particular relationships of power (political, economic, bureaucratic and so forth). As a result, illness experiences are enmeshed in and inseparable from social relationships. (p. 7)

The meaning a given culture assigns to certain behaviours and beliefs affects how individuals view themselves and their relationship to the environment. This collection of beliefs and attitudes affects in turn how behaviours and beliefs related to mental disorders will develop – whether a mental disorder is regarded as a limited episode in the person's life or as a chronic illness leading to exclusion from one's social network or to being forced to assume a given role in that network.

A social perspective

So, there are quite a few studies showing that cultural and social factors can play a significant role in determining the course of mental illness and whether or not the patient will be discharged, irrespective of symptomology.

Waxler (1979) suggested that the search for an explanation of the positive outcome for patients in third world countries should concentrate on the cultural domain:

We must look at the social experience of the patient within his culture, at his experience with family and neighborhood, with doctors and hospital, to find explanatory variables of good outcome. (p. 156)

Harding et al. (1987a, 1997) have pointed at social factors as a possible explanation for the remarkably good results they found in their Vermont study. One of the hypotheses suggested to explain the patients' good outcome is that they were discharged into a rural environment where there were relatively few stress factors (Zubin 1985). The same hypothesis has been suggested to explain the differences in outcome found in the WHO study between patients in industrialised countries and those in developing countries. Harding rejects this hypothesis in the case of Vermont, however, pointed at the state's high level of alcohol abuse and high suicide rate. Eisenberg (1988) makes a similar criticism of the notion that life in third world countries is marked by a low level of stress because of an assumed high level of acceptance:

It is tempting to suppose that the toleration for impaired behaviour is greater in developing countries (…). This, however, grossly underestimates the complex role demands stemming form caste, kinship, religion, sex and age stratification in such societies. (p. 4)

The hypothesis offered by Harding et al. (1987a) to explain the well-documented favourable outcome and low drop-out rate in their study is in line with Waxler's approach. The aftercare of patients was the responsibility of a small team of five persons. These psychiatric workers followed up the discharged patients from the beginning of the project while all the patients were still in hospital, to when they were discharged, and later when several of them were readmitted on occasion. The continuity of contact remained in tact even when the official support programme was concluded ten years later:

This continuity of contact persisted during the second 10 years, as people changed their roles from clinicians and patients to friends and neighbours. (p 724)

This suggests a social explanatory model of recovery, which does not deny the possible role of genetic and biological factors, but which also assigns a central role to cultural definitions, socio-economic conditions and human interaction.

The perspective that the work of Eisenberg (1988), Harding et al. (1987a, b) Warner (1985) and Waxler (1979) opens up is the possibility that social interventions could alter the course of illness, that social encounters could contribute to the recovery process regardless of the prognostic variables (se also Barham 1984). In the last analysis, this approach could in effect mean the dissolution of the illness model. It is not simply that treatment and other factors "have an effect" on the illness; the illness, its cultural meaning and how it is received and treated are actually inseparable elements. This approach shifts the focus from "disease" to "illness", from a possible somatic process to

> ... how the sick person and the members of the family or wider network perceive, live with and respond to symptoms and disability. (Kleinman 1988, p. 3)

Patients' own efforts in their recovery

Most recovery research has in common the idea that both the onset of and recovery from severe mental disorders occur as a result of the interaction between the individual and the psycho-social environment. The underlying conception of the self in this view of recovery was seldom problematised – that of a self that observes itself and even creates itself through relationships with others. But in recent years this a rather outdated conception has been problematised (see Danzinger 1997, among others).

The self is often described as the product of a continuous negotiation between internal and external demands and as divided into a private and a public sphere. Regardless of psychological school, we meet this division between internal and external, private and public, subjective and objective (Estroff 1989). In most cases there is some overlap between these two sides of the self. But if the distance between them gets too wide, the self breaks down and we have difficulty conceiving of the mentally disturbed person as rational and interactive:

This lack of agreement or constructive interaction between self and others about self may also result in an incomprehensibility of person identified (…) as the hallmark of psychosis. (Estroff 1989, p. 190)

Strauss (1989) describes psychosis as the breakdown of the self's way to deal with reality, either as a result of internal conflicts, biological tension or stress generated by external sources. He describes a course of development that corresponds to the three phases of a crisis, which Rakfeldt and Strauss (1989) call "the low turning point" – an original organisation of the self that collapses in order to be reorganised again in a new way. Persons who have entered the first phase of psychosis experience mounting stress caused by the inappropriateness of their way of coping with their overall situation. As the tension rises, they become increasingly rigid in their way of handling their life situation. This leads in turn to even greater stress and finally to a psychotic breakdown. Thus, psychosis is defined as the deorganisation of the self. This may lead to a reorganisation of the self to enable it to function more flexibly, but the personality may also become chronified at a more rigid level of functioning.

Deegan, a psychologist who has a long history of repeated hospitalisation, describes the onset of illness in these terms:

What initially had seemed like a fleeting bad dream transformed into a deepening nightmare from which we could not awake. (…) We experienced time as a betrayer. (Deegan 1988, p. 13)

Contrary to the old adage, time does not heal all wounds; patients soon realise that their friends and peers have moved on in their lives while they themselves have come to a standstill in what appears to be a dead-end. The lack of hope is the motor that drives the vicious circle of chronification.

The self's struggle with itself

Estroff (1989) discusses two possible notions of schizophrenia: as something a person either *has* or *is*. The initial assault of the disorder on the individual's identity becomes protracted as a result of various stigmatising processes directed towards the individual following upon the illness. She concludes that even if schizophrenia were defined as an illness, as something a person *has*, the consequences of the diagnosis for the person's social identity are so all-pervading that in our culture it is regarded as something a person is, an "I-am illness" (p. 189).

However, the findings of a number of studies indicate that psychosis seldom invades the whole of the self. Podvoll (1990), for example, talks about "islands of clarity" and Lally (1989) says that often patients refuse to accept the symptoms as a part of themselves.

In an early study, Sacks, Carpenter and Strauss (1974) described patients' way out of the state of delusions and hallucinations as a complex three-stage process. These three stages can be seen as steps in a recovery process where particular symptoms are focused on. At first, patients are almost completely at the mercy of their delusions. They comprehend the world in terms of these delusions, which are the point of departure from which they try to deal logically with the world. From this position they begin slowly to test reality and a phase of "dual awareness" sets in. During this phase patients become better able to put their delusions into perspective. In their thoughts and actions they can both act on the basis of their delusions and at the same time question them. They become better able to seek the support of others when testing the viability of their own ideas and are more open to what other people say about their situation. This helps to bolster their self-confidence. As the delusions begin to recede, "they now confront the anxieties that attend resumption of the responsibilities of non-patient life". (Sacks et al. 1974, p. 120) This period is often marked by depression and a sense of loss at the retreat of the psychotic symptoms. Certain traces of delusions can still be noted, but they are now integrated as parts of the personality.

The process of moving away from the so-called positive symptoms of delusion and hallucination can in some cases precede the patient's social recovery. But it can also occur after a period of time when the patient has been functioning adequately in social contexts. People with psychotic symptoms can even live a normal social life with little inconvenience from their symptoms. (Romme & Escher 1989)

The hypothesis that patients during the first phase are capable of logical thinking within the framework of their delusions and that this is followed by a period marked by dual awareness means, in extension, that patients with severe mental disorders are not really so very "different" from the rest of us. It means that they can recognise their symptoms as being foreign to the self and that they try to manage them in some way. It means that they are not inaccessible to attempts by others to communicate. It means that what from the outside might seem to be incomprehensible utterances and actions can be understood within the framework of the patient's delusions.

The self's recovery

In a later study Breier and Strauss (1984) broadened their focus to include a longer period of time in the patient's life and to study how patients relate not only to their symptoms but also to their whole life situation. Through interviews every second month, they followed up a group of 20 persons for a whole year after discharge from hospital. They found that the way back for these persons could be divided into two phases: first came a "convalescence" phase, followed by a "reconstruction" phase.

Convalescence is marked by anxiety about leaving hospital, which is the first environment that one learns to manage in the capacity of psychiatric patient. During this phase discharged patients see themselves primarily as "former patients" and maintain contact with persons whom they met on the ward and who know what they have experienced. During this phase the former patients' relationship to the surrounding world is one-sided and marked by their dependence on the continued support and assistance of others.

In the reconstruction phase, persons who are recovering begin to regard themselves more as ordinary citizens than as former patients. The personal relationships they formed on the ward begin to thin out. Instead they seek to renew contact with people they knew before they were hospitalised and to form new relationships with people not connected with psychiatry. These relationships tend to be more reciprocal than those that existed in the preceding phase. The former patients begin to make their own plans in life and, after a while, set about realising them.

In an article on the contribution of patients to their own recovery, Strauss, Harding, Hafez and Lieberman (1987) distinguished three levels of activity. Initially, patients can collaborate by accepting the prescribed treatment and avoiding stressful situations. The next level, which for the patients means continuing to participate in programmes others have devised for them, requires a greater measure of self-generated activity on the part of the patients. On this level, patients participate in rehabilitation programmes to train various functions that had been affected by the illness. The third level proposed by Strauss and associates implies a radically new role for patients. On this level the patients' own contribution is much more creative than before. They begin to formulate their own definitions of their problems and work out solutions; they formulate their own goals and try to find meaning in what they have experienced. What is known about this third level is not systematised knowledge but mostly anecdotal knowledge.

This descriptive model ascribes to patients a central role in their own recovery. When Strauss and his associates (1987) talk about the recovery process, they use concepts seldom found in modern psychiatric terminology: force of will, courage, hope:

> Thus, by selecting environments and involvements, by controlling symptoms or choosing not to, and possibly even by force of will influenced such factors as courage and hope, it is possible that the patient has a major role in the recovery from psychosis. (p 164)

Davidson & Strauss (1992) studied a group of 66 patients with various psychosis diagnoses to determine how a sense of self develops during recovery. Their investigation extended over a period of between two and three years after the patients had been discharged. By following the course of daily life of these persons, the study gives a close-up picture of the recovery process. It describes parts of the self that were not affected by psychosis and how these parts expanded to eventually encompass greater parts of the self. The four phases found by Davidson & Strauss can be regarded as a refinement of what is known about the "dual awareness" phase. (Sacks et al. 1974)

The first step in the recovery process is that the person discovers that he/she is not simply nor wholly an illness, that *parts of the self have remained uncontaminated by the illness*. These may be parts that one recognises from one's past life or parts that are discovered for the first time in connection with psychosis. This discovery – that a measure of competency in certain areas has been retained – opens the way for persons on the road to recovery to begin to regard their illness and the devastation it has caused as having certain boundaries. This in turn becomes the basis for the emergence of a new self-image that is not reducible to only illness. An important factor contributing to this discovery seems to be the presence of other persons who believe in the individual's ability to be or become something other than wholly and only an illness, even when that individual has done everything in his/her power to refute the reasonableness of such a belief. A recurring concept in this context is hope (Davidson & Strauss 1992). At first, other persons are the bearers of hope, one or more persons who have seen and believe in the patient, even when the patient has done everything to prove his/her worthlessness to all concerned. A hopeless case. Deegan (1988) gives this picture of vicarious hope:

> We do remember that even when we had given up, there were those who loved us and did not give up. They did not abandon us. They were powerless to change us and they could not make us better. They could not climb this mountain for us, but they were willing to suffer with us. They did not overwhelm us with their optimistic plans for our futures, but they remained hopeful despite the odds. Their life for us was like a constant invitation, calling us forth to be something more than all of this self-pity and despair. The miracle is that gradually (...) we began to hear and respond to this loving invitation. (p. 14)

The second phase of the reconstruction process consists of *making an inventory of this self, of the parts of the self that have not been contaminated by the illness*. One of the subjects in the study described this period as one of putting together all the ingredients and cooking utensils needed to make a cake. The inventory is not always wholly realistic and is dependent on the support of others. The individual is still rather vulnerable to the judgements of others and becomes easily distraught by overly critical comments. This period may continue for a long time before any results become apparent.

During the third phase, persons in the process of recovering begin to *put the self to use*, incorporating various parts of their personal inventory in the process. In a very short time, they may make great strides in certain areas of their lives. That the self has moved into an active phase can sometimes be expressed in ways that psychiatry may not recognise, as it concerns what appear on the surface to be simple everyday situations. Davidson and Strauss (1992) give the example of a patient who announces with pride that she is now able to turn on the radio *herself* and choose a radio station that plays the kind of music *she wants* to hear. This simple act was for her a momentous step in her recovery.

Persons on the road to recovery "pull themselves together" and are no longer simply recipients of the good will and support of others; they begin to have an own impact on the environment. The self once again becomes the source of desire and possesses an independent will that can be expressed in concrete terms and that leaves its mark on the environment. The independent will is free from both the power of psychosis, the therapist and the family. Davidson and Strauss (1992) point out that during this phase the efforts of clinical staff to get patients to accept the course of treatment planned for them may have the opposite effect in that the treatment perpetuates external control at a time when the individual is trying to become established as an "own" person.

The persons' actions and the outcome of their actions are integrated with the self as tangible evidence for and confirmation of the areas in which they used to have some measure of competence. Positive experiences prepare the groundwork for improving one's self-image. As *the person's self-image becomes increasingly more positive, it becomes a resource for coping with symptoms* and the stigma that the person now has to contend with. The new self-image begins more and more to function as a protective shield against residual signs of illness and detrimental aspects of the environment and living conditions.

The insight that one can influence one's environment provides a foundation for managing the illness.

And once there is a sense of self that can be seen as responsible for managing the illness, it then also becomes possible for the person to take a more active and determined part in his/her social and vocational rehabilitation, developing, copying mechanisms and learning to exercise self-control over symptoms. (Davidson & Strauss 1992, p. 140)

For persons who are struggling with the effort to manage their lives in relation to psychotic episodes and psychiatric treatment, it gives them proof that they are still persons with a will of their own who can direct their lives toward goals that they themselves have set up and have the competence to attain.

Active attempts to manage

In research on the recovery process, the individual/patient is not presented as helpless and completely at the mercy of the disorder; regardless of whether the roots of the helplessness are thought to lie in genetic factors, chemical imbalance or a disturbed personality.

In recent years there is a growing body of research into how persons, with varying degrees of success, manage their symptoms, their so-called "coping strategies" (see Brenner, Boker, Muller, Spichtig & Wurgler 1987, Carr 1988, Falloon & Talbott 1981, Cohen & Berk 1985, Lee, Lieh-Mak, Yu & Spinks 1993) and "self-help" (see among others Boker 1987 and Chamberlin 1978). Even before the 1950s, Bleuler (1950) and Freud (1959), in their respective studies of Chief Justice Schreber, interpreted certain of the magistrate's symptoms as failed attempts at self-healing (see Boker 1987).

As part of the follow-up study of 20 patients, cited earlier, Breier and Strauss (1984) investigated how the individuals in their study controlled their own symptoms. Eighteen of the 20 patients had developed various coping strategies to manage, first of all, such symptoms as generalised suspicion, feeling "high", depression, disjointed thinking, hallucinations, delusions, deep-seated exhaustion and anxiety. Breier and Strauss classified the coping strategies described by patients in a model consisting of three elements:

- *Self-management*, which entails being on the lookout for situations and behaviours within oneself and others that trigger or precede the psychotic symptoms
- *Self-assessment*, which has to do with comparing one's own behaviour with the behaviour of others, such behaviour that is generally regarded as acceptable. Other persons become role models
- *Self-reinforcement*, which Breier and Strauss do not define

A prerequisite for self-control is that the individual can identify the behaviours and situations that are to be controlled. In the work of identifying these, the person comes to study himself/herself in relation to the environment. The control mechanisms patients develop can be divided into three categories:

- *Instructing themselves*: When the undesirable behaviour or threatening situation had been identified, the patients could admonish themselves. One patient in the study told herself firmly to "act like an adult" and "take responsibility" for her own conduct.
- *Reducing their own level of activity.* The patients withdrew from the threatening situation or discontinued the stressful activity by taking a walk or sitting down and relaxing.
- *Raising their own level of activity.* To get away from the distressing symptom, some patients scouted around for other activities to get involved in. They could get so caught up with what they were doing there was no room left for the symptoms. These activities need not be simple ones; they could demand a high degree of stress tolerance and autonomy.

Romme and Escher (1989, 1996) describe still other means of coping that can be added to Breier and Strauss' categories. They investigated 48 persons, both psychiatric patients and people who had never come into contact with psychiatry, all of whom heard voices. Several of them had found successful ways to manage their voices and developed various cognitive strategies of their own. *They entered into a relationship with their symptoms.* Instead of trying to escape their voices, they tried to get closer to them, "to get to know them", and in various ways structured their contact with their voices and tried to work out compromises. One person, for example, made a contract with her voices that she would give them her full attention at a certain time every day on condition that they did not disturb her for the rest of the time. Other persons reported that they could distinguish between good and evil voices. They then concentrated solely on the good voices and could even use them as advisors.

Throughout the research on patients' coping strategies, it is the individuals themselves who identify what symptoms they want to become more adept at managing. This is the basis upon which they devise a variety of ways of relating to their voices. The work of mastering such a situation shows that often people with psychotic symptoms relate actively to their symptoms and to their own lives.

An important consideration in this context is the meaning that the individual and the environment attach to the symptoms and to the situations that arise as a consequence of the symptoms. Strauss (1992b) pointed out, for example, that situations are seldom stressful in themselves, but can become stressful depending on how the individual and the environment react to them. What is stressful for one person need not be so for another. And what is stressful at a particular time in one's life need not be so at another time. A situation is stressful depending on how the person interprets and assigns meaning to the situation. The search for and construction of meaning in the patient's experiences are repeatedly cited as factors in many patients' recovery accounts.

How we interpret our environment and thereby create the world we live in is not the concern solely of patients or psychiatry. Negative symptoms are included in the criteria for a schizophrenia diagnosis. By negative symptoms are meant the absence of normal functions. They are symptoms of the patient's reduced productivity, reduced mobility, fewer social contacts, fewer words and fewer expressions of emotions. Negative symptoms are considered more difficult to combat because they develop so slowly and are therefore regarded as chronic (Strauss et al. 1974). In an article on the psychological and social aspects of

125

negative symptoms, Strauss et al. (1989) offered a hypothesis that has later found support in research (see for example Corin & Lauzon 1992); namely, that negative symptoms can also be interpreted as reasonable ways for patients to manage threatening psychological and social situations.

Withdrawal can be the person's response to having experienced repeatedly that the demands of life in the community lead to a relapse into psychosis. Because of these experiences the person loses hope and has increasing difficult to find an identity as a non-patient. The danger of the withdrawal strategy is that it reduces patients' possibilities to come into contact with other people and situations that might help them to find a better way to solve the problems to which their "negative symptoms" are a response. Withdrawal may result in a vicious circle. Psychiatry's attempts to "protect patients" from external stress by creating stimuli-deficient environments may contribute to such a vicious circle by preventing patients from learning to master troublesome situations in a more rewarding way. On the other hand, the opposite strategy of "activating patients" may instead disrupt the delicate balance that the individual may have succeeded in achieving.

Journey of recovery – standstills and forward leaps

The course of recovery described here does not follow a straight line; it occurs by stages with leaps forward alternating with seeming stagnation. The model outlined by Strauss and other research scientists places an active self at the centre of the recovery process. This model may help to redefine the meaning of behaviours that have customarily been interpreted as symptoms of mental disorder.

There are long periods of time when the patient seems to be at to a standstill. In the previous section describing the course of recovery, we saw how such a period may in fact be a façade behind which the person is gathering strength. Strauss (1989) has aptly called these periods "woodshedding", referring to the habit of some jazz musicians to seclude themselves in a woodshed to practice new melodies and new ways of playing their instruments. From the outside, these seem to be periods of apathy and withdrawal and often occur when the patient is discharged from hospital. Psychiatric staff tend to interpret these external signs as "negative symptoms"; that is, as signs that the person is still in the grip of psychosis.

> The woodshedding periods appear to involve no change; in fact, there is often minute practicing. Subtle changes occur that would not be recorded on most rating scales. On close inquiry it appears that the patients are becoming used to being in the community again, talking with people a little more, gathering their self-confidence, and recovering a familiarity with non-psychotic life. (p. 23)

From the perspective of the self as active, this withdrawal can be seen as an active choice made to avoid situations and social inter- actions which the person fears could lead to heightened so-called positive symptoms (hallucinations, delusions, etc). It may be a way to gain insight about oneself after the experience of a psychotic episode, which is a radically new event in life that the individual must take into account in the conduction of his/her life.

These periods of woodshedding have also been described in terms of a moratorium (Strauss, Hafez, Lieberman & Harding 1985). Periods of moratoria alternate with periods of sudden change, or what Strauss calls "change points". Change points may come about through the patient's own efforts or as a consequence of external pressure; they may lead to continued recovery or to a new psychotic episode. Breier and Strauss (1984) describe the transition from convalescence to reconstruction as a critical period that may lead to an increase of psychotic symptoms, in which case the individual may once again be hospitalised. But it could just as well lead to a noticeable improvement in how the person manages his/her life. The improvement might occur immediately or after a short period of intensified psychotic symptoms, which could result in hospitalisation during the most turbulent phase of the change.

In the work of managing the demands of daily life, patients in the process of recovering use a method which Strauss (1992b) likens to mountain climbing. This means securing one's foothold before taking the next step. It means taking one step at a time, a procedure that sometimes conflicts with the demands of the environment. For example, in certain forms of supported housing provided by the local community or public health authorities, new residents are expected to participate in planned activities from the very first day; for some persons this might mean having to take on far too many new tasks at one time.

In those cases where the changes lead to improvements in how patients relate to life and in their symptomology, a new plateau is reached at a new level of functioning. This new level becomes for a period of time the "ceiling" (Strauss et al. 1985) for the person's functional capacity. These improvements in the person's functional level (the ceiling) can in time come to be regarded as a new period of moratorium or stagnation. The ceiling has now become the floor or foundation for new changes.

The pattern outlined by the above-cited researchers points to an uneven development with periods of apparent stagnation to which the environment may respond by making new demands for change. Persons on the road to recovery may experience these demands as adding to their stress or as a sign of hope and confirmation that other people believe in their continuing ability to deal with life. New demands may bring the person to either a higher or a lower level of functioning.

Few studies on recovery deal with such questions as: How far can a recovery process reach? What can we learn about total and social recovery processes and how long they can persist? Is there a given pattern of rise and fall within the framework of the disorder or do these processes point at the possibility of a life beyond the reach of the disorder?

Instead of dealing directly with these questions, most of the research on recovery cites the epidemiological literature referred to earlier where it states that between 20 and 30% of the patients with a schizophrenia diagnosis were judged to be socially recovered and a further 20 to 30% totally recovered. Deegan (1988) treats this problem in a different way. She describes recovery not as a condition, but as a process. This point of view is not without its problems, unless normality is also regarded as a process. If not, there is a risk that persons who have suffered a psychotic breakdown can never regard themselves, nor be regarded by others, as completely normal; they are constantly in a process moving towards normality. Anyone can suffer a psychotic breakdown. But for persons who have previously received psychiatric treatment, a new breakdown is regarded as a "relapse". People who have earlier had reason to be in contact with psychiatry are subjected to added stress just because of their psychiatric history. A relapse is regarded as indicating that the disorder is chronic and constantly present, even through the person seems normal, at least on the surface.

The importance of social relationships

A recurrent theme in several of the studies mentioned above concerns the importance that persons who have recovered attribute to other people in their surroundings.

Estroff (1989) makes the following summary of one of the main tenets of symbolic interactionism, a theory which studies in this field often take as a starting point; namely, that the self is formed and develops in relation to other people and that for this development to take place, a non-self must be present. The interplay with other persons gives patients an opportunity to orient themselves, first in relation to their experience of psychosis and to being a patient, and then, in a later phase, to the stigma so often associated with having been hospitalised as a mental patient. Estroff (1989) discusses two dilemmas first-time mental patients face where the role of other persons could be decisive. The first dilemma arises when the symptoms do not disappear of themselves and the first-time patient must now cope with a situation where not being oneself is virtually to be oneself. The second dilemma arises when family and close friends tend to forget or misrepresent the person's former self prior to the onset of the disorder so that even the patient begins to doubt whether that former self ever existed.

A third dilemma, which Estroff does not discuss, is likely to arise if and when patients begin to leave their symptoms and patient state behind them and both they and persons close to them are faced with the challenge of imagining that change could indeed be a possibility.

The literature on recovery points out four possible functions that other persons could fill: as an intermediary in the provision of material support, as a unwavering and vicarious source of hope, as an object of identification and as a poser of challenges.

Deegan (1988) points out that other people can be *bearers of hope* and is supported in this view by Frank's (1963) earlier research on successful therapeutic interventions.

Belin (1994) discusses the importance of other people as good *role models* who can provide "scope for play" where patients have the opportunity to test themselves in relation to an environment that is favourably disposed toward them. Bleuler (1963, 1978), in a longitudinal study of patients with a schizophrenia diagnosis who developed in a positive direction, concluded that an essential principle of treatment was

> ...a steady, quiet appeal to the healthy within the morbid, to the patient's sense of human responsibility and dignity and to his membership of human society. (1963, p. 31)

In their follow-up of 20 patients hospitalised for psychotic disorders, Breier and Strauss (1984) explored the importance of social relationships for the recovery process. The patients described twelve ways by which people in their surroundings had helped them.

During the convalescence phase, which coincided with the patients' discharge from hospital, the most important functions that social relationships filled were:

- *Ventilation of thoughts and feelings*: that patients have people with whom they can talk about what has happened to them and to whom they can express their feelings was valuable for relieving tension and anxiety.
- *Testing of one's notions against others' reality*: through the interplay with other people, the patients had help in sorting out which of their experiences were delusionary, hallucinatory or real.
- *Confirmation and integration*: many patients were worried about what reception they would be given after their psychotic breakdown and hospitalisation. To be met with understanding and support played a large role in reducing their anxiety and

reaffirming their hope of being reintegrated in the community and once again becoming part of a normal social context.

- *Continuity*: closely related to receiving confirmation and being reintegrated into the community was experiencing that the social relationships formed before the psychotic breakdown and subsequent period of hospitalisation were still in force. These personal contacts served as a reminder to the patients that they had once upon a time been "healthy", and could be so again.
- *Material support*: a functioning social network made it easier for the patients to deal with many situations in everyday life, including housing, transportation and the need for financial assistance.
- *Problem solving*: other people were able to offer concrete advice on how to manage situations involving housing problems, work and recreational activities and personal relationships.

These functions were still of some importance in the reconstruction phase, when patients began to seek out and establish more balanced relationships and their patienthood state had begun to fade. However, new functions came to play a more prominent role:

- *Motivation*: in their relationships with other people, the patients found support both for the progress they had already achieved and for making new advances. As we saw earlier, it is a question of achieving a balance in the relationship between support and making demands, between respecting pauses in the person's development and encouraging new progress. The balance between these poles varied from person to person and situation to situation.
- *Reciprocity*: as the patients progressed toward recovery, their personal relationships changed character. From having been the recipient of the care and concern of others, it became increasingly important for them to be someone who had something to share with others and who could even offer support and assistance.

- *Warning of symptoms*: in the reconstruction phase, other people were in a position to warn patients about changes in the number or nature of their symptoms. This helped patients to manage their symptoms better and avoid situations that could cause problems.

When the patients had reached the point where they were ready to make plans for a life after psychosis, and sometimes even began to carry out these plans, social relationships filled still new functions:

- *Empathy*: other people's understanding of what the person had experienced helped patients to accept themselves after the psychosis. Being understood and accepted generated a sense of well-being.
- *Modelling*: observing and imitating how others behaved helped some patients in situations where they tended to belittle themselves or make too great demands on their own performance. One person in the study related how he practised being as nice to himself as the people he socialised with were to him.
- *Insight*: insight is a further refinement of ventilating thoughts and feelings. Conversations with other people helped patients to have a more balanced self-image.

In a later article Strauss (1992b) discussed still another function that social relationships could fill; namely, to help patients have more reasonable expectations for themselves by showing them that other people have shortcomings and problems too. This awareness has helped them to develop a more realistic self-image.

Social relationships are no guarantee that there will not be relapses. Of the 20 patients in Breier and Strauss' study (1984), five were readmitted to hospital. However, upon conclusion of the follow-up two years after the first discharges, 17 former patients could be said to be in the process of recovering.

The population in this study is too small to allow for any far-reaching conclusions. But it can be worth noting that all the patients followed the same development course regardless of their individual diagnoses. Of the three persons in the population who were diagnosed as schizophrenic, two were in the reconstruction phase at the end of the study. The social relationships of these two people did not differ from those of the patients with other diagnoses.

Characteristics of the other

People who have recovered from severe mental disorders have pointed out several key qualities of others who have helped them in their recovery. Because these others are real-life people with their own shortcomings and problems, persons recovering from mental disorder are able to identify with them. They observe and adopt some of the ways in which other people manage their problems. A permissive accepting attitude is another quality often found among these people. A non-judgemental attitude allows patients to test the validity of their thoughts, ideas and roles under non-threatening conditions and thereby eventually move beyond a one-sided patienthood. (See Beiser 1995)

Other people can offer alternative interpretations of the breakdown that help patients to make some kind of sense of their experiences in relation to their own life histories. Other people can even present patients with a range of transitional rites and positions to adopt when they are on the verge of leaving the life of a total patient (see for example Lally 1989 and Zarifan 1988).

In ways such as these, persons in the process of recovering were helped to build up their self-confidence and form a sense of self that successively became less dominated by symptoms of mental disorder and social exclusion.

Another side to social relationships has to do with getting help to manage situations in everyday life. People who have been treated for a mental disorder experience being together with other people and receiving help in managing daily life situations as a sign that they are accepted, just as the persons they are. The paradox is that just by accepting the person where he/she is at present creates an opening for possible changes to the better. Deegan's (1988) analysis of her own recovery process shows that when other people remain hopeful, it can stimulate the return of hope in the patient and thereby initiate a recovery process. But it is a question of maintaining a precarious balance. The hopes of other people must not lead patients to feel that they fall short of the expectations. Their hopes must be based on an acceptance of the patients just as they are, with all their failings and shortcomings while, at the same time, sowing the seeds of trust in the possibility of change. The return of hope is in turn the source of the patients' growing confidence that they will be able to steer their own lives, even if only in small ways at first, so small that most people would hardly notice them. (See also Strauss 1989)

In a research overview entitled *Psychoterapins effekter vid psykos* (The effects of psychotherapy on psychosis – our transl.) (The National Board of Health and Welfare 1989), the suitable characteristics of therapists are described as follows:

> Whereas for neurotic clients it is the therapist's understanding and authenticity that seem to be important, for schizophrenic patients it is the therapist's acceptance and authenticity. (p. 11, our transl.)

Cullberg and Levander (1991), in their review of patients who recovered with the help of psychotherapy, noted that:

> In the reports given by the former patients, the human and empathetic qualities of their therapists were, as expected, much more than the technical/methodological aspects of the therapies. (p. 259)

> One of the former patients in the review regards the therapist today as "a good pal" and several others report that their therapist had "promised" them support and relief if they co-operated in the therapy. They experienced this as a real support and decisive for forming a "therapeutic alliance". (p. 259)

Cullberg (1996) emphasises the importance of the good relationship, of being seen and regarded as a living subject to entice the patient out of a "psychotic regression". In a Norwegian study of patients diagnosed as schizophrenic, the patients referred to similar qualities in their therapists as having helped their recovery: confidence (faith, trust), acceptance, understanding and empathy.

> The patients often mentioned that they had trust in their therapists and that the therapist accepted them unconditionally and were empathetic. (Rund 1990, p. 135)

The opinion of practitioners of the psychodynamic school is divided as to whether therapists should use exposing strategies and concentrate on the patient's childhood experiences or whether they should work with the patient's current situation and immediate future (Lamb 1976). However, today many therapists seem to be of the opinion that therapists/caregivers can and should present themselves to severely disturbed patients as a much more realistic person than would be necessary for less disturbed patients; as a person who can offer concrete advice and express an own opinion. The goal of the therapy should be to help patients to manage everyday situations, but most of all those situations that both patient and therapist find could lead to increased tension for the patient and might foreshadow the beginning of a new psychotic episode.

Also Harding et al. (1987a, b, Harding 1997) refers to the special quality of the relationship that had developed between staff members and the discharged patients whom they followed up. As mentioned earlier, long-term relationships had developed which persisted even after the follow-up had officially ended. In time the quality of these relationships changed from one-sided dependency to reciprocity and genuine friendship.

Many social scientists together with their interview subjects reiterate the importance of social interaction in everyday situations where the other person (staff member, close relative or friend) expresses caring and friendship in a concrete way. Strauss (1992b), for example, talks about "fast-food therapy" wherein a staff member and a patient leave the grounds of the institution to take a meal together (See also Topor, 1993, 1995, 1996.) Strauss finds:

> That we generally do not consider actions such as taking someone out to lunch as therapeutic may have more to say about the inadequacy of our theories and focus than it does about the efficacy of one modality compared to another. (1992b, p. 230)

A possible explanation for why we so often disregard such situations is that they are commonplace and that they are not the special privilege of a particular professional group, thereby disqualifying them as possible therapeutic situations.

Specific and non-specific factors

Researchers have been interested in what patients with mental disorders consider to be of importance in their contacts with their caregivers, by which is usually meant the therapist. Until recently, however, the patients interviewed were almost exclusively persons diagnosed with a neurosis disorder. During the 1960s it became evident that the different kinds of psychotherapy generally had the same rate of success with this group of patients (see Bregin & Lambert 1978). Since then there has been considerable research on what has come to be called specific versus non-specific factors. The point of departure in the search for specific factors was the assumption that changes in the patient's condition were brought about by specific techniques and that the task of theory was to explain the correlation between technique and change. In extension was the idea that it was possible to prove that one theory or technique was superior to another and therefore more true. (Butler & Strupp 1986)

Research into non-specific factors emphasised, on the other hand, factors which in their practical application were common features of all forms of psychotherapy. One of the factors suggested as an explanation for changes in patients was the personal characteristics of the therapist. The efficacious aspects of the psychotherapies were equated with the placebo effect and several researchers pointed at the similar success rates for placebos and the psychotherapies and for psychotherapies undertaken by experienced therapists and those by laymen (Strupp & Hadley 1979).

Various hypotheses have been launched to explain these results. One has to do with the personal qualities of the therapist, another the patient's type of problem. A third hypothesis is that certain forms of therapy are better suited for certain types of diagnoses. A fourth hypothesis focuses on the interaction between the personal characteristics of both therapist and patient in combination with various external factors.

The hypothesis that all forms of psychotherapy have certain operative features in common, besides their obvious differences, has been elaborated further through the corresponding hypothesis launched by Frank (1974) that also all types of mental disorders have certain features in common. It was on these common features that the various psychotherapies had an effect. Frank described the success of the different forms of psychotherapy as "the restoration of moral"[4]. He ascribed the decline in patients' morale as resulting from their own and the environment's repeated failure to manage their problem. What characterises a low morale are feelings of inferiority, isolation and hopelessness, which lead in turn to low self-esteem. The most common symptoms of patients in psychotherapy, i.e. anxiety and depression, are direct expressions of this decline in morale ("demoralization", p. 271). The symptoms tend to add to the demoralisation and this in turn inhibits the person's capacity to manage his/her symptoms, which in turn leads to further demoralisation.

Frank (1971) has analysed six features that are common to all forms of psychotherapy:

1. *A strong relationship between the help-seeker and the helper.* The relationship is one of high emotional arousal and is based on trust in the helper's capacity to help. The qualities of the therapist mentioned in this context are empathy, warmth, acceptance and respect.

2. *The creation of meaningfulness*, which both explains the cause of the patients' suffering and points at how to overcome it. In talking about "myths" in this connection, Frank throws light on the importance of the meaningfulness of the explanation for the patient compared with the claim of therapeutic schools that they work with the truth. Frank writes:

> Although many rationales of Western psychotherapies do not invoke supernatural forces, they resemble the myths of primitive ones in that they cannot be shaken by therapeutic failures. That is, they are not subject to disproof. (1971, p. 356)

Meaningfulness is a support for therapists in that it provides them with a framework for interpreting what happens in therapy and a language to convey this interpretation to the patients.

3. *The imparting of new knowledge by the therapist to the patients* about their problems and new ways of understanding and managing the problems.

4. *The awakening in the patient the hope that help is available.* Several researchers have described hope as the main ingredient in the success of the therapy. (Frank 1963)

5. *The conveying of experiences of having successfully managed problematic situations.* These experiences reaffirm the patients' hope and feeling of being capable of achieving something with their lives.

6. *Emotional arousal,* which prepares patients to be open to other solutions to their problems than those they have used earlier. The emotional arousal between patient and therapist is an acknowledged component in several forms of therapy. Even in forms of therapy that deny its importance, the patients have attributed much of the positive outcome of the therapy to this factor.

Butler and Strupp (1986) see the result of the therapy as being contingent on the interaction between the patient's interpersonal style and the therapist's ability to handle the patient's style; in other words, it is the therapist, not the form of therapy, that is the important variable. However, the therapist's words and actions do not have an effect on their own, but rather hinge upon the importance that the patient ascribes to them (and vice versa). The patient's experience of the therapist as "empathetic" or "warm" can only be understood in context, that is through a close study of the actual interaction between patient and therapist:

> Disembodied or decontextualized "factors", whether specific or non-specific, are unlikely to yield a clinically relevant understanding of therapists' influence on patients. (p. 38)

In a report by the National Board of Health and Welfare on the effects of psychotherapy on psychosis (1989:4), a commonly held distinction was made between patients diagnosed as neurotic and those as psychotic:

> The more the patient in therapy experienced the therapist as empathetic, the more the patient's schizophrenic symptoms were reduced. When the patient experienced the therapist as having a low capacity for understanding, the symptoms of schizophrenia tended to intensify. But apart from this, it does not seem to be so important for schizophrenic patients to seek self-understanding as it is for neurotic patients. While the therapist's understanding and authenticity seem to be the qualities that are most important for neurotic clients, for schizophrenic patients it is warm acceptance and authenticity. Schizophrenic patients seem to focus on forming a relationship rather than on understanding themselves. They seek a relationship that they can rely on, a reliable person who cares. (p. 11, our transl.)

An example of this kind of study is Frank and Gunderson's (1987) study of the personal characteristics of therapists and of patients diagnosed as schizophrenic who stayed in therapy. Frank and Gunderson chose a number of factors based on their studies of the literature and on their own clinical experience. This approach gives us a good overview of the ideas that are common to this field of study:

> We hypothesized that the therapists who would be the most successful in keeping schizophrenic patients in psychotherapy would be 1) optimistic about the schizophrenic's capacity for recovery, 2) active and energetic, 3) personally open (self-disclosing), 4) "facilitating" (empathetic, warm, unconditionally accepting, genuine), 5) comfortable dealing with issues of dependency and aggression, 6) inclined to limit regressions and expressions of primitive impulses and demands within therapy, 7) guided by a coherent treatment philosophy, and 8) highly experienced. (p. 393)

Interestingly enough, the results of the study show that:

> ... regardless of the type of psychotherapy provided (RAS or EIO[5]), patients were more likely to continue with therapists who were more

willing to share their own personal experiences, feelings, and reactions with their patients and who showed little interest in or tolerance for the expression of primitive impulses and demands. They also were more likely to continue with therapists who had a strong commitment to a well defined treatment ideology, no matter what the type. (p. 400)

It appears, then, that the facilitating factors in recovery do not hinge upon the therapist's theoretical orientation, although the therapist's trust in the efficacy of his/her method and theory is important. Besides this, what seems to work best is concrete relationship where the self-disclosing therapist (who thereby apparently breaks several of the rules applicable to his/her theoretical orientation) is fairly reality-oriented.

We should bear in mind that Frank and Gunderson's work is concerned with patients who stayed in therapy and not with patients who recovered. That is to say, patients might choose to continue with the therapy for the very reason that it does not challenge them, does not help them, and that they thereby establish an alliance with the therapists to ensure that nothing will change (see Racamier 1973). On the other hand, a continuation of therapy could be seen as a way to achieve recovery.

Comprehensive studies with the user perspective

In several cases service users were brought into the investigation already at the study's initial phase in which the key processes and concepts were elaborated. In these studies adaptations of the focus-group method were used. A common characteristic is that they tried to encompass the whole recovery process and not limit it to given themes chosen by the researchers. Two studies that used open-ended questions to people about what had facilitated their recovery are Sullivan's *A long and winding road: the process of recovery from severe mental illness* (1994) and the study by Tooth, Kalyanansundaram and Glover, *Recovery from schizophrenia – a consumer perspective* (1997). Seven factors in the first study and eight in the second were found to be associated with recovery from a user perspective. The findings are summarised in Table 3 below. As the table shows, six of the factors were common to both studies. The content and meaning of the various factors tend to overlap; they have to do with the person's sense of self, medication, support from public authorities and his/her informal social network.

Table 3. Significant factors in the recovery process, a comparison between Sullivan (1994) and Tooth et al. (1997).

Sullivan	Tooth et al.
Medication	Medication
Community support service	Process
Self-will, self monitoring	Self
Vocational activities (including school)	Activities
Spirituality	
Knowledge about the illness/Acceptance of the illness	
Mutual aid groups – supporting friends	Environment
Significant others	Network
	Hospitalisation

The factors that tend to overlap are:

- *The persons themselves* report that they have contributed to their own recovery. A central feature of the role of individuals in their own recovery is described in terms of regaining power over one's own life. Not so seldom recovery was described as a one-person effort: "I did it myself". (Tooth et al. 1997, p. 36)
- *Other persons* in the individual's social network are significant in that they offer material support and their continued presence and companionship helps the person to feel accepted, thereby strengthening his/her self-esteem.

    Other persons who can contribute to the recovery process are fellow patients who meet in self-help situations, both situations that are arranged and the more informal situations that occur among users in supported housing settings, at day centres or in occupational projects. There is a positive effect in meeting other people in the same situation as oneself – one is not the only one – and in giving one another advice and tips.

- *Medication* is mentioned by many of the patients as a positive factor. In both studies, however, the patients also expressed their frustration at the reluctance of professionals to discuss medication with the patient, the appropriate dosages and the advantages and side-effects of different drugs.
- *Professional support and treatment* is mentioned in both studies. The role of hospitalisation is discussed only in the study by Tooth et al. (1997). Both studies discuss community-based interventions with respect both to traditional forms of treatment (medication and therapy) and social interventions like case management, supported housing and recreational and occupational activity programmes. Tooth and her associates classify professional help under "the non-specifics of psychotherapy". Sullivan (1994) makes the same observation, both when it comes to planned activities and to individual professionals who have contributed to the work of recovery:

> ... much of the power of helping still comes in the form of a relationship. However, the manner in which the professional helps is not by being dispassionate, detached, or objective. Rather, the professional helps when s/he joins with the consumer, engaging in partnership and treating the individual in a respectful and normalized manner. (p. 22)

The factors appearing in only one of the two studies are:

- *Spirituality*, most of all in terms of traditional religions that offer both a meaningful framework for the person's experiences and support by the congregation and religious leaders.
- *Knowledge about the illness and/or acceptance of the illness*, which means that the person has gradually begun to recognise the early signs of becoming ill again, takes the prescribed medication and has reduced any drug misuse. "Accepting the illness" means, according to Sullivan, that the patients accept the limitations caused by the illness. One of the questions in the discussion on the meaning of acceptance is what is it that patients have to accept. What message psychiatry wants to con-

vey to the patient depends on the professional in charge; it often implies that the patients must accept that he/she is suffering from an incurable disease. The patient's role is to submit to the treatment which, for the moment, is considered to be the optimal one. This kind of acceptance can be likened to internalising a stigma, which in some of the literature is seen as a factor that could lead to chronicity. Sullivan says that for some users the recovery process means challenging the limitations that they have experienced in their lives and thereby, for a certain period, raise their level of stress.

- *Hospitalisation* could be a help to recovery in that it could interrupt a downward trend.

Despite their concentration on the positive factors, Tooth and her associates also felt called upon to discuss *factors that obstructed recovery*, as these were mentioned spontaneously by persons in the study. The most negative factors included the side-effects of the medication (slower thought processes, jerky body movements, feeling stupid) and the professionals' attitudes towards the patients (the assumption that the patient is incapable of anything, failure to involve the patient in the treatment, autocratic mannerisms, lack of interest in the patient's experiences, pessimistic view of the treatment):

Sixty-one per cent reported their interaction with health professionals to be not only negative but detrimental to their recovery. Whilst many participants had positive interactions with specific health professionals, the general impression of health professionals was none the less poor. (Tooth et al. 1997, p. 49)

Tooth and her associates (1997) actualise the contradictions between the user and the professional perspective: "Whose story is valid?" (p. 21). A main difference between the two stories is that "... health professionals and consumers do not talk about the same things." (p. 21) The way patients are presented in the professional literature focuses on their failings and shortcomings whereas users, in their life stories and writings, emphasise their own abilities and strengths. Other differences between users and professionals mentioned by Tooth et al. concern language usage and how the concepts used by both groups are defined. Lastly, the users emphasis the past and current support they have had from other patients.

In an arranged dialogue between professionals and users who recovered from mental disorders, there were three main areas where the two groups were in disagreement (Blanch, Fisher, Tucker Walsh & Chassman 1993). The first concerned *the social distance* between professionals and users. Professional caregivers had difficulty accepting that users described it as two separate worlds and that they experienced care as mostly negative. In the discussion some of the professionals questioned whether the users were truly representative of their group, but this question was never explored further in the study.

A second area of disagreement concerned *medication, diagnostics* and *compliance* (i.e., accepting the prescribed treatment). The professionals regarded these features of care as essential tools in promoting recovery, whereas the users regarded them as factors that made them powerless because they left no room for alternatives.

The third and last area where there was controversy concerned *time*. The professionals' demand for effectiveness and quick results conflicted with the users' experience that recovery is a time-consuming process and cannot be rushed. The users felt that it took time to get to know them well enough to devise an individual treatment plan and that interventions that were designed to quickly reduce their suffering could instead inhibit the recovery process.

Factors in the recovery process

The article by Young and Ensing from 1999 is one of the few attempts (perhaps the only one at present) to shed light on the factors that contribute to the recovery process and explore how they are related to one another. In Young and Ensing's study of 18 patients diagnosed as suffering from a variety of illnesses including bipolar disorder (six persons) and schizophrenia (four persons), they found that the recovery process could be divided into three main phases:

1. Start of the process – overcoming "stuckness":
- acknowledging and accepting the illness
- desiring and having the motivation for change
- having or finding a source of hope and inspiration.

This phase is described in the study as being the most difficult one as it means admitting to certain limitations that one has earlier denied. A source of hope and inspiration that was frequently mentioned in the study was spiritual experiences.

2. Intermediate phase – finding what had been lost and moving on:
- discovering and developing self-empowerment
- recovery as a process of learning about and re-defining the self
- a return to basic functions

What happens in this phase is that a good cycle is put in motion. Small step by small step, the person begins to get back some measure of control over his/her life, which bolsters the person's self-esteem. This in turn provides the groundwork for taking new steps towards achieving even greater control. Gradually the person becomes better able both to control the concrete circumstances of his/her life and the various symptoms of the disorder. It is here that coping strategies enter the picture. As a result the person discovers a self that he/she thought had disappeared for all time and develops new components of that self. A feature that Young and Ensing (1999) highlight in their study as being a specific contribution in their research on recovery is the importance of self-care in everyday life such as keeping oneself clean, cleaning house, eating cooked meals:

> The important unifying concept of the basic self-care category was the conscious effort to re-establish a routine of basic self-care activities that constitute 'normal' functioning. (p. 226)

Lastly, the authors mention the importance of participating in activities outside the home and of having social contacts, especially with other people who also have mental problems. Many of the users in the population of their study had little contact with their family and felt abandoned by them. For this reason family members had an insignificant role in their study of the recovery process.

3. *Later phase – improving quality of life:*
- recovery includes aspiring to achieve an overall sense of well-being
- recovery includes aspiring to reach higher levels of functioning

The re-creation of a positive self-image is a powerful driving force in the recovery process. Many of the persons in Young and Ensing's study (1999) said that they had found their way to a better self-image by becoming involved in a spiritual movement: "... spirituality is not only viewed as a source of hope but also as a source of meaning in one's life" (p. 228). Another source of well-being mentioned in the study was reduced symptomology, which appeared either as fewer symptoms, as a reduction in the intensity of the symptoms, or as a combination of the two.

The patient in his/her context

A common feature of much of recovery research is that the individual is perceived in his/her social and cultural context. This simple shift of focus constitutes a radical departure from common practice in traditional psychiatry where the illness is thought to prevent the person from participating in social life, an idea which for many years was substantiated by the practice of isolating patients in mental asylums. Davidson and Strauss (1995) have criticised traditional psychiatry for its one-sided emphasis on the patients' illness, symptoms and failings, and suggest instead what they call a "life-context approach" (p. 48). The framework for understanding the patient should be the whole of the person's life course, which thereby invalidates any division between healthy and sick:

> This entails describing illness no longer as an absence or deviation, but in terms of its particular configuration of features and their impact on the person's life as a whole. It also entails describing aspects of a person's life

outside of illness such as strengths and areas of health, rather than defining the person only in terms of what it lacks. (p. 49)

Davidson and Strauss outline four areas that are central to understanding an individual's life context:

1. Intentionality:
Intentionality has to do with human beings experiencing themselves as capable of steering their own life in a chosen direction – the ability to plan, choose, make decisions and carry them out. Intentionality does not disappear completely during a psychotic episode, even though they may be limited at times to situations that other people find to be trivial.

2. Temporality:
This concept refers to the necessity of seeing each situation, each action, as occurring in a time dimension, as a moment of time in a life course. It has to do with understanding that patients with diagnoses that bear the stamp of chronicity each have their own history, a past and a future. Acute mental distress occurs but for a limited period of time in that history. It is an event that most certainly has an impact on the individual's continued life course, but in no way does it constitute the end of the individual's personal history. People continue to play a role in their own life histories, not merely as helpless victims but as active subjects.

Perhaps the reduction in the number of hospitalisation admissions, the existence of a social welfare system and a network of so-called intermediate forms of care have indeed created alternatives to the forms of chronicity that developed behind the walls of the psychiatric hospital.

3. Meaning:
People do not see their lives as consisting of uncomplicated chains of events occurring one after the other without rhyme or reason. They choose from among a multitude of events in life and try to give them meaning, try to sort them out and place them within an overall life context. Experiences contribute to but also consist of stories that people compose about their own lives. The meaning that

people attribute to events in life and the events that they place special value on are easily lost in the historiographies that psychiatry creates about and for patients. The meaning that psychiatry offers patients often consists of discouraging reports of brain damage, genetic defects, traumatic childhood experiences and life-long illness and incapacitation when in fact the reinterpreting of a person's life experiences may pave the way to recovery.

4. Competency and dysfunction in co-existence:
It is extremely rare to find a person who consists only of dysfunctional behaviours and illness. Usually people suffering from a severe mental disorder do not only have areas in their life that are affected by their symptoms but also areas where they function quite adequately, at one and the same time. In rehabilitation contexts we encounter expressions of this approach in interventions that focus on the patient's so-called "healthy sides".

By observing these four dimensions in the attempt to understand persons with mental disorders, patients can continue to be treated as real-life human beings – not as beings who, because they are mentally ill, are strange and incomprehensible to us, whose words and actions require other kinds of interpretations than ours, who lack a will of their own, whose only life context is one of illness and who are incapable of steering their own lives.

Psychiatry has consistently endeavoured to reduce the individual to a given set of symptoms, an illness syndrome, in order to be able to establish a diagnosis and plan a course of treatment. An alternative approach, as summarised by the work of Davidson and Strauss, has as one of its goals:

> ... a more realistic complexity in our descriptions of patients and (to) avoid simplistic reductions which sacrifice key data. (p. 53)

Such an approach could provide a good foundation for studying the phenomena of self-healing and spontaneous cures.

When mental illness ceases to be regarded as a condition whose development follows a given course and is unaffected by outside influences (except for perhaps a hypothetical breakthrough in the future); when people with mental disorders cease to be regarded as helpless victims or moral degenerates, but as persons with the ability and will to affect their own destinies; when we cease to regard professional groups as the only ones who might be able to affect the course of the illness; first then will it be possible to regard people with mental disorders as part of a social structure and as participants in forming personal relationships and by which they are formed.

Structural conditions provide a framework for the reproduction of those publicly sanctioned practices and bodies of knowledge that are possible at a given point in time; micro-social, everyday situations where individuals, in their interpersonal relationships, have a possibility to break with the most probable patterns of behaviour by using to advantage the ambiguities that are inherent in all social situations.

Such a constructionist perspective would make it possible to move beyond concepts like schizophrenia:

> Becoming a schizophrenic is essentially a social and interpersonal process, not an inevitable consequence of primary symptoms and neurochemical abnormality. (Estroff 1989, p. 194)

Despite how it is described in psychiatric textbooks, the diagnosis schizophrenia is not an objectively given reality, but rather an attempt by psychiatrists to summarise various observations they have made under certain circumstances. And although these circumstances actually help to create the object under study, they are seldom accounted for. In other cultural and institutional contexts than those that dominate in Western society, the schizophrenia concept has outlived its usefulness because it deviates too much from the reality it was meant to describe, understand and treat.

Contacts with other cultures and the closing of the psychiatric hospitals have helped to create other possibilities for conceptualising, relating to and understanding mental and emotional distress. The encounter with people who have a mental disorder and exploring how they manage their lives under such altered circumstances creates a need for new concepts to replace the traditional vocabulary of psychiatry:

In mental disorders, there may be discontinuities in the evolution of disorder and recovery processes, e.g. as in insight/delusion formation or in the notion of phases of recovery. But the notion of abnormal thinking as discontinuous from normal thinking, of one symptom as discontinuous from another, of one diagnostic category as discontinuous from another, seems likely to be erroneous and to have misled us in terms of our thinking about treatment and aetiology. The postulating of possible erroneous discontinuities has left much clinical practice unnecessarily separated from theoretical and research efforts. However, it is at least possible not to begin to develop a more advanced model of human functioning in both health and disorder. (Strauss 1992a, p. 25. See also Bleuler 1969, 1978; Ciompi 1984)

Summary – conclusion

Our way of understanding mental disorders has confronted us with a paradox: a sizeable share of patients whose diagnoses can be regarded as chronic do in fact recover, either totally or at least enough to allow them to live satisfactory lives outside the psychiatric hospital. Severe mental disorders are not a final judgement, neither in terms of mental illness, handicap or functional disability. The illness and the functional disability can be overcome. Research has been unable, however, to show that there is a significant correlation between specific treatment programmes and patients' recovery. All forms of treatment across the whole field of psychiatry can report cases of patients who have recovered while being treated by methods that fall within the respective school's theoretical framework. Many patients recover without any connection to specific forms of treatment.

A number of research studies have focused on severely disturbed patients' recovery process, regardless of whether or not the recovery is attributed to specific forms of treatment, and regardless of the content of the treatment. These studies show that even severely disturbed patients remain active in relation to their social situation. Even in the case of deeply psychotic patients, some parts of the self remain in tact. These parts of the self act in order to manage the new situations and experiences that have become part of the person's current life. Even while under the influence of psychosis, the person enters into social relationships and can be influenced by what other people say and do.

Although the research presented here has generally focused on the schizophrenia diagnosis, the findings seem to indicate that there are no significant differences between this diagnosis and other severe forms of mental disorders when it comes to recovery. (See for example Schreiber 1996, Young & Ensing 1999)

The knowledge that recovery research has produced is often confirmed in the everyday practice of psychiatry. It is reflected in the anecdotes that staff members relate to one another on the ward, at mental health clinics and in community-based programmes. Mental health workers and social workers alike have been astonished to find that patients can function adequately under the right circumstances. Despite years of hospitalisation, despite extreme suffering, they have retained a large measure of their initial competency (see for example Crafoord 1987 and Szecsödy 1989). Patients who received community support after discharge from hospital were able to get on with their lives, demonstrating abilities and resources that far surpassed what their hospital records showed them to be capable of. Nevertheless, there are problems when this body of knowledge is to be put into practice in a more organised way by psychiatry and the social services. In especially the psychiatric branch of medicine, there is a contradiction between, on the one hand, the low status accorded to qualitative research, and on the other, the central role played by the doctors' observations and the high value they put on their patients' statements in connection with making the diagnosis. That qualitative research has a low status can be seen, for example, in the title Strauss and Hafez (1981) gave to an article in which they advocate the use of anecdotes as research material. In the article "Clinical questions and 'real' research", they write:

> Clinical observations and reports, especially if developed with careful attention to the nature of the evidence and proof and elaborated by the study of several subjects, can provide qualitative data for which measurement may not be available or even feasible. (p. 1592)

The dominant image of the severely mental disturbed patient is that of a helpless victim of his/her childhood or of biological/genetic factors, or the patient is described as a morally weak person who should try to pull himself/herself together. Closely related to these images is the idea that a cure may perhaps be possible only through specific treatment interventions provided by professional groups who possess the right specialist knowledge. Nevertheless, research on the recovery process indicates that the person's own efforts often depend, not so much on the support of professionals as on the support of the people in his/her immediate surroundings who provide material support, assurance, hope and acceptance.

The way back to a more positive self-image is often described as depending on what happens in everyday situations. But as these situations are so commonplace, they are often overlooked. How could "fast-food therapy" ever be a serious challenge to the hegemony of psychotherapy and neuroleptic medicines, particularly when such daily interventions are administered by friends, family, mental health workers, home-help personnel and even by the patients themselves?

The advantage of unbiased research into the question of how severely mentally disturbed patients recover is that it is even able to build on these daily experiences of improvement.

With the deinstitutionalisation of psychiatric care, patients who would otherwise have spent their whole lives in psychiatric hospitals have been given the possibility to make a way for themselves in the community. Outside the psychiatric hospital many of them have been able to build up a life of their own with the support of others. New institutions have evolved to support them in their home environments. A growing number of professionals now meet these former patients under circumstances that differ from the conditions of the hospital ward or mental health clinic. These more complex conditions create a whole new scope for action, an open space for both the suffering individual and the professional caregiver in their encounters with one another and the surrounding world (Topor & Schön 1998).

Several researchers (among them, Androli 1986, Bleuler 1991 and Boyle 1993) have found that many of the symptoms that used to characterise the most common forms of mental disorders have either changed or disappeared altogether. Research on how people with severe mental disorders manage their suffering and recover may give us a good basis for understanding this development.

The new circumstances under which persons with mental disorders come into contact with psychiatry and the social services have brought about a change in their formal status. They are no longer be obliged to do what others have decided they should do, or to live in the way that others have decided is best for them. As a consequence of this newly acquired freedom, both research, the mental health system and health care may have to ask themselves some new questions, questions like what constitutes a mental disorder and how to help people who have a mental disorder? Perhaps the new order can generate other answers instead of the traditional ones provided by psychiatry?

Challenges facing research

Today there is a good deal of epidemiological research on the "outcome" of severe mental disorders and recovery from such disorders. This research has certain limitations with respect to how it defines its basic concepts and what terms apply in many of the follow-up studies (number of patients and length of time of the follow-up). Nevertheless, there are a sufficient number of studies where the definitions are generally accepted and that have large patient groups and a long follow-up time where the results show that a significant share of patients who were diagnosed as schizophrenic have recovered.

As for learning more about the course of the recovery process and the important factors that contribute to that process, we have access today to a comprehensive autobiographical literature presenting self-experienced descriptions of the recovery process. There are even a few meta-studies of these autobiographical accounts that could also be an important source of knowledge. (See e.g. Coyne Plum 1987)

In the research presented above, regardless of whether the studies have focused on individual factors in the recovery process or have taken a more comprehensive approach, certain factors turn up time and again. Important recurring factors are the continuity of the self through and beyond the psychosis, the person's own efforts, the importance of other people and the symbolic value of everyday situations. Several of the studies mention, in addition, hope, spirituality and experiencing empathy – the feeling that one is noticed, heard and respected. Acceptance of the illness; the respective roles of professionals, family and friends; the need to be active; and medication are also mentioned in a number of studies as important contributory factors. In other studies, however, they are regarded more as deterrents, and in still others their role was ambiguous.

This research thus clearly indicates that recovery from severe mental disorders is possible. Furthermore, we know something about the factors that contribute to recovery. Nevertheless, Strauss and Estroff's observation from 1989 still applies:

> There is something seriously missing in the field of mental illness that does not attend *closely* and *broadly* to patients' subjective experiences and sense of self. (p. 177, italic mine)

Furthermore, the recovery research to date falls short on two points in particular:

1. The factors that have been found to be important for the recovery process are somewhat superficial. It is easy to understand that anyone, and especially a person who is suffering from a severe mental disorder desires empathy, does not want to be locked up, wants to have a reason to hope and wants to have friends. But so far research has not investigated such factors and therefore offers answers to questions like:
    *   How are these factors expressed in practice? As concretely as possible, what was the chain of events that led up to a person being able to say that he/she has been noticed, when that same person has been defined as an annihilated self?
    *   How do these factors actually work? In what way can personal relationships promote the recovery of a person who has been given a chronic illness diagnosis? What generates hope and how does it affect the diagnosis of schizophrenia?

If not firmly grounded, these concepts risk becoming increasingly ideological, where anyone is free to assign them meaning in terms of his/her own preconceived theoretical allegiances.

2. A second shortcoming of recovery research is that it tends to produce a growing list of positive factors that are simply added on to one another. At best, an attempt is made to relate the factors on some time axis, but this seldom leads to improving our understanding of the process. Neither does this growing list of contributory factors tell us why some people recover more than others whereas others do not recover at all.

Research on the recovery process still has some fundamental questions to address. Estroff, who has for some time studied the life of severely mentally disturbed persons lead in the community and their self-image, summarises the challenges facing recovery research today:

> To conclude, I have argued here that we have failed to pose and pursue several essential questions about the subjective experience of schizophrenia. How do the pervasive cultural, clinical, and personal symbols, metaphors, and meanings of schizophrenia influence prognosis? How do individuals with schizophrenia understand and locate themselves in relationship to their symptoms, labels, and responses? What contributed to a person's ability to separate himself or herself from this sickness, and does it facilitate or even constitute recovery? (Estroff 1989, p. 195)

Strauss and his associates formulated one of the most basic questions in this context as well as the reason it has not yet been answered:

> One of the major features inhibiting research on the evolution of disorder and recovery is the complexity involved. What characteristics should be studied? (Strauss et al. 1985, p. 295)

The subject's complexity cannot be properly addressed with the methods normally used in medical research. We stand on the verge of a new era of discovery, an era in which we are called upon to explore a largely uncharted territory, an era when we are in great need of carefully documented accounts of personal experiences and practice.
Against this background, the empirical study of this uncharted territory should be directed toward:

155

- Important factors in the recovery process. As most of our current knowledge of this process is based on studies conducted in the USA, a country that has its own history of institutions and its particular system of social security, it could be interesting to see if corresponding studies in the Nordic countries yield comparable results. If so, the similarities between the different studies would probably help to validate their findings.
- Of what do these factors consist? With clear and concise descriptions of situations where these factors come into play, we should be able to achieve a better understanding of their nature and beneficial components.

How do these factors work in conjunction to promote a process of recovery? Recovery research has made a major contribution in uncovering factors that promote recovery; the task now is to articulate and elaborate these findings. A possible goal for the present study is to help define the first step toward designing such a project.

---

[1] By positive symptom is meant such symptoms as hallucinations and delusions. By negative symptom is generally meant signs of withdrawal.

[2] Although there is much valuable knowledge to be gained from the study of autobiographical narratives, this topic does not fall within the framework of the present study.

[3] These figures need to be clarified in that an undetermined part of this reduction can be explained by trans-instutionalisation, i.e., the transfer of responsibility for patients, staff and whole wards to other public authorities.

[4] The Swedish translation of the word "moral" is "morality" but also spirit, courage, fighting spirit, perseverence and discipline. (Läromedel 1969)

[5] The study compared two types of psychotherapy in combination with psychopharmaceutical treatment: EIO = Exploratory-Insight-Oriented and RAS = Reality-Adaptative-Supportive

Part II

5
On the empirical study

Psychiatry's notion of chronicity is based on several core premises:

- that chronic conditions have a biological basis
- that the pathological state does not change. If it does change, it is not for the better; rather, pathological states follow a degenerative so-called natural course in accordance with the pattern characteristic of the illness
- that medication is the only way to ameliorate a chronic course
- that any improvement not brought about by medication is temporary at best. But medicines have no lasting effect on the downward direction of the natural course of the illness. Nor should signs of improvement change our conception of the illness.

Chronic mental disorders or illnesses differ from somatic illnesses in that they are a double assault on the individual's identity:

- The very illness can be likened to the dismantling of the social and psychological processes upon which human identity is built. Mental illness intrudes upon the will, emotions and cognition. Persons so afflicted become unlike themselves, and unlike the rest of us.
- And like somatic illnesses that have become chronic, the very fact of being chronically ill changes the person's self-image. The assault on the person's identity becomes even more deepseated as a result of the stigmatism attached to being a patient under psychiatric care.

Certain criteria have been formulated for determining and measuring the occurrence of a chronic condition or illness course: hospitalisation, diagnosis, duration of the disorder and an accompanying functional disability. None of these criteria is without problems, however, in that researchers and clinicians cannot agree among themselves about which criteria are viable and in what combination or to what degree. Furthermore, certain criteria have been shown to be connected, at least to some extent, with social conditions rather than with the individual's state of ill health.

Recovery from a chronic condition or illness course is a paradox. Recovery constitutes a radical departure from the notion that certain psychiatric diagnoses are associated with a permanent state of ill health or an irreversible degenerative process. The progression from chronically to recovered, by definition a contradiction in terms, has resulted in recovered patients being assigned a new diagnosis.

The occurrence of recovery from certain psychiatric diagnoses is, of course, dependent on how the diagnoses are defined. This definition is a crucial factor when determining whether recovery is at all possible or, if possible, how many patients with a particular diagnosis will eventually be classified as recovered. The criteria for recovery also determine the extent of the recovery. A common practice to distinguish between total and social recovery.

The criteria for recovery found in the literature are the absence of symptoms and of treatment interventions, a normal social life, insight and long-term duration of the measured recovery. However, there is a lack of consensus regarding which of these criteria are to be applied, in what combinations and to what extent. Another problem is determining what these four criteria actually measure. Regarding the absence of symptoms, for example, whether or not the person is judged recovered may hinge upon the psychiatrist's competence in uncovering hidden residual symptoms. Another factor that is likely to affect the recovery appellation is the treating psychiatrist's attitude toward the idea that all human beings are apt to display some psychotic symptoms at one time or another.

Also a problem is the third criterion, the ability to lead a normal social life. If this is taken to mean the person's return to a mental state prior to the onset of the illness, how is that former state determined and is a return to it always desirable? Psychosis is an overwhelming experience; to have recovered implies that the individual has had to integrate that experience into his/her personality.

The insight criterion is also problematic. The problem here is that determining whether a patient has achieved insight has been shown to often depend on the professional care-giver's particular theoretical frame of reference. It is easy to confuse insight with the patient's viewing the world with the same eyes as the professional. And as we know that professionals have different explanations of severe mental disorders, the insight of the one might not be the insight of the other.

The last two criteria raise the problem of deciding how to define treatment intervention – are community-based support measures and psychotherapy to be regarded as treatment interventions? How much time must have passed since the last intervention? To what extent are these interventions regarded as belonging to the normal world and not a sign of mental disturbance? The criteria for recovery concern not only the particular individual's state of health but also how society is organised and its cultural values.

In recent years both sections of the research community and the user movement have focused on the recovery concept in conjunction with the user perspective. What both groups share in common is an emphasis on the psychological and subjective aspects of recovery. If severe mental disorder is defined as the loss of central social and psychological functions, then recovery must be its opposite: the feeling of having regained control over one's symptoms and over particular aspects of one's life. This means that the person has regained not only control over certain functions, but also a sense of purpose and meaning.

In this context, recovery is seen as a process; the risk is that the recovery process becomes as long-lived as chronicity. The former patient may become fixed in a permanent role as someone who used to be mentally ill and is still struggling with its effects; psychiatry's counterpart to the notion of "once an alcoholic, always an alcoholic", even if a "sober" one. Furthermore, by emphasising the individual's assessment of his/her own recovery process, there is the risk that the professional's subjectivity will simply be replaced by the patient's.

Another central problem with the concepts of chronicity and recovery is that they claim to be judgements pertaining to the individual patient's condition. In fact, when used in practise, they mostly measure conditions external to and beyond the control of the individual; for example, the length of stay in hospital, the labour market situation and the treating psychiatrist's theoretical allegiance. The concepts of chronic disorder and recovery came into being as a way of describing and summarising observations made under clinical conditions. It was observed that some patients were hospitalised for long periods of time but that other patients who had been expected to be institutionalised for the rest of their lives could be discharged to a life in the community. However, both concepts have come to live a life of their own and occur independently of the situations in which they were initially devised. Instead of characterising given situations (referring to the individual or patient, the treating psychiatrist, the clinical environment and/or culture, psychiatric expertise, level of knowledge of the society at large, and the dominating social conditions), they are presented as an objective measurement of an person's "internal state".

The occurrence and prevalence of the chronicity and recovery concepts in psychiatry are wholly dependent on how they are defined. The only foolproof way of determining chronicity is after the fact; i.e., after the patient has died while in a state of persistent mental illness. Ambitious efforts to delimit a diagnostic field for predicting chronicity have has little success. In fact, the chronicity concept in psychiatry is to some extent an artefact. What we have been able to ascertain is that a not insignificant number of people afflicted with a severe mental disorder do in fact recover, regardless of predictions and expectations to the contrary.

Conclusions prior to the empirical study

This review of chronicity and recovery, the two central concepts of this study, has shown both concepts are somewhat problematic. The problems in connection with how they are used in psychiatry are summarised in the following questions:

- What are the criteria for determining chronicity or recovery?
- What are the possible combinations of these criteria?
- What measurement scales are applicable to the different criteria?

One approach to the problem of defining and applying the concepts of chronicity and recovery is to first clarify the basis on which we choose our definitions (see Borgå 1993), and then to treat these concepts, not as separate variables, but as descriptions of situations. This means viewing chronicity and recovery as points of intersection between a series of approximate assessments of a person's condition, on the one hand, and his/her social conditions, on the other; or as points of intersection between the professional's clinical experience of patients' life-long suffering and the research finding that a significant number of patients within the same category progress beyond their mental affliction and totally recover, or at least recover socially.

In the following empirical study, I use a combination of the criteria discussed above (Borgå 1993). The relevant criteria in the definition of a chronic mental state are diagnosis, need for treatment, duration and extent of functional disability.

Diagnosis: all the subjects in the empirical study have received a diagnosis corresponding to what the National Board of Health and Welfare (1996) has termed "severe mental disorders": "schizophrenia and other psychotic states of ill health, manic-depression, profound depression and anxiety and "pronounced personality disturbance".

Duration: the minimum period for the duration of the diagnosed symptoms of illness has been set at six months. The basis for this time limit is the six-month minimum duration given by the DSM-handbook for establishing the diagnosis of schizophrenia.

Functional disability and *hospitalisation*: the criterion I use as an indication of functional disability is hospitalisation. Although this is a somewhat ambiguous criterion (it might have more to do with handicap than functional disability), a long-term stay in hospital is undeniably indicative of a social problem.

For the definition of recovery in this study, I have chosen a combination of no hospital stays for a certain length of time and assessments of the person's state of health and social situation.

Hospitalisation and treatment: To be classified as recovered, the person must have remained out of hospital during the preceding two years (Bott 1976, Sullivan 1994). To be classified as totally recovered, the person must not have been a recipient of outpatient care of any kind, nor of any form of community support designed specifically for people with functional disabilities. This latter criterion does not apply to persons classified as socially recovered.

Professional assessments: At the time of the interview, the interview subjects were regarded by professionals as being capable of engaging in functioning social relationships, which include working, studying and/or participating in other forms of organised social activity. In those cases where residual symptoms were in evidence, these were regarded – based on the statements of the persons concerned – as causing few disruptions of the person's daily life. The persons assessed as being totally recovery reported and displayed no residual symptoms of any kind. The professional assessments were then discussed thoroughly in the research team before a final decision on each person's status was reached.

Own assessments: The interview persons' own judgement of themselves as recovered or in the process of recovering is the third criterion we used for determining recovery.

To participate in the study, the subjects must fulfil all the criteria for both chronicity and recovery. The choice of criteria combines several ways of regarding the two basic variables. That this choice is open for criticism is inevitable, as would be any other choice of criteria. The reader has been presented with the crucial arguments and should now be in a good position to judge the reasonableness of the study's design.

The interview subjects

The group of respondents (see Appendix 2) consists of 16 persons –
eight women and eight men, ranging in age from 29 to 63. At the time
of the interview, four were married, two were unmarried but living
with a partner, three were divorced and seven had never been married.
Five of the respondents had children. Fifteen were living in their own
homes and one was still lived at home with his parents.

Nine of the respondents reported schizophrenia as "their" diagnosis.
Of the remaining seven respondents, two reported their diagnosis to
affective psychosis, two "schizoid", one paranoid psychosis, one personality disorder and one borderline psychotic personality.

At the time of the interview three of the respondents had no assistance of any kind from the social services or psychiatry. The remaining
thirteen were receiving support of some kind from psychiatry and/or
the social services. For two persons, their only form of support was, in
the one case, continued sporadic contact with her psychotherapist and
in the other sporadic visits to the day care centre. Eleven respondents
were receiving medication for their mental problems, ranging from
daily doses to taking a medicine only when needed. Two persons were
receiving counselling at the outpatient clinic, and two were receiving
psychotherapy outside the clinic. Seven respondents were receiving
support from the social services for their housing, work and/or recreational needs. One person was receiving treatment in primary care in
connection with her mental problems.

The division between total and social recovery is not an easy one to
make. But applying these concepts to the group according to the criteria in the analysis (see Chapter 2), we can make the following
assessments: four of the respondents can be regarded as totally recovered. The other twelve had functioning social lives (work/vocational
activity, housing, social network) parallel to undergoing continued
treatment, primarily medication (in all cases "much less than before")
but also some therapeutic counselling.

6

In search of meaning
Truth and meaning

"The destination and map I
had used to navigate before
were no longer useful."
Judith Zaruches, in Frank 1995

What do people do to recover from severe mental disorders? What helps this process along? These two questions are the focus of this study. But all of our interview subjects have told us a larger story, they have accounted for a broader personal history. They have been able to make sense of their recovery only by relating events to their earlier situation in life, a kind of alienation work. Thus, in addition to the information the respondents have given us that has a direct bearing on their recovery effort, we have also obtained considerable biographical material. This need to contextualise their recovery, to construct a coherent account where all the elements are interconnected, has helped us to better grasp our interview subjects' recovery work. This "extra" result gives us further insight into the recovery process, but it also obliges us to clarify the interconnecting links in the life stories.

What we have observed consistently throughout the material is that these accounts of recovery follow a classic pattern for life stories. Another consistent observation is that throughout the whole process, from the onset of the disorder, during the psychotic episodes and through to recovery, our interview subjects see themselves as being on a quest for meaning. Furthermore, these accounts of recovery follow culturally sanctioned forms for constructing meaning.

With reference to both of these observations, it is evident that the interview subjects have used given cultural patterns in assembling their material, even though the stories they construct from this material are their own. But people who have been diagnosed as having a severe mental disorder face special problems when it comes to recovering and to telling about the struggle it has entailed. There are no culturally sanctioned elements at their disposal by which to construct such a narrative. Since it is considered to be impossible to recover from severe mental disorders, there are no readily accessible action sequences and life story models upon which they can build when constructing an own life story.

It is perhaps a self-evident observation, at least for those who discount the psychiatric literature's definition of people in the situation our interview subjects find themselves, that these accounts of recovery are largely coherent and have been constructed from certain key elements of narration that are common to our culture. The stories are logically constructed and conform to generally accepted conventions; they are not the incoherent products of insane minds. Bruner (1987) had Sartre in mind when he wrote:

> Life stories must mesh, so to speak, within a community of life stories; tellers and listeners must share some "deep structures" about the nature of "life", for if the rules of life-telling are altogether arbitrary, tellers and listeners will surely be alienated by a failure to grasp what the other is saying or what he thinks the other is hearing. (p. 21)

The life stories recounted in the interviews can be understood as culturally adequate products, not only with respect to their internal qualities (where in contemporary imagery creatures from the films Alien I, II, III or implanted datachips might take the place of archaic descriptions of Satan and hellfire), but also as logical constructs. This problematises the image of madness as a primitive force that is alien to cultivated people and modern society.

Two aspects of the life stories will be studied in this chapter: their structure and the meanings and contradictions with which the persons concerned are struggling. In contrast to the chapters on material

167

conditions, the self and others, which build on stories of practice, this chapter is concerned for the most part with the narrative level.

A classic narrative structure

The object of the inquiry, recovery, has an inherent structure that we could expect would determine the direction of the responses of the persons we interviewed. Recovery implies the idea of turning points, turning points in a positive direction, from suffering to some kind of improvement. But it is impossible to reach such a turning point unless one has first experienced a turning point for the worse. The idea of turning point is often associated with separate incidents where something of vital importance to the individual changes. But as this study shows, the situation is quite the opposite. In most cases, a turning point has consisted, not of a single event, but of a sequence of events, like a string of pearls which, in the eyes of the teller, depict how he/she came to be a psychiatric patient and how, sometimes after years of deep emotional distress, he/she has finally left the life of a patient behind and found relief from deep mental anguish.

Gergen and Gergen (1988) reduce the four classic forms of narrative – comedy, romance, tragedy and satire – to three types of sequences:

- *Stable*, wherein the individual or situation remains largely unchanged (persistently healthy, persistently unwell)
- *Progressive*, wherein there is an improvement, a positive development over time (from unwell to healthy)
- *Regressive*, wherein the person undergoes a process of deterioration (from healthy to unwell)

In tragedy the main thrust of the narrative is regressive, whereas in comedy and romance an initial regressive sequence is often followed by a progressive one. The organisation of a story thus depends to a large extent on where the beginning and end are situated in time. Naturally, recovery accounts contain both regressive and progressive elements, which may be combined to form stable sequences if the illness or the recovery process remains stable long enough. This is what has occurred in the case of several of our interview subjects. In most of the interviews, the subjects end their stories in the progressive phase. Had they been interviewed at an earlier (or perhaps later) point in time, we may have been shown only the tragedies, the regressive narratives.

Because their stories concern recovery from severe mental disorders, most of our story-tellers are aware of the temporality of the ending of their stories. They have internalised the culture's doubt about the possibility of a real, in the sense of permanent, recovery from severe mental disorders.

Uniqueness within a shared culture

Our collection of life stories are, thus, incorporated within a given culture. They are built up from a repertoire of elements that are socially constructed and available to each and every person in the culture. (Bruner 1987) The underlying idea of the stories is the person's perception of his/her life from a point of time in the past that is termed "the recovery". But when it comes to the concrete elements of the recovery story – Bertaux's "How did that happen?" – people who have recovered from severe mental disorders find themselves in a vacuum. Their odyssey is considered impossible; it could not have taken place. Their history can be understood only as a tragedy. The transition to a comedy therefore lacks recognisable phases and sanctioned cultural content.

Stimson and Oppenheimer (quoted in Castel 1992; see also Blomqvist 1996) found in their study of drug abuse that there are four obstacles drug misusers must overcome in their search for a way out of their predicament:

1. The lack of a recovery model, of a culture that could show a person how to overcome addiction. "To stop would mean *being part of a unique experience*, charting a course that no one had ever travelled before". (p. 217, italics mine)
2. Uncertainty about one's strength of will. How can we be sure that a drug misuser has really stopped using drugs? Can we rely

on his/her determination, when the lack of volition is thought to lie at the core of the problem?

3. The difficulty of finding an alternative to drug misuse.
4. The necessity of severing all ties, physically and symbolically, with the drug environment and finding alternative activities to fill the time that used to be devoted to drug misuse.

People who are recovering from severe mental disorders face the same kinds of obstacles. Severe mental problems affect most parts of the person's life, both with respect to time (the suffering itself but also all the accompanying activities connected with care and treatment), and the person's social network, which tends to be limited to professionals, other people with mental problems and whichever family members have remained on the scene. To return to ordinary activities and reconstruct a social network beyond the realm of psychiatry is an arduous undertaking. Also the question of the real extent and duration of the recovery is problematic in that recovery is associated with unknown biological processes and not with the individual's volition, which by definition has been grievously incapacitated.

Most important in this context is the lack of accepted models of recovery from the severe mental disorders that characterise our interview subjects' situation. On the contrary, we are more accustomed to "atrocity stories" about patients who are mistreated both within and outside psychiatric care (homelessness, physical and mental abuse, abandonment, abnormally high death rate) (see for example Steinholz-Ekecrantz 1995), or about patients who are dangerous to themselves and others (suicide, criminality, a burden on their families, etc.).

The few widely known cases of people who have recovered are cited as special cases from which it is impossible to draw general conclusions. In Sweden there is perhaps only one well-known case, Elgard Jonsson. In Jonsson's case, his association with Barbro Sandin, an unorthodox therapist who is reported to have a very special personality, has played a much discussed crucial role in his recovery (Jonsson 1986).

Thus, to paraphrase Castel, the stories of recovery from severe mental disorders imply that the tellers have had a unique experience;

they have wandered along a road that no one has travelled before. The interviews confirm this quality of uniqueness in a number of ways. As mentioned earlier, several of the persons we interviewed stated that no one had ever asked them the kinds of questions we asked in the interview. A possible explanation for this oversight is that progress toward recovery is considered so unlikely that psychiatry has not found it meaningful or instructive to inquire more penetratingly. On several occasions the persons we interviewed exclaimed that we were discussing situations they had forgotten all about. The interview stimulated recollections of situations and incidents that were not included in their standard repertoire of stories about their time as psychiatric patients. It was as if their life stories were unfolding as the interview progressed. Our interest in obtaining descriptions of recovery practice in context made it necessary for them to view past events in a new light, whereby even long-forgotten incidents came to light.

To be an "ex"

We can better understand the problems connected with stories of recovery from mental disorders if we compare them with what we know about other groups of people whose station in life has changed. Fuchs Ebaugh (1988), a researcher who has done considerable work on "role-exits", asserts that there is a basic pattern for this phenomenon that applies to a different groups of people. Her definition of role-exit is:

> The process of disengagement from a role that is central to one's self-identity and the reestablishment of an identity in a new role that takes into account one's ex-role... (p. 1)

As examples of the kinds of groups to which this pattern applies Fuchs Ebaugh mentions nuns who leave the convent, transsexuals who undergo a sex change, people with drinking problems who join Alcoholics Anonymous, mothers who give up custody of their children in a divorce, doctors, air-traffic controllers, police and seamen who more or less change their professions more or less of their own volition. Might not this pattern also apply to patients who have recovered from severe mental disorders? A comparison between this group and those referred to above can help us to determine what, if anything, is unique in the situation of people who have had or still have severe mental disorders.

The phases of role-exiting

Fuchs Ebaugh divides the role-exiting process into four phases ranging from 1) the person's original identity to 2) a period of "disidentification" and "disengagement", and further to 3) a time when the person's identity bears the imprint of his/her role as an ex-patient, and 4) to a new identity through "identification" and "engagement" in a new role. She then subdivides the actual transition, phases 2) and 3), into four steps:

1. *Growing uncertainty*. This stage entails questioning one's present role (spouse, alcoholic, doctor). Furthermore, the person unconsciously displays "cueing behaviours" that signal a readiness for change. Further development depends to a large extent on how the environment reacts to these cueing behaviours.
2. *The search for alternatives*. If others react positively to the cueing behaviours, the person is encouraged to believe that he/she has some free choice. The next step is to develop a more conscious cueing behaviour repertoire and to seek out people and reference groups who can reinforce the kinds of changes the person is contemplating.
3. *The turning point*. Gradually or, as in most of the cases in this study, suddenly a situation occurs that proves to be a turning point. Fuchs Ebaugh describes five types of turning points: special events, the straw that breaks the camel's back, time-related factors, excuses and either/or factors or alternatives. A turning point occurs when the new role is made public, which in turn reduces the person's feeling of cognitive dissonance. Reaching a turning point leads to a mobilisation of new resources both internal and external to the individual; however, at the same time the person may experience him-/herself as "hanging in the air" before a bridge to a new identity is brought into place.

4. *The creation of a role as an "ex".* The person must now assert his/her new identity in front of other people who knew him/her in the former role. To create a new role entails entering into new relationships, meeting other people who are unaware of one's former role, as well as people who have made the same role-exit and others who have fastened in the old role.

In our attempt to apply Fuchs Ebaugh's hypothesis of stages to the life stories we collected from people who have had severe mental problems, we found that her claim to have uncovered a general pattern for this transformation process is somewhat problematic. In some of the interviews we can find traces of the respondents' cueing behaviours. If the change begins with an interpersonal encounter with one or more persons, we can see how the parties in the encounter might signal to one another that they can imagine how the patient's situation could be modified. In such cases, the patient is already hopeful and thus open to the idea that the environment could envisage and react positively to possible alternative roles for the patient. This in turn nurtures the person's hope for a life other than that of a chronic patient. But patients' cueing behaviours are often met with scepticism, and even deep concern, from the environment. (See Strauss & Rakfeldt 1989, on the downswing that may precede a turning point upwards.)

The next step is more problematic for people with mental disorders who are struggling to recover. First of all, for a long time there were no other groups to whom they could turn to win support for their hopes of recovery or to find concrete alternative roles they could begin to fill. Furthermore, the turning points described in the interviews differ from the pattern envisioned by Fuchs Ebaugh. A main factor in her description of the process of becoming an "ex" is that the person makes the change public and begins to seek out new social contacts. None of the people in our study have reported that they have publicised their role-exit. Rather, because our culture has little conception of possible ways back to health, to publicise one's recovery entails instead the risk of being defined once again as a mentally ill person. It is like being a recovered alcoholic in AA, but without having access to a movement like the AA. They are, and remain, in the process of recovering, but as it is a process without end they remain for all time anonymous mentally disturbed persons who, for the moment, seem to be functioning well enough to get along in society. But even such "good" periods can be subsumed under a traditional conception of chronicity. Several of the interviews show that the person's social network continues to consist mostly of professional carers, other people with mental problems and family members, even after an extended period of recovery. One reason might be that the majority of the interview subjects had recovered only "socially" and thus were still in need of social interventions; but, in fact, even some of the persons we interviewed who had recovered totally had similarly limited social networks. A change of role is difficult to accomplish when the person's social life takes place in surroundings that bear the imprint of his/her former identity. Several of the persons in the study whom we find to have completely recovered moved from the district where they had earlier received psychiatric treatment, thereby breaking with their former social network. So, judging from our interview material, taking the final step in Fuchs Ebaugh's developmental stages toward a new identity, that is of becoming an "ex" and assuming a new identity unassociated with the role of psychiatric patient, seems to be a very difficult undertaking indeed.

Special features of the role-exit process

Fuchs Ebaugh describes several main features of the process of becoming an "ex". One is the "social desirability" (p. 39) of the role change. Another possible feature, to which, however, she does not refer specifically, is whether the role change was anticipated. It is reasonable to expect that this feature would be associated with desirability as well as with a third feature which she also does not mention, the "degree of institutionalisation" (p. 39). All of these features are to a greater or lesser extent associated with so-called "rites of passage". To form a couple, set up house together, get married and have children are all socially desirable and expected forms of behaviour that are arranged more or less in sequence and expressed in certain rituals (house-warming parties, bachelor and bride-to-be parties, marriage ceremonies, christenings, and so forth).

Many institutionalised roles and role changes are given their own designation: a person becomes a divorcée, widow or widower, spouse, parent and so forth. Less institutionalised role changes have an "ex" prefix or the word "former" attached: ex-convict, former alcoholic and so forth. People with severe mental disorders who live out of hospital are sometimes referred to as ex-patients or former patients, without this term signifying anything about their present state of mental health.

User organisations have tried to coin a term for people who have been or still are under psychiatric care. One that has been proposed is "survivor", but this term refers more to what the person has experienced, or perhaps still is experiencing, than to a new identity. Referring to oneself as a survivor does not by itself mean that one has undergone a role change. There are other groups as well for whom there are no words for referring to their role change (transsexuals, for example, is a term that highlights the state of transition rather than a new role). Even the term "user" or "service user" as a substitute for "patient" underlines contact with and use of support and care services. The use of unambiguous terms in this context indicates that society regards such role changes as highly probable. The absence of such terms implies that they are improbable. This clearly applies to people with mental problems. It is as if neither psychiatry nor the user organisations themselves can conceive of the possibility that some patients may not only become ex-patients, but also acquire a whole new identity. Normality is given a new dimension – as signifying an unattainable utopia.

Fuchs Ebaugh discusses the implied paradox of *socially desirable role changes that are not institutionalised in the society*. These are exits from roles that the community at large finds reprehensible: criminality, prostitution and drug abuse, for example. Interestingly enough, Fuchs Ebaugh does not include the role of mentally ill patient in her study. What is paradoxical in the role changes these groups undergo is that, although their role changes are considered desirable, they have to contend with difficulties that far exceed the problems usually associated with role changes. Their role changes are considered improbable and therefore lack credibility, or the change is seen as being temporary at best. It is as if it were impossible to leave one's

175

former role once and for all, which puts people who have undergone such a role change in a difficult position:

> However, in these instances, role residual, or the "hangover identity" from a previous status, often impacts current expectation and evaluations. (...) The ex-con is in a continuous dilemma because not to admit to a previous identity can be prosecuted as fraud; however, to admit to a previous felony jeopardises his or her chances at current employment. (p. 156)

Alcoholics Anonymous has institutionalised this "hangover identity" in the expression "sober alcoholic". The illness is chronic but the sick person can resist and counteract the symptoms. We see a similar phenomenon in the USA among users of psychiatric services. There is incipient awareness within the movement that severely mentally disturbed persons could possibly recover, but here recovery is framed as a life-long process. Regardless of how long people have lived a life free from symptoms, in the final analysis they are still ill, in the sense of being "vulnerable"; they are still "chronics".

Still another feature of the role-exit process outlined by Fuchs Ebaugh, "sequentiality" (p. 39), is missing in the case of people with mental disorders. By sequentiality is meant that the role-exit occurs in preordained steps, often with respect to both their order and duration. Sequentiality both steers and is a source of security for persons going through the process. Others have wandered along this path before and their collective wisdom tells us that painful emotions like sorrow, insecurity and doubt are appropriate reactions (this is how one should feel in this phase) and will pass in time.

For persons in the process of exiting from a role, and for people in their surroundings, sequentiality (see for example Cullberg's crisis and development model, 1975) supplies the process with a beginning and a – happy – end. However, for persons diagnosed as severely mentally ill, psychiatry recognises only one sequence, chronicity; in the long-run there will be no long-lasting change in the person's condition, other than perhaps a change for the worse.

Still another aspect of the role-exit process concerns the extent to which a person's own volition can steer the course of the process, what

Fuchs Ebaugh terms the role-exit's "voluntariness" (p. 35). This refers to the possibility to choose, to the person's "degree of control" (p. 38) and "degree of awareness" (p. 39). These features are concerned with the process's "reversibility" (p. 37), whether or not the role change is reversible.

Inasmuch as mentally disturbed persons must overcome their lack of control over their own lives and actions, they differ from all other groups, except drug misusers. Because it is their own volition that has failed them, like other people many of them continue to doubt their ability to break the downward spiral of chronicity. The spectre of "relapse" bears down on them with the whole weight of clinical psychiatric expertise. Furthermore, also as discussed earlier, a false idea can have very real consequences. To believe that one is feeling better is, in fact, merely a prelude to feeling worse. The relapse can occur at any moment, in ways that cannot be explained for the explanation lies in "the natural course", which research has yet to chart. The person's only recourse is to accept his/her illness and submit to the evidence-based treatment that research has produced, a treatment that may offer, if not a cure, at least fewer relapses.

A final feature of Fuchs Ebaugh's analysis of the role-exit process concerns the "centrality of the role" (p. 36). Closely connected with centrality is another feature: "single versus multiple exits" (p. 38), that is, if in exiting the role the person leaves behind more than one role and has to recreate several new ones. The more central the former role is, the harder it is to exit it. One of the reasons for this difficulty is that the more central the role is, the more "secondary roles" are involved which are affected by the role-exit process.

People with severe mental disorders tend to be reduced to their diagnoses. A large part of their lives are affected by the illness. Their social network tends to shrink to a minimum, consisting, as mentioned earlier, of family members, treatment staff and other patients (see Ewertzon & Forssell 1999).

In the recovery process, even family members, who also tend to be reduced to the role of "concerned family", must go through a role change, not only in relation to the patient – who is no longer a patient – but also in relation to their own lives and to their own social networks.

177

Recovery also entails breaking off contact with the treatment staff, which former patients may experience as threatening, both because the staff may be the only "normal" people they were in contact with while patients and because individuals among the staff may have played a significant role in their recovery. Total recovery often means that one's relationship with those who have aided the recovery process ceases, and perhaps prematurely. One of the persons we interviewed told us that she has not had voice hallucinations for the last two years prior to the interview, but she implored us not to tell the staff at the outpatient clinic she still visited from time to time because these visits were a large part of her social life. She feared that if she no longer showed any symptoms, it would no longer be possible for her to visit the clinic. She also said that she sometimes told the staff that she still heard voices because they then became more attentive toward her.

Several of our interview subjects have found ways to remain in contact with staff members who have been specially important to them long after treatment was terminated. Harding (1997) mentions as a possible explanation for the positive results she obtained in her study (Harding et al. 1987a, b) that friendship-like relationships had been formed between certain "ex-patients" and members of the rehabilitation team who followed them up after the rehabilitation project was concluded.

After close study, we find that Fuchs Ebaugh's claim to have found a general pattern for role-exits is difficult to apply to persons with a history of severe mental disorders due to the nature of the problem they are said to suffer from and to social circumstances. People diagnosed as having severe mental disorders cannot recover. This is the role they are able to fill, and no other. The advances made in psychiatry can offer them only symptom reduction and fewer acute relapses with recurring hospitalisation. From this perspective, the question of recovery is irrelevant, except in cases of "spontaneous cure" which, as the term implies, cannot be initiated and from which we have nothing to learn. Spontaneity is by definition a unique occurrence and impossible to reproduce, for that would make it a contradiction in terms. Thus recovery characteristics such as own volition, desirability and control are also irrelevant.

People who begin a process of recovery, which we would expect to be a socially desirable phenomenon, are met with scepticism and their progress is looked upon mainly as a temporary state of affairs circumscribed by the limits of the illness. They can expect little support from psychiatry, or from the user movement, at least if they intend to follow through with the recovery process, complete their role-exit, and cease being a patient (or an ex-patient), someone with a severe mental disorder. The most people in this situation can expect is to become an "ex", a term that implies the continuing existence of a latent problem; they remain an "ex" with no possibility to become anything else. They are trapped in a social and conceptual vacuum between people who are "actual patients" and "normal" people. This vacuum is reinforced by the rules and regulations surrounding society's support. Erik's situation is a case in point. He had progressed so far in his recovery process that he was able to obtain employment on the ordinary labour market. When he received his first salary, however, he discovered that certain deductions had been made. During the 20 years of his illness, he had accumulated a substantial debt for unpaid child support. These were deducted from his salary, which left him with as little money as he had before he started to work. Consequently, he quit his job and went back to being an ex-patient, where once again dependency on social support, visits to community day care centres and occupational therapy became his foremost social arenas (Estroff, 1985, has studied the same phenomenon in the USA).

Exiting from the role of psychiatric patient necessitates a total role change. But as the dominant medicalised culture in the Western world regards severe mental disorders as an attack on the very core of the personality, consciousness, volition, emotional life and identity, a role-exit entails a total transformation. It is hard to see how such a process whereby a non-existing person is transformed into a person, or becomes a different person, can occur without outside help. But by definition, no one is in a position to offer such help because the person is thought to lack the capacity to establish and maintain interpersonal relationships.

So, for people who begin to recovery, there are no established forms for institutionalising the process (it is hardly common practice, for example, to celebrate the homecoming of a person who has spent time in a mental hospital), for acknowledging its sequences or for exiting a role in group. People have to create each step on their own, who thereby become masters in "*bricolage*", do-it-yourself experts (Levi-Strauss 1962). They must use the materials at hand, regardless of their original purpose, and become "jacks-of-all-trades", not only when it comes to the art of narrating but also in the art of living their own lives.

Metaphors of illness and recovery

The persons we interviewed in the study use several recurring metaphors when describing their experiences. In the centre of these scenarios is the individual, a self. The most commonly occurring metaphor, corresponding to the basic structure of several of the recovery stories, is that of a journey: A lonely journey to a place that lies off the beaten track. A descent to the absolute bottom:

> I have plunged much deeper into my inner life than your average Joe does. The moon is inside me and the moon has a dark side that is terrifying, and it's inside me as much as outside me.
>
> What I mean by the moon's dark side is what happened with Apollo 13; for a while there, they were totally cut off from the world, and that's what happens in a psychosis. You're all alone in a terrain where no one has ever been before. And no one ever asks you about it or has the courage to take that journey with you. You enter a territory that psychiatry just won't help themselves to. They're afraid people are going to get stuck in psychosis, that's why they only talk about healthy things. But if you really want to learn something, then you've got to dare to go along on those journeys. If someone would only go with you, you could transmit certain things. Otherwise it's only us patients who talk about these things among ourselves. (Jan)

What is being described here is the feeling of being completely alone, which is underscored by the imagery of a desolate landscape:

> Well, I remember one drawing in particular that meant a lot to me... The assignment was to draw a picture of yourself in relation to the outside world. And what I drew was a picture of myself inside a bubble...'cause I

felt... one of the notions I had was... that I was living in a glass bubble, cut off from the world around me... I had this weird feeling that I was surrounded by a bubble. So I drew myself sitting inside a bubble with my back turned... I sat and read a book with my back turned against the world, which was on the outside... And inside the glass bubble everything was grey and black and the book was all grey and black, but outside there were all these colours and people and lots of light... (Susanne)

The metaphors often allude first to cold and isolated places followed by places of warmth and fellowship. In such cases recovery has to do with undertaking a journey within oneself and to one's self in order to find out how to leave the cold and come into the warmth.

I had a longing to come back to myself. I had almost left my good house for good, to see it as such, so to speak. (Richard)

Another common metaphor alludes to not having the necessary tools for dealing with life. Here too, there is clearly loneliness and remoteness from others.

There was this psychologist who I heard on the radio who said that we human beings each have our own tool-kit, but that people with problems like mine have fewer tools in their kit than other people have. They don't have as many tools to deal with what life hands out. I thought then that maybe this somehow applied to me. And then I thought afterwards that I could just as well make my own tools, I could somehow make or get hold of the tools that would make me better, so that I too could deal with things. Then maybe I could wind up with a good tool-kit, too.

A fragile normality – a turn for the worse

The life stories begin from the time when the person lived a more or less ordinary life. At the same time, however, several of the respondents could point to certain traits within themselves and situations that at an early stage were undermining the façade of normality, but which they were able to manage for a time.

The first breakdown occurs either as a result of increasing tension and contradiction within the individual or through external events, or as a combination of both where the external events aggravate problems that the individual is already experiencing:

> The psychotic experiences had a lot to do with the trauma of the divorce and all that, but that's not the whole story. Because when I was a little kid I didn't love life at all. I could see it for what it really was. That life is hard to live, and I must have been about ten years old when that thought first occurred to me. (Jan)

The breakdown is seen as resulting from the failure of this earlier way of trying to cope with one's situation in life. It means that the patient has made a crucial break with the illusion of normality he/she has maintained for so long. As a consequence of the breakdown the person comes to the attention of the public authorities, first and foremost psychiatry. The initial contact with psychiatry can play different roles in the recovery stories. Some of the subjects described a fear of being hospitalised, whereas others saw it as a possibility to get help. For some, the first contact with psychiatry may have actually marked a turning point to the better. Here the person has already hit bottom by the time he/she comes to the attention of psychiatry. To seek and be given help and to acknowledge the painful experiences of one's earlier life is the first step towards progress.

For the majority of the respondents the first contact with psychiatry represents a further turn on the downward spiral. It is confirmation of one's worthlessness, an extension of the experience of neglect in early life.

In Sven's case, his contact with psychiatry was a last resort from the start:

> I guess a lot of it has to do with when I lived at home with my mum and dad, and it suddenly occurred to me to tell them to lock the door because I didn't know what I might do, you know. It was terrible. I felt so rotten. It was horrible not knowing if I could stop myself from doing my parents an injury. It was pretty tough in fact.
>
> And when I realised that was my situation, I knew it just couldn't go on, there was something crazy going on. I just knew it. And so I let them decide what would happen next. And they were real good to me, my mum and dad and the doctor. They stayed calm, they took it easy with me and

told me that I should go into hospital. So I did what they said because I knew there just wasn't any other way. And I was having a really tough time, something was really sick inside me. (Sven)

In Richard's case as well, contact with institutional care was mainly a positive experience:

It has to do with three things: there's the hospital staff; there's peace and quiet, friendliness and security in how the staff treat you, what you think about when you go to bed at night or when you're sitting around drinking coffee... a chance to think about things; and then the third thing was the medicine. (Richard)

The effort to be noticed, to draw attention to the problems one is struggling with is a recurrent theme during this period. Seen from this perspective, the breakdown is "a relief" because it is often associated with the feeling of finally being noticed and the hope of getting help.

It was clear to me then, too, that I wanted someone else to take over the responsibility. I couldn't do it on my own. I desperately wanted someone else to do it. And it was... it became so absurd, too, because I started acting out in all destructive ways possible... so much so that everyone around me could see it. I acted like that so that others would see it, but I wasn't in the kinds of places where anyone did anything about it. (...)
    I mean, what actually got me to ask for help was my sister. She said that things were getting completely out of hand. Yes, so she said, "Seriously, this can't go on". She caught me trying to cut myself... and that got her really scared. So she said she could contact an outpatient clinic for me... but that I had to promise to keep the appointment. I was so glad she did that. That's just what I wanted, for someone to take responsibility for me and make me do something like that. Maybe I wasn't all that glad about it at the time, but I felt relieved. I felt, like, "at last". (Susanne)

The feeling of finally being noticed may turn out, however, to be a false hope. The encounter with the psychiatric system can be a disappointment that intensifies the feeling of being invisible. In such instances, it is not a turning point upwards, but rather another turn in a downward spiral.

Well, so I made an appointment and went to... one of those. Five or six sessions with a psychology student... It was really frightening. Yes. But I think it mostly had to do with the person I was seeing. He wasn't in such good shape himself. I hope with all my heart they dropped him before he graduated. (Susanne)

By coming into contact with psychiatry and the social services, the person's deviant position becomes apparent. But this acknowledgement does not necessarily result in getting help to regain one's self.

The marginalisation process in Irene's case began with the divorce of her parents and was confirmed in her early teens when she was raped but no one seemed to take the incident seriously. Shortly thereafter her father dies:

And then my father died in July and I so went back there. And got through the funeral and everything. And then I started the 7th grade. By then I was already smoking grass and hanging out with that crowd, and skipping school of course. I guess it was in the spring term when I ran away from home the first time. I just packed my stuff and marched off to [names two cities] with my friend. After that, I ran away lots of times.

And that's when they brought in social welfare. An officer from the child welfare board came and asked me how I could do such a thing? What was wrong with me?

The encounter with the social services confirmed Irene's worst fears: It's my fault. I'm what's wrong. The people who finally did notice Irene are unable to distinguish between the role she was playing, the function of which was to get attention, and Irene herself who needed to be noticed. To get attention is to be reduced to a role, one that corresponds to the diagnoses and assessments of the social services and psychiatry.

The downward spiral – hitting rock bottom

The personal accounts unfold as life stories in which the individual, in order to find his/her self, is forced to relinquish everything, forced to make the descent to hell. The descent is usually marked by a series of way stations and can be understood as a radical demolishing of an alien identity.

The bottom level is characterised by a feeling of a total loss of power and sense of identity. Premature attempts to rise from the bottom fail because the demolition process has not been completed so that the new identity rests on a false bottom. It is this state of total hopelessness that provides a firm foundation from which the person can gain momentum. Rock bottom is namely also a take-off point in several of the recovery stories:

> One thing's for sure; something helped to calm me down after I had gone through that process, had become crazier and crazier – for years I just kept getting crazier. I've learned a lot from that. I've learned that you have to get a lot more crazy before you can climb back up again. And that idea doesn't scare me anymore. (...)
>
> In a way I guess I felt that I didn't dare dream or believe in the future because they seemed so unattainable, so remote. I think that for at least two-thirds of the time I was in therapy, things just got worse and worse, and it has to do with, once you get entangled in a lot of weird systems, you know, well you got to burrow down to the bottom before you can begin to climb up again. (Susanne)

The distinguishing feature of hitting rock bottom is that the person cannot descend any further. Some of the stories relate how every now and then a turn for the better occurred and things started looking up. Whether or not a particular turning point constitutes rock bottom can only be determined in retrospect.

An example of a situation in Irene's life which many people might regard as being negative but which in one particular case became a positive force concerned her becoming pregnant. For a while the pregnancy and life after the birth of her son constituted a crucial turning point in Irene's life:

> The day I turned 16 I'm supposed to get my period, but it doesn't come, instead I'm pregnant with my oldest boy. My first thought was to get an abortion. I thought: Sweet Jesus, how am I ever going to take care of a child on top of everything else. (...) But at the same time, I came to think

about the money I inherited from my dad. I'm pregnant and could just leave home and get away from those jerks [by which she means her mother and stepfather]. And that's what happens. I move out in March already. I have my own apartment. I'm still in the 8th grade. [The child's father] was a confirmed hash smoker. He never quit. As for me, I actually take time-out. Stop smoking hash and cigarettes during the pregnancy. Conduct myself really well. Can't start the 9th grade because my son is born in October. I get help at home with English, French and maths. I feel real lousy in the hospital. I don't get a real psychosis, but just want to throw myself out the window. I couldn't feel he was mine. (...)

When I came home from the maternity ward, there's my fantastic grandmother and she lived [here] for three weeks and helped me all day long. She's always been my lifesaver. Fantastic. So, with her help I settle down to be a mother and do my best.

In the spring I start the 9th grade. I graduate with a 4.7 average and start high school. I smoke a little, but not much, I really give it my best shot. Try to be an intellectual, stop painting my face... become the first female leader of the student union, write lots of stuff for the school newspaper... (Irene)

In Irene's case the metamorphosis seems total, but evidently the groundwork of her new self is unstable: "It goes on like that until I turn 18." The downward spiral continues until she she really does hit rock bottom, overwhelmed by feelings of death and annihilation, four years later:

I'm overcome by a feeling of dread that's out of this world. Death anxiety. I've always felt... existential anxiety, but this is something different. Panic, I'm dying. (...) So now at the clinic they get to know me in a whole new way. (...) This leads to my drug abuse getting even worse. During all those years I was on a pretty powerful mix of amphetamines, alcohol and loads of pills and fags. There wasn't a day I wasn't high. Not one. More than anything else I was on Esucos that I got on prescription...

Life was just pest, pest, anguish, anxiety... When I was about 21, 22 I began thinking about giving up. I couldn't take it any more. I couldn't see any way out. The only problem was, I was too chicken to jump or slit my wrists, so I thought if I increase the abuse even more, it'll happen on its own. (...) I entered a phase in my abuse when amphetamine didn't do anything for me anymore. No kicks, no high, no nothing. It was just a way to keep up the status quo. You drank and you... Nothing helped to put a lid on things anymore.[Year], it's spring and I'm so tired all the time. I've had hepatitis B several times. They had me in the infection ward. My whole body's worn out... In May I take more than I can handle and don't notice it until that evening when I take my usual mix of pills and *wham-bam*. Then I get over the chock from the overdose and I get huge pains in my liver, kidneys. I swell up like a balloon, so my boyfriend phones for an ambulance and I end up on the infection ward again. I'm 22 years old and already a regular customer. So they say to me: "That there's not worth it. You won't even make it to 25."

I'm lying there, like, sick as hell and they contact the hospital because they think I should get a disability pension because I've got three years at most to live. That's when social welfare gets into the picture in full force. I'm lying there sick as I can be and they're going to take my child away from me.

In several of the recovery stories, the downward spiral is described as having been the result, at least in part, of the person's own conscious choices. Drug abuse and what is regarded as symptoms of mental illness can have a similar function:

The funny thing is, I don't know if it's possible to do what I did, I mean, to consciously or subconsciously tear down, I mean, really tear down everything inside you, pull it all down and go stark raving mad, just to see what it's like. (Sven)

Often there is more than one downward turn towards the "true" bottom. People who have hit rock bottom stand completely uncovered. The façade that had covered over the emptiness has collapsed. The gulf between the role and individual can no longer be bridged.

In such a situation hospitalisation could be experienced as a form of security. It allows the person to just let go:

Yeah, but somehow I wasn't able to act the way I saw some of the other patients doing, just drifting along, showing the world that they can't cut it. I couldn't do that. When I got to the point where I couldn't keep up the façade any longer, that's when I went into hospital. They gave me sick leave first time around, but I had already decided I wanted to be admitted. I wanted 24-hour care. (Susanne)

Besides feeling naked, unmasked, which may be an indication that the person has hit rock bottom, another indicator often mentioned in the recovery stories is an overwhelming feeling of hopelessness:

I saw everything as being completely hopeless... I didn't have much faith that I could ever come out of it as a whole person... but I didn't have any choice either... Stopping therapy and going back to the way it was before wasn't a real option for me... because I had already moved on. I couldn't go back... so I felt, like, all I could do was keep going ... to the bitter end. (Susanne)

That last time I was sicker than ever before. Because I threw myself off the porch. I was having such a hard time that I simply gave up, just gave up altogether. I stood there at that railing and just gave up, and so I climbed over the railing and dropped straight down the slope, several meters down. And of course it hurt. But I remember saying, and I meant it too, that the pain of a couple of broken ribs is nothing compared to emotional pain. (Sven)

The turning point(s) upwards

The ascent from rock bottom can begin in several different ways. The turning point may occur after a relatively short time, but also after decades of being under psychiatric care. The stories describe the turning point as having been reached either as the result of the person's own decision, of a fortuitous external influence in the form of a purposeful effort by another human being, or of a series of coincidences and random incidents and events.

Although reaching the turning point is often presented as a consequence of one's own maturation process, several of the recovery stories mention an unexpected change of circumstances that forced the person to make a decision. The catalytic role that these events (or persons) come to play in the person's life story cannot be discerned from the event itself. In fact, one could expect such events to have primarily negative consequences, but instead they are depicted in the life stories as being a push in the right direction. The person may even have met similar people or situations earlier in his/her history as a patient without the encounter having had any significant impact.

The fact that these earlier situations did not have a catalytic effect suggests to us that change, as envisioned in the life stories, has to do with a genuine encounter. External circumstances are not enough. These catalytic persons and/or situations do not simply exist in an external objective sense; rather, they are just as much an inner subjective invention as they are a function of the role ascribed to them in the individual's autobiography. The person notices them, realises they are opportunities and assigns their own special meaning to them. The encounters become a mutually creative process.

A turning point does not have to be a dramatic event. A central aspect of a turning point is that it represents a change in how people perceive themselves in relation to their own lives, symptoms and condition. The ascent from rock bottom occurs in small steps. Often, these small steps involve recapturing what we earlier called power with respect to taking part in the decisions about one's life. Irene talks about how important it was for her to make the ascent in small steps. One step at a time is described in several of the recovery stories as a successful tactic:

> I was in such bad shape that I couldn't even think straight thoughts, I can tell you. I lay on the bed, and I couldn't imagine for one minute that I was capable of thinking, for example. I can now, don't you agree? I understand now that I'm capable of having my own thoughts, I can think most of the time. But I couldn't then. I remember lying in bed, I was in almost complete despair. I got out of bed and went out on the ward. And I called out, 'I can't even think a single thought'. It was the only way I could get it through my head, by shouting it out that to the whole room. I couldn't think it through for myself. That's how uptight I was. I was so uptight, like all tied up inside. It was... nothing was moving around in there at all. And not because everything was dead inside, but because something was wound up so tight that I... nothing could move inside. But then I thought to myself: I got to try to do this a little bit at a time. I just got to try to loosen the knots inside a little at a time, take small steps, so maybe I can get somewhere, that's what I thought to myself. That maybe I could

loosen the knots if I just did it a little at a time every day. And that's what I did. And things have loosened up. And I did it a little at a time, like. I succeeded in loosening the knots, I mean. (Sven)

Although a turning point per sé is a radical shift of attitude from hopelessness to the idea that perhaps one's situation could change, in practice a turning point is achieved through many small steps.

The way up

The upward journey is not a straightforward linear process. Cosmetic changes that are concerned only with the material conditions for the self's growth (a job, a place to live) and do not affect the sense of the self may lead to apparent changes, for a time. But in the long run there is a risk that superficial changes merely serve to enhance the original "façade/true self" dichotomy and result in a loss of ground. Relapse is a recurrent theme in the recovery stories and the explanation given is that the person tried to live a normal life too soon. The problem is not an inability to assimilate the external attributes, but rather that these attributes were not grounded in a complete turn-about at rock bottom:

There was a person I got to know at the gym who helped me get a job as a nursery school helper. And I took the job. An ordinary job, to keep up the façade, that there's nothing wrong with me... In a way I was right back where I started from when I went into hospital, going to work and keeping up a façade and going home and being all by myself. Now I was trained for it. (Susanne)

And after a while I got a new psychosis. You could say it was my own fault. I had been doing too much for the user movement and got too involved and didn't get enough rest and so it got all mixed up. I overdid it and wore myself out. (...) I think I spent too little time on myself. So I'm much more careful about that today. Somehow I've kind of felt that there's a point to all these psychotic experiences. They're not completely meaningless. If I'm suffering, it can't be pointless, it's got to have some meaning, some purpose. Looking at things today, I'm better at talking about them especially since I had that relapse because it reminded me that something's going on inside all the time. I can never say "now it's all over", that it was just something that happened during the eighties; this is something that goes on all the time. (Jan)

Jan's explanation for his relapse is that he had not thoroughly dismantled his alien self before he started to build up a new self:

> I thought I had finally got some order in my life. I had talked through a lot of stuff and now I had my life in order and could put all that stuff behind me. But it turned out that everything was still there. All the baggage was just as untreated now as when I put it aside. I thought I was finished with all that, but it was as if nothing had been done. (...) There was nothing for it but to unpack all the goods again. (...) In my psychosis I sunk to the level of a three-year-old. That far, but no further. (Jan)

This is where Jan had finally hit rock bottom. To ascend from rock bottom does not mean to return to square; the self that is regained or unmasked is not the same as the original self. The road back goes forward. Some interview subjects describe it as rebirth. A new self is born:

> Yes, I feel that part of me is gone forever... it's just gone, like, and in another way I think it's like a long drawn-out rebirthing. (Susanne)

Constructing meaning and context

Attention is given in much of the literature on narratives, which derives it images from the textual domain, to the coherence of life stories. The story organises the intrigue in a logical way, in temporal sequences and with a common theme throughout that binds the different parts of the story together.

Many "recovery-tales" and theories on recovery from a range of human conditions (Greenberg 1994, Plummer 1995) offer coherent explanatory models for how the condition arose and, on the basis of this explanation, what the way out of it looks like. The point of departure is a recovery strategy or programme that aims to minimise the diversity and plurality of experience. Even in the case of less serious mental problems there is an array of psychotherapeutic methods that offer coherent theoretical explanations. These methods stem from a common model, that from the cause there is a path leading to relief from the symptoms or at least to greater insight.

Plummer (1995) has formulated a ten-step model based on the recovery literature: the first step is to identify a new problem and then to frame a new concept for the problem. At the core of what makes the problem new are life stories where the initiators of the new movement have often had personal experience of the problem. From these life stories a personality profile is sketched where readers can recognise their own situation in the description of the problem. The personality profile engenders a diagnosis, just like in the manuals in psychiatry. Many of the life stories seek to situate the core of the problem in the person's childhood, such as growing up in a dysfunctional family or having been subjected to abuse and maltreatment. From such sources a series of stages is derived leading to the actual/current problems.

> Finally, the solution is proposed, most commonly as a form of "spiritual growth" thought of as a series of stages. Out of suffering, a new self is born. (p. 105)

The solution, in the main, lies in the person's acknowledging the problems and beginning to talk openly about them; that is to say, in reproducing the same life story as was first presented in the literature.

The recovery theme is ideally suited for the classic life history genre. We have the hero who after having lost something of great value embarks upon a lonely journey in search of it, becoming even more forsaken along the way; he goes through dreadful ordeals until finally, made stronger by the ordeals (overcoming them has given him greater self-knowledge), he returns to the starting point of his journey. But now his position is different from the one he could easily have been his had he not been forced to challenge his fate. Most of the life histories we have collected in this study follow this pattern. But recovery from severe mental disorders creates special problems for those who have gone through it, as discussed earlier. Recovery histories are met with considerable scepticism in our culture and there few such histories that could serve as models.

Perhaps this explains somewhat the rather meagre responses we received to the opening question in the interviews, before we came into the concrete questions where we asked the respondents to describe in concrete terms situations they referred to in the open-ended part of the interview. In several instances the respondents seem unclear about how they began to feel unwell and display various symptoms, and then why the symptoms eventually disappeared. They seemed to lack a coherent model for explaining their experiences. There was a risk that our constructions of meaning might have more to do with our analysis than with the actual responses. We have tried to limit this risk by retaining the separate categories of meaning side by side without reorganising them into comprehensive wholes.

In several interviews, the respondents seemed to apprehend various contexts for the first time during the course of the interview itself. It was as if we were the first persons with whom they discussed their experiences, and as if they, in their conversations with us, examined for the first time a diversity of events and found ways to link them to each other. Several of the comments show that we were, in fact, the first. The interview subjects experimented with four explanatory models in their search for meaning: the psychotherapeutic, the medical, the spiritual and the interactional.

The psychotherapeutic model

The interview subjects who had undergone psychotherapy were those who constructed the most clearly coherent categories of meaning in their life histories. Childhood experiences had led to increasing problems during adolescence, finally resulting in a breakdown. The recovery is seen as being closely linked to a psychotherapy that extended over a period of years. There were persons who had not had psychotherapy who also constructed corresponding categories of meaning in their stories, but in these cases they did not associate their recovery with psychotherapy.

Where the former group has absorbed a way to interpret their experiences through their often long psychotherapy, the latter group has been creative in how they use the building blocks of meaning that are available in our culture. This creative effort (*"bricolage"*) can also be found among the respondents who have had psychotherapy. All of the respondents have built up their stories using components derived from the other possible categories of meaning.

The medical model

All the interview subjects had been treated with various neuroleptics. Many had conflicting experiences of these medicines. In the case of several of the respondents, the medical explanatory model constituted a main component in their effort to find the meaning of their experiences. However, none of the respondents used the medical model to explain what caused their problems. On the other hand, they described the medicines as being an important factor in their recovery. None of the life stories contained an exclusively medical model of explanation; when it occurred, it was in connection with one or more of the other alternative explanatory models.

The spiritual model

Several of the life stories refer to spiritual experiences as a source of meaning, not so much as an explanation of what caused the onset of the disorder and thereto accompanying experiences, but rather as an important element in the recovery process. It seems that spiritual experiences and the ability of religious groups to provide a means for interpreting and managing one's life could constitute a functioning explanatory model illuminating the path to a communality beyond the world of psychiatry.

The interactional model

While the earlier categories of meaning have a well entrenched position in our culture in that they are institutionalised in various organisations, the fourth explanatory model is less well known. There are no groups or organisations that represent, formulate, defend and develop it. It can, however, be considered to have a certain foothold in the everyday thinking of our culture. All of the life stories contained descriptions of interactions with other people that explained, if not all, at least a part of the onset of the illness, the person's experiences during the period of disorder and the recovery. In several life stories everyday interactions with other people constituted the main explanation. Of course, the psychotherapeutic explanatory model has interactional elements as well, but in the interactional category of meaning what was being referred to was the importance of the direct interaction. In essence, the interactional explanatory model concerned the person's spending time in the company of "ordinary" people, by which they also meant low-ranking mental health staff in the professional hierarchies of psychiatry and the social services.

These four categories of meaning do not occur in a pure form in any of the interviews. One of our male respondents relates, for example, that he had traumatic experiences in his childhood (psychotherapeutic model), but associates his first psychotic crisis with tension in his marriage and being overworked at his job (interactional model). In explaining his recovery, he mentions his close contact with someone in his family and a doctor with whom he had a good relationship (interactional model). Further, he mentions his faith (spiritual model) and that he was finally prescribed "the "right medicine" (medical model).

There is nothing in the interview to indicate that these components are not interconnected. Through analysing the transcripts of the interviews, it is possible to interpret the apparent incoherence between all these components as attempts to construct meaning from a multitude of diverse experiences. But perhaps we should be satisfied that the emerging picture is sufficiently coherent to give the person who is telling about these experiences (and the one who is listening to the telling) a satisfactory context.

Hydén (1995b), based his article on the rhetoric of recovery on a interviews of a number of patients who had undergone psychotherapy. The article does not specify what kinds of problems they had sought help for, but from the text it is evident that they had not been diagnosed with a psychotic disorder. Perhaps it is because of these two factors (psychotherapy and a non-psychotic problem) that Hydén found a fairly unambiguous and coherent structure embedded in his material:

> What is striking in the interviews is that they are all largely built up around a central dramatic plot; from a life of torment before therapy, a

breakdown, to finally undergoing psychotherapy and obtaining "release" and achieving "a good life". (p. 77)

The life stories are organised in a way that corresponds to the rhetorical elements Hydén found in the literature on successful forms of treatment. These rhetorical elements encompass, first of all, the person's demonstrating *a predisposition* for a particular method of treatment. Then the storyteller must show that *the treatment really worked*, and as a third element, the *process of change itself must be presented*. Lastly, it must be clearly evident that a *reconstruction of the person* has taken place. The recovery must be proved.

Such linear coherent rhetorical structures are difficult to find in the actual life stories. Hydén points out that the storytellers are perhaps more ambiguous than the rhetorical model would seem to indicate and that there can be several "story lines" (p. 78) gleaned from diverse sources for the purpose of moving the story forward. Nonetheless, it is possible to assert that the rhetorical structure found in our group of interviews differs in a significant way from Hydén's model. In most cases (with the possible exception of the respondents who had psychotherapy) there was no connection between a particular method and the achieved changes. Our respondents were not engaged in trying to prove a point or a method or a model that had helped their recovery.

Again with the possible exception of the persons who had psychotherapy, our respondents were not predisposed for a particular method of treatment; they did not undergo any special or successful forms of treatment, although in some cases a combination of several treatment interventions played a role in their recovery. Of course it is a recovery process they are describing, but the process is complex one.

As for the ultimate result, recovery, in some of the life stories it is other people who make that judgement, while in others the fact of the recovery is "discovered" and comes to be "accepted" first during the course of the interview itself.

Although telling about one's recovery entails "looking back" over one's life, the occasion of the interview is not a given end point that rounds off the story in a clear-cut way. Insofar as the person has not had any symptoms, or only mild symptoms, for several years, has not been hospitalised for mental illness in the last two years, has an own place to live, a job or meaningful occupation and a social network, he/she is in a situation or state which, because it has no name, is difficult to organise a life story around.

Ultimately, the interviews are descriptions of the person's current situation or condition and a number of other situations that have no clear-cut narrative interrelationship. Insofar as they constitute fragments of explanations, it is difficult to integrate and lift them to the rhetorical level purported by Hydén (1995b).

Anne, who has long experience of psychiatric hospitalisation, presents a tentative explanation for the onset of her disorder, but then immediately retracts it:

> At first I thought this voice thing was really weird. I had heard that people who were schizophrenic heard voices. I had read a book about it and thought that my hearing voices was because I had read that book. That it was just my imagination. Maybe I had read it too closely and it had, like, been absorbed into my head. But then I thought that was just nonsense.

Later she describes as a central factor in her recovery undergoing a brain scan where she assumed that the person she thought was inside her head would show up on the X-ray. Finally, once and for all, the psychiatric staff would be convinced that what she was experiencing was real. When the brain scan did not show any trace of such a person, she began to think that perhaps the staff were right in their assertion that she was only imagining things:

> *What do you think made him disappear?*
> That I ignored it. That I didn't fantasise. They said that it was me, myself who... I was the only one who heard and saw him... and I've thought about that a lot. That it's only me imagining things. It's me making a fool of myself and trying to get attention. To get people to pay attention to me because I feel so lonely. So I say "I hear voices. Help me!" That gets me attention from the staff, and like... And I got it too. I wasn't alone then.

As the interview progresses and comes into the actual recovery, another explanation is introduced, an interactional explanation suggested by the psychiatric staff and which the respondent took to heart and developed further. But here we have strayed far from a description of a predisposition for a specific form of treatment and a description of the administering of that treatment. Nevertheless, the life story ends with a new self emerging into the light of day, but it is a much more concrete and poetically formulated self, without any of the connotations found in the psychiatric literature:

> *You've told me how your appearance has changed in the last two or three years. Have you changed in any other way?*
> Yes, I have. My soul is red now. It used to be black. Everything is easier now. I can breathe. I can't explain it, but I feel happy. I'm satisfied with myself.
> *Red is an intensive colour...*
> I'm burning with a love for life. I accept life now.

The diversity and complexity of the categories of meaning that emerge from the life histories makes the question of how insight is discussed in the literature and applied in practice a problematic one. Insight is thought to refer to a truth about why and how a person came to be mentally disturbed. But there is no such consensus in psychiatry and the people who enter this domain formulate their insights on the material they find within, and outside, that domain. The categories of meaning we have found among the persons who have recovered create an opening for the possibility that the crucial factors may have little to do with how well the explanatory model conforms to scientific explanations. Rather, they have more to do with the extent to which particular explanations are able to create a context that is acceptable to the persons concerned and others in their surroundings. Meaning acquires the power of truth insofar as it makes life comprehensible backward in time and predictable forward in time.

Not either/or, but both

A central element in the recovery process is the reconstruction of a context, a main thread connecting the diverse parts of one's life, of one's self, to form a coherent whole. The context provides a meaning, one that has been extracted from all the earlier breakdowns of meaning in connection with the illness.

Meaning before, during, and after the psychosis

The attempt to construct meaning is a main theme running through the life stories. Preoccupation with trying to find a meaning to one's life may be the first sign of a disorder. Even while in the throes of the psychosis the effort to construct a context for understanding one's experiences goes on – one often realises that there is something wrong with having such experiences – proceeding from what is defined as symptoms to the care and treatment that is administered as a consequence of the symptoms.

> And when I come home there's my dad with one of his pals and they're drinking. I fall behind in my studies and start thinking that in the summer that's when I'll catch up, but then it starts: such anguish. I go around and wonder what the hell is wrong with me? I'm 25 years old and my life is going nowhere. That's what it can be like. I've read Hesse and been influenced by Siddharta and revolted against the performance demands at the university. And that's going to be my salvation, the inner way. Because it's not about performing and because action is about satisfying needs, so action has no value in itself – you act to satisfy needs – and when your needs are satisfied you achieve equilibrium and equilibrium is balance and you shouldn't upset balance, and that's what makes excessive actions a sin. That's about how I get it to fit together. They're my own ideas and I stick by them. And I carry them out with the same firmness of principle as Siddharta did. (…) But then I find a medicine against worry and anxiety. One day I'm lying on my bed in my little room. I'm lying there looking at the ceiling. I had better eyesight then than I have now, and I stare at a spot on the ceiling and, the more I look at that spot, the more I notice that my worry and anxiety go away. Concentration gives security. It's a kind of meditation, but I didn't know that then. (Sören)

It is not so important that the meaning that is constructed while the person's life is dominated by the psychosis may seem to us to be strange and poorly anchored in reality. What is important is that, because these attempts to manage and understand painful feelings and experiences are regarded by others in the person's surroundings as additional symptoms, the work to construct meaning occurs under increasingly isolated conditions.

It is difficult for other people to accept the idea that although the result of the effort to construct meaning may seem strange in the person's own eyes as well as in the eyes of others, such a meaning may be better than having no meaning at all or than accepting the meanings that are generally available. Sören, whom we met in the above interview excerpt, describes this duality:

> I'm aware of what I'm doing. I think it's interesting. I'm discovering things. They see it as an illness, but it's just as much a technique. It's a technique for solving a problem and that's how I've reasoned the whole time: "OK, maybe it's looks weird and I know people around me think it's weird, but I know what I'm doing." It's a technique that enables me to cope. And I bloody well find inner peace, even if what's on the outside is still going on. (Sören)

What is being described here is a kind of dual consciousness which Sacks et al. (1974) among others, have described as characteristic of the second phase in the process of recovering from a psychotic breakdown. The person still has delusions and hallucinations, but is aware at the same time that these *should not be happening*.

Acceptable/unacceptable constructions of meaning

The overarching structures that provide meaning in the life stories consist often of the conventions and accepted explanations to why people fall ill with psychosis and, perhaps, what could be conducive to their recovery. Medical explanations are wholly accepted. Psychodynamic explanations engender scepticism. On the one hand, they are still given credence in institutional settings, but on the other they are not considered to be "evidence-based" (National Board of Health and Welfare 1997). Powerful interest groups in psychiatry regard them as being ineffectual and therefore without explanatory value. Nevertheless, psychodynamic structures of meaning are deeply rooted in the culture outside the realm of psychiatry.

Interactional explanations are considered to be layman explanations with little or no scientific value. Possibly interactional elements can be linked to some social-psychological school such as symbolic inter-actionism. But symbolic interactionism is not anchored in psychiatry nor in the culture at large. Interactional explanations are summarily treated as anecdotes and, as such, do not contribute to knowledge development.

Lastly, the fourth explanatory model, spirituality, is probably con-sidered in psychiatry to be the tip of the iceberg of underlying symp-toms, and thus is proof that persons who hold with this type of explanation have not recovered from their disorders. However, spirit-ual explanations have a strong position in institutional settings outside the domain of psychiatry in a variety of religious congregations.

Hope

Undoubtedly, psychotic crises can be experienced as the breakdown of all meaning. At the same time, people in crisis expend considerable energy in looking for and constructing a meaning that would give shape to the chaos that arises when an alien force enters into and appears to take command over a person's life.

All of the four explanatory models found in the life stories have the capacity to generate hope. Insofar as they create some kind of order, they offer a possibility to imagine a continuation of the story. The medical model is the most pessimistic of the four; it is also the pre-dominant one. It is the model most frequently adhered to by personnel who have the responsibility of providing assistance and treatment. As we saw earlier severe mental disorders are defined in this model as life-long illnesses for which the model can provide treatment to alleviate the symptoms (but with certain side-effects). Furthermore, the model offers some hope that a future breakthrough in medical research will solve the riddle that still lies at the base of every diagnosis.

In many of the stories, rock bottom is reached when the person is treated as being long-term ill, is deprived of the links that connected him/her to a normal life and "comes to realise" that the future consists of spending his/her life on the ward of a psychiatric hospital or in moving back and forth between hospitalisation and limited stays out of hospital supported by medication. This, too, can be a category of meaning, but one in which all that makes life meaningful has been removed. What is perhaps missing in the medical model is what Frank (1995) describes as the life that exists parallel to the healthy life, a "remission society" (p. 8) where people with various illnesses live, perhaps not as cured (or temporarily healthy) but well. As examples of the inhabitants of this parallel society Frank mentions cancer patients who no longer have pathogenic cells and people who wear a pace-maker, to name just two. People who have recovered from severe mental disorders can be considered citizens in this hidden society, as well.

> The triumph of modernist medicine is to allow increasing numbers of people who would have been dead to enjoy this visa status, living in the world of the healthy even if always subject to expulsion. The problem for these people is that modernist medicine lacked a story appropriate to the experience it was setting in place. (Frank 1995, p. 9-10)

Hope is always directed towards something. Hope provides a foundation for desire. Desire is in turn the starting point for changes, even if these are associated with great uncertainty about goals and the means for achieving them.

Mattingly (1994) writes:

> The presence of desire brings with it a readiness to suffer. Our desire causes us to take risks (or pay a price when we fail to take risks) and this in itself causes suffering. Often our object will not be attained, or when attained it will not give us what we hoped for, and these things also cause pain. Our desire for something we do not yet have strongly organizes the meaning of the present and makes us vulnerable to a disjuncture between what we wish for and what actually unfolds. (p. 818)

This desire, the idea that one's fate is something other than chro-nicity, is a source of hope. Hope does not spring from an inner well, even if it seems to be able to survive with little help from the outside.

When we got to [city 4] there was no direct connection to [city 5]. I would have to sleep in a cell at the airport. A flight attendant who worked for the airline felt sorry for me... Sometimes I've been incredibly lucky and met such nice people in the midst of it all... She convinced the authorities to let me sleep at her place. A 15-year old girl shouldn't have to sleep in a detention cell at [the airport]. They let me go home with her. What a person! Really. I'm sorry I don't have her name and address so I could write 25 years later and thank her...

Even back then I was so awfully grateful. Even if you're only 15, it's humiliating to be treated like a criminal. Everyone spoke over your head and treated you like a whore. A hardened criminal... (Irene)

What we can see from the above is that people may be barely aware that they are harbouring hope; instead, they may have accepted the life of a chronic as a less worse option, even if thoughts of suicide and actual suicide attempts show the full extent of this existential dead-end.

...it became more and more hopeless. I was more and more depleted by all the new medicines and such. I got injections so my whole body was stiff even though I was discharged. It was hell. But I wanted to live and then I had a son, I used to say he was my life insurance. I had to live for someone else's sake. (Jan)

It seems that the construction of meaning during the recovery process can begin when the person is joined in this effort by someone else, someone who realises that even if the person's own explanations are hardly tenable, they are not merely symptoms of illness. They are both, not either/or:

... I guess, too, it was his way of not giving me advice but every now and then coming in to where I was sitting and saying things by asking me questions... (...) The memory of his staying, that he didn't abandon me, that he didn't say, like the psychologist I had before him said: "Don't think that I'm going to mother you." (...) I got the feeling that he wouldn't leave me in the lurch. Maybe that's where some of the answer lies. (Nils)

In this interaction, the person's efforts to construct a meaningful context more closely resembles socially accepted models of meaning. Both the individual and the individual's conception of a personal meaning can win acceptance and be a convincing force.

Where for Bourdieu the biographical illusion is an ad hoc construction of the whole person erected from a mélange of events, modern man tends to perceive himself and his history as a more or less coherent entity.

If 16th century and earlier Europeans has no conception of a personal identity or self, the self is a firmly entrenched social reality in our part of the world today. Having a soul gave humankind a foundation to stand on; with the emergence of a personal identity, a self, humankind came into possession of an object, an own self, for which it was the sole caretaker.

Extracting from the myriad of events in life and from one's own sometimes incoherent actions a "good enough" whole constitutes a central project for modern man. The construction of the self in daily life has been aptly described by Kaufmann (1996):

> Faced with a sociality that is both integrated and disconnected, the individual can only be himself by creating an identity, that is to say by spinning the thread that will give his live meaning. The principle of a unique truth is absolutely central if daily life is to function well. The individual reworks this thread day after day, using it to construct a person by implementing its uniformity. This effort is made more difficult because the entity being formed is uncertain and changes constantly. The idea is thus not a simple mirror image, it is a crucial moment in the dialectical process of constructing reality. The very moment when comprehension of sociality enters into individual consciousness, where sociality is sorted out and worked through to bring about certain behaviours from among the thousands of possibilities; that is to say to select that which will be concretised and thereby become a part of sociality. The subjective is not in contradiction to the objective, to reality; it is a moment in the construction of reality, the only moment when the individual has scope for invention, a moment that is characterised by the necessity to choose and the obligation to uniformity. (p. 59-60)

In the life stories, but also in the everyday practice of recovery, we have evidence of the effort to recreate an own coherent self. And even if the idea of an own self is a social construction that stems from the breakthrough of modernism, it is nevertheless real for contemporary actors of today.

Mattingly (1994) introduces an important consideration when she describes the rendering of an intrigue not only as a narrative reconstruction but also as a creative effort that occurs during the very act:

> Being an actor at all means trying to make certain things happen, to bring about desirable endings, to search for possibilities that lead in hopeful directions. As actors, we require our actions to be not only intelligible but to get us somewhere. We act because we intend to get something done, to begin something, which we hope will lead us along a desirable route. (...) Because we plot, as actors, the structure of lived experience already contains a (partly) plotted shape. Even if our actions are taken up, reworked and redirected by responses to other actors, we still have some success some time in working towards endings we care about. (p. 813)

The constructions of meaning that occur in the life stories in this study are clearly rooted in the common cultural capital of a Europe at the start of the millennium. The study's interview subjects have a firm footing in the modern tradition and their stories draw sustenance from other stories where elements of comedy and tragedy are combined.

When we consider the concrete micro-situations that our respondents have participated in within the framework of their recovery, we find that some widely culturally dispersed sources are missing. The absence of both meta- and micro-stories of the process of recovery from severe mental disorders and the interview method's concentration on concrete events presented in their context have very likely forced the respondents to look back over their lives and re-examine their earlier experiences.

The stories of practice in context that constitute the basis for the analysis in this study provide a tool that can help us to see out of the opaque window that Öberg mentioned (see above).

7
Material conditions
When, where and with what?

The material conditions we are referring to here are broadly synony-
mous with Burke's concepts "scene" and "agency", where "when and
where" corresponds to scene and "with what?" to agency.

What Burke calls the scene is treated in various ways in the literature, two of which appear to be diametrically opposed. Bruner (1987)
has pointed out that the scene is usually absent in psychological and
psychiatric literature: "Most psychological theories of personality, alas,
have no place for place." (p. 25)

Neither geographical location, historical time nor characteristics of
the institution play a major role in these theories.[1] Rather, people
appear to exist in a sociological vacuum. Their thoughts and actions
emanate from biological processes, or from abstract internal motives
and drives, or else are rooted in a given context, usually the family, a
context that is so limited that it too could be reduced to an abstraction.

On the other hand, there are authors, found mostly in sociology, for
whom the place is where everything starts. Asplund (1980) cites
Goffman as providing the clearest example of this viewpoint:

> Goffman tries consistently to reduce all human activity to scenographic
> conditions. (…) Goffman [declares] the scene to be the basic element –
> everything consists of and emanates from the scene. (p. 129)

Later in the same work, Asplund returns to Goffman and his article
"Role distance" (Goffman 1972). In this article Goffman seems to be
arguing that it is in the actors' power to conduct himself in ways other
than what the conditions of the setting seem to dictate; actors have a

swingroom for their action which they decide on for themselves. It is this wedge between the actor and the role as determined by the scene that Goffman calls "role distance". Here, Aspund argues, Goffman seems to be emphasising that actors have freedom of movement. But, he continues, Goffman is actually doing the opposite because he puts back into the scene the conditions for determining what, on the surface, seemed to have been a certain freedom of movement in relation to the scene:

> ... also the dissonance between expected and actual behaviour, or the wedge between the role and the individual, is according to Goffman a *scenic* condition. (Original italic, p. 167.)

Without such scope for action there can be no actor. Since the actor is reduced to the scene, there is no real need to posit the existence of categories behind the scene. All life stories are strictly determined by their material conditions. The conditions restrict the scope for action or the possibility of free movement; material conditions determine human conduct.

Certain of the topics discussed below are not treated in any great detail in the interview material. Two such topics are the social insurance system and the interview subjects' housing situation. Although these topics are mentioned, sometimes specifically sometimes indirectly, in most of the interviews, it is mostly as background material. A third topic that is only briefly mentioned is the historical context. Here we are reminded of Bourdieu's remark about the risks inherent in tape-recorded sociology.

In this chapter we discuss the social insurance system and the interview subjects' housing situation in connection with a macro-analysis of their life situation. Although both the social insurance system and the interview subjects' housing situation are commented on as necessary conditions for recovery, their role is hardly given the same importance it tends to have in macro-analyses.

Historical changes in scene and agency

Scene and agency are both historical constructs. The life stories in this study take place at different points in time during the past few decades and in two different countries; they take place in cities and in rural communities, at different types of residential institutions and outpatient facilities and in various social environments that lie outside the domains of psychiatry and the social services. So the situations recounted in the stories have no single clear-cut background. Nevertheless, the respective scenes do have certain characteristics in common. In both Norway and Sweden, psychiatric hospitals continued to be built even after modern neuroleptics came into widespread use. However, all of our interview subjects had their first contact with psychiatry after the inception of the deinstitutionalisation movement in psychiatry. In both countries the first modern neuroleptic medicines were introduced in the mid-1950s. In Norway psychotherapy was already being practised (if on a small scale) for this category of patient. Psychotherapy in Sweden achieved a real breakthrough first in the 1980s in connection with the reorganisation of psychiatry into sectors. One of the differences often pointed out between Norway and Sweden is that Norwegian psychiatry has a clearer humanistic tradition whereas in Sweden psychiatry is said to be oriented more towards techniques and natural science. (Cullberg 2000b)

Generally speaking (but with some important exceptions), it could be said that in both countries the sectorisation of psychiatry has been based on a compromise between these two traditions, where the medically oriented psychiatric tradition predominates in the hospitals whereas the psychotherapeutic tradition lay behind the expansion of out-patient clinics. For a time the clinics duplicated the work conditions of therapists in private practice; for example, time units were an important therapeutic instrument (hours by appointment only, waiting lists, fixed length of the sessions), talk was the main instrument for change and voluntary participation was emphasised as the basis for the therapy contact.

Social-psychological interventions, both in ideological and methodological terms, play a subordinate role on the theoretical level during this period of development, despite the rapid growth of vocational and socio-therapeutic units in many psychiatric hospitals in the years after the second world war. It is first towards the end of the 1980s that social interventions were introduced, such as community centres and vocational and occupational programmes which operate outside the hospital setting.

The division into sectors became the predominant organisational principle in psychiatry. The prestige words here are continuity, accessibility and comprehensiveness. Continuity requires that psychiatric programmes be firmly grounded in the local community. Continuity is established between individuals and their social networks and requires the co-ordinated efforts of various public authorities. However, the emphasis on specialised interventions for separate diagnoses was re-introduced at the end of the last century in connection with the launching of so called evidence-based psychiatry. (National Board of Health and Welfare 1997)

At the end of the 1980s and into the 1990s, a new generation of neuroleptics was introduced. These medicines have fewer known side-effects, which is one of the reasons suggested for their more widespread acceptance by patients.

In both Sweden and Norway, the number of hospital beds began to decline toward the end of the 1960s, and has continued to do so ever since. The actual extent of the decline (deinstitutionalisation) is hard to assess because a form of transinstitutionalisation has occurred parallel with deinstitutionalisation. By transinstitutionalisation we mean the transference of inpatient resources (beds, treatment interventions, budgets, staff and service users) from the county council to the municipalities. (Stefansson 1991, Topor & Karebo-Larsen 2000)

At the end of the last century several important changes occurred in psychiatry. The ambition to clearly distinguish the separate functions responsible public authorities together with the introduction of a handicap perspective resulted in the transfer of the greater part of the socially oriented outpatient programmes from psychiatry to the social services. Psychotherapy's reputation in the publicly financed health care sector was called into question and evidence-based methods began to make inroads in health care. (National Board of Health and Welfare 1997)

The closing down of the psychiatric hospitals began to be criticised in the mass media. Homelessness in urban communities was seen as one of the results of deinstitutionalisation. The psychiatric hospitals were once again looked upon as possible places of asylum that offered protection to society's most vulnerable groups (Heilig 1999a, b).

In summary, the last 30 years could be described as an era when social and psychological explanatory models and treatment forms were introduced in psychiatry and their status consolidated. After the 1980s the ambition has been to draw a sharper line between medical and psycho-social interventions. As a result, there has been a renewed medicalisation of both psychiatry (that is to say, its organisation, practical applications and explanatory models) and the public discourse. The social services' responsibility for an increasing share of interventions for persons with severe mental disorders has often been criticised for poor quality, too little quantity and questionable content. The social services have had difficulty finding a language to describe and explain their interventions.

Ways and means for promoting recovery

Of the various "ways and means" or agencies recounted in the stories, the discussion in this section is limited to five of them: psycho-pharmaceuticals[2], the social insurance system, language usage, talk and actions. Two additional ways and means in connection with the recovery process are mentioned here only briefly. Both presuppose a relationship with one or more persons and will therefore be discussed in more detail in Chapter 9.

Psycho-pharmaceuticals and social support, primarily in the form of monetary benefits, have often been described in the interviews in connection with the scene, in either-or terms. They are described either as being a life-saver or as wholly without merit, even counterproductive. In the stories they are presented rather as ways and means, the effects of which depend on how and where they are used.

Social insurance system

An prerequisite for the deinstitutionalisation process that took place in the industrialised world, one that is seldom discussed, is a well-functioning social insurance system. At an elementary level, the social insurance system ensures that the most basic needs of patients will be met after they are discharged from the total care provided by the psychiatric hospital.[3] In one of the few textbooks in psychiatry that mention the importance of the social insurance system, Mosher and Burti (1989) point out that the discharge of patients from psychiatric hospitals in the USA has been closely linked to such social insurance measures as Medicaid and Medicare.

Both Sweden and Norway have a comprehensive publicly financed social insurance system for the continued care and social support of persons discharged from psychiatric hospitals.

Nevertheless, a study undertaken within the framework of the evaluation of the reformation of psychiatric care showed that the living conditions of young people with functional disabilities connected with mental illness were considerably worse than for those with physical disabilities or with no disability at all. (Official Reports of the Swedish Government 1992:37)

Each of the respondents were receiving, or had received in the past, some form of disability allowance or disability pension at the time of the interview. Each has had, or still has, access to publicly organised and financed social support and treatment. It is possible that the social insurance system and the various incentives offered for the person to re-enter the labour market could in fact build bridges. But they could also have the opposite effect. Ruth, who used to attend a community-operated day care centre, is now in the process of returning to working life. In the meantime she is still drawing a disability pension. The pension gives her a measure of security, but it has since also become something of a problem for her:

Right now a few good things are happening. I've heard that there is a job I could have, but this creates a problem with the social insurance office; but it would be fantastic if... (Ruth)

The majority of our respondents have not yet re-entered the regular job market and their present financial situation is insecure. Many of them manage only because they receive gifts from their social networks. Eric, who has made considerable progress toward recovery, gives the following example:

I like working only half-time. I have one day when I clean the house, one day when I just relax and take it easy... but I'll have to go back to full-time. As it is now, it doesn't cost my employer anything... But I want to work full-time, too, to earn more money. I have very little to live on as it is today. When I've paid all the bills I have maybe 3000 kronor [about 300 USD] left. Cigarettes cost about 700-800 kronor and food about 1500, so there is not much left over for clothes, instead I get clothes from other people. I have some really nice clothes... I have a debt that I have to pay off at 1000 kronor a month. It's for the child allowance I didn't pay when I was sick. So I owed all that money. It's a lot of money, but in two years' time I'll have paid it off and then I'll have an extra 1000 a month. That'll be great.

The allowances paid out by the social insurance system are often quite small, which means that people in the process of recovering often have to live under the added strain of financial insecurity, which in turn is counterproductive for the recovery process. Later in the interview Erik talks about an aspect of recovery that is seldom brought to the fore and problematised; namely, that the illness can also mean a care-free existence with few responsibilities:

Are you happy today?
I feel I've gone through a test of some kind. But I'm glad it's over. Most of the time when I was ill I lived in a world where I was ecstatically happy. A world where I didn't worry about paying the rent; I was so extravagant, bought tapes and cassettes and listened to music and was wholly absorbed by the music, more and more... (Erik)

Several of the interview persons report that they were offered opportunities for work training, but in none of the instances does this seem to have affected the recovery process, nor has it facilitated entry into the regular job market. Such programmes can, however, be a temporary solution to financial problems, an opportunity to test oneself and to keep in touch with the world outside the realm of psychiatry:

> I didn't know what I wanted to do... I had done a course in social anthropology... Eventually I got a supported vocational job out at the university. (Sören)

Several of the respondents found having a disability pension to be an advantage because then they no longer had to exhibit symptoms in order to continue receiving social assistance. When people no longer feel financially insecure, they may be able to begin managing their own life with renewed vigour.

If social welfare recipients in general are required to remain accessible to the job market, the opposite is true of people receiving disability allowances or a disability pension. The regular job market is not designed for them. To have a job entails the loss of certain benefits. Thus the step from unemployment to entering the regular job market for people on the road to recovery is a big and risky one. For this reason people engaged in a wide range of vocational and occupational programmes provided by the social services and psychiatry receive no payment for their efforts. As a result it prevents them from bettering their economic situation and their position in the social insurance system. Their efforts do not lead to raising their pension or sick allowance status. Social welfare benefits and sick allowances for persons who have been absent from the job market provide basic financial security but, as mentioned above, are seldom sufficient to give the person access to the normal range of cultural events and consumer goods enjoyed by others in the society. The only places the person can afford to visit are the arenas of organised normality (Hansson 1993), where people in the same vulnerable situation as themselves gather. There is a risk that a parallel society will be created and that arenas which could have been opportunities for transition turn out to be deadends instead.

Another aspect of the welfare state that comes to light in several of the stories is the possibility to obtain state loans to continue one's schooling beyond upper secondary level.

But after that my contract with AMS wasn't renewed anymore. I'm wondering what I'm going to do next. I liked being at the library and thought that maybe library school wasn't such a bad idea. But first I had to take 80 credits. I chose cinema history and theory and got accepted. It was really a Marxist stronghold. We did a lot of group work and had lots of parties; it was a lot of fun, things opened up a bit... that's where I learned what dialectics means. But all this has to do with having a good feeling about life. I've been trying to find a word for that feeling... something more profound... a kind of sensuality. It's also the basis for what happened after that. I know what I mean now... I collect myself. I've become one with my feelings. I've become self-evident. That's awesome. To discover life. (Sören)

The social insurance system provides a material base which in certain phases of a person's life can open up new and important arenas.

Medicine

Medication is a topic in all of the interviews, where the respondents compare the advantages and disadvantages of various medicines. Most of the stories contain a detailed discussion of medication and the procedures for its ordination which the respondents have experienced throughout the years of their contact with psychiatry. Prescribing medicines is usually the first procedure when a person has sought treatment for psychiatric problems. The patient feels unwell and is treated accordingly.

Not only is medication the first treatment patients receive, many of our respondents report that it was the only treatment they received throughout the whole time of their hospitalisation:

Eventually I get a chance to talk with the head doctor and she's optimistic. "We'll make you well in two weeks." In that sick place. I get some medicine. That's what I get. Two weeks pass, yet I'm not discharged. I'm allowed to continue with my education. I go to school direct from the hospital and I try, but I can't do it. I fall behind and taking all that medicine has broken me down and made me weak. (Ruth)

The focus on medicine, i.e. on determining what medicine or medicines to prescribe, administering them and then waiting for them to have an effect, is combined with the promise that the medicine will put an end to the patient's suffering. But with a one-sided focus on medicine there is no reason to talk with patients about what they have been through and what they are currently experiencing, such as the symptoms themselves and their contacts with psychiatry and the stigmatisation accompanying such contacts. None of the persons we interviewed believed that they had been given the "right" medicine in the "right" dose from the onset. Even in those cases where patients experienced some reduction of symptoms, the problems remained, as did their questions about what had happened to them.

There are especially two features of psycho-pharmaceutical treatment that are mentioned in connection with the recovery process; one is medicine as a chemical substance, the other is medication as social interaction.

Medicines as chemistry

One aspect of medication that is reported in the stories is medicine as a combination of chemicals that are introduced into the body and cause certain intended effects to the person's metabolism. This aspect of medication has to do with quantity and type. Several of the respondents are convinced that there is a *"right dose"* for them:

I think that the foremost reason why I'm getting better is that I get the right dose of medicine that sort of puts me in the right corner therapeutically, so to speak; that makes me more receptive. (Tina)

The right dose is associated in the interviews with having few or no side-effects and is often mentioned in connection with a phenomenon that we shall return to in a later context: the possibility to negotiate about one's medication. Receiving the right dose is for the most part associated with the second aspect of medicines as chemical substances: the right dose of the *right medicine*:

> And so I came to [the hospital] in the fall of [year]. I had stopped taking my medicine and got sick again. I came to a different ward and got a different doctor and he said that the medicines I was taking were making me sluggish. "We're going to try something else", he said. And those are the medicines I'm still taking.
> *They worked?*
> Yeah, they worked. I was there seven weeks. And I began to work immediately afterwards. And I worked for about 10 years. (Maria)

In Maria's case a specific medicine or combination of medicines is considered to play a central role in her recovery, but respondents report that medicine alone is not enough. In these stories receiving the right medicine in the right dose is often connected with other factors, such as social and psychotherapeutic interventions and the situation surrounding the decision to prescribe medication and its ordination.

> I think it was that I finally got a medicine that enabled me to get through this. It helped me get a grip on a whole lot of things. Since the medicine didn't smother me, didn't take away my energy, instead it gave my inner driving force a chance to work. Without knocking me out. Another thing, I guess, was that I could manage it all by myself. I didn't need to be injected, I could take it by myself. I think giving me that responsibility was what helped me get control over myself; not like before. I was the master of my own medication. I didn't have to go through the humiliation of pulling down my pants and having them shoot it in, something that was put into your body whether you needed it or not. (Jan)

Medication as social relationship

Many of the interview subjects who report that the right medicine in the right dose has been an important factor in their recovery regard medication in a social-psychological context, as an occasion for human interaction. Jan, says above that the right medicine "didn't smother" him, didn't "knock me out". At the same time, he points at how important it is that he take the medication himself, not as an injection administered by someone else, but as his own carefully considered action: "...giving me that responsibility". Here Jan turns the focus on the issues of responsibility and power for reasserting one's own life.

Other respondents raise the question of medication in connection with other important factors in their recovery process; primarily that of having a social network consisting of both family and professionals, but also medication as a complement to their own abilities.

> ... medicine has worked for me and I don't have any side-effects. The support apparatus has also worked – doctors, psychologist and the day centre and so my friends and... Somehow I have a feeling that I'm more noticed today than before. It was important just to be there in person, because I was in a silent period when I didn't say very much, and was just there among company and was accepted. (David)

> I feel I have such a good supportive apparatus in my own doctor and the psychiatrists and mental health nurses at the out-patient clinic that I feel sure of getting help when I ask for it. Having that security has helped me endure. And these people know that. I wrote a long letter to the nurse because I think they've been really nice to me. So I'm very conscientious about taking my medicines myself. I don't fool around with my medication when I'm feeling good, like many I know do. They talk about it at the day centre, then when they're better they stop taking their medicines. I prefer to talk to the doctor. (Ester)

A main, but paradoxical, theme that recurs in several of the life stories is the importance of being a part of the decision-making process regarding one's own medical treatment. The "psychotic patient" and the "scientist" enter into a negotiation relationship where the latter, in practice, acknowledges the former's experience as a kind of expertise. This theme has two aspects that are emphasised in varying degrees in the life stories:

- medicines, dosage and change of medication to bring about the optimal benefits to the patient

217

- acknowledging the patient as a person who possesses broad knowledge and experience and allowing them some degree of hegemony over his/her own life

Through this recognition a special relationship is formed between the therapist and the patient and between the patient and his/her self-image. Both of these aspects affirm that the patient is in need of help but *at the same time* is someone who should have a say in what this special help should consist of. The patient remains an active agent in relation to others and to his/her own life, to his/her own self.

It is in this "both the one and the other" situation – at the same time both psychotic and capable of participating in decision making – that medicines seem to have a positive effect, over and above their purely chemical effects. Conversely, it is in situations where this kind of relationship is missing that medicines are reported as having a devastating effect.

Here at [the treatment home] no one sits in authority, there's no autocrat who prescribes pills. Here you get medicine after a consultation, in mutual understanding. Patients have a lot to say here. The patient knows how a certain medicine works. How he feels. The doctor here has great respect for my wishes. For example, I asked to change Cipramil for something I read about called Soloft, which is a similar medicine. (…) when I suggested it, she said: "Sure, we can try it. Let's make an experiment." (Lars)

[The therapist] respected some of the choices I made… For example, that I didn't want to hand in urine samples… He respected that I didn't want to take any medicine.
So you've never taken any medicine?
I've tried once or twice, but for me to take medicines that make me even more a stranger to my own body is a bad solution.
So you were allowed to choose…
Yes, he respected that, not just by letting me get out of it, he respected it also by letting me come to therapy often every week instead. That's strong stuff. Unique actually. (Susanne)

Out of the close contact between patient and therapist can grow an awareness of the meaning of one another's behaviour and of certain events. Rakfeldt & Strauss (1989) point out that when approaching a turning point certain patients display additional or more severe symptoms. This temporary "decline" risks resulting in increased medication instead of supporting the process the individual may be going through.

Negotiating about medication does not necessarily mean granting the patient's every wish – nor the doctor's. Adequate information is important for a successful negotiation. Adequate information also presents alternatives to the treatment being suggested. Lastly, adequate information acknowledges its own limitations: the limitation in the body of knowledge in psychiatry. (See di Paola 2000b)

> The only conversation I can remember clearly, even I can see by my patient records that they did talk with me, is when I was with the psychiatrist, and so he says: "What you're describing now, that's a side-effect of your medication". I was taking Hibernal first, but then they put me on Haldol. And so he went on: "We can do this two ways. Either you can have a second medicine that will take away the side- effects or we can reduce the dose. What do you want to do?" So I chose to try and reduce the dose. I can see in my records that it was a cautious reduction, but still, they had given me a choice. And straightforward information, that all my discomfort was from the medicine. (…) Getting that information was important because then I knew that the discomfort wasn't because of me, but because of the medicine. It helped me to accept the lower dosage and not just refuse it and condemn them, but to keep on the medication without having so much discomfort. I was looking for a dosage that I thought I could put up with.

Adequate information concerns not only the information that treatment staff give patients about the treatment's effects and side-effects, but also the corresponding information that patients can give the staff. A negotiation in this context implies the right to have one's suggestions given serious consideration, the right to look for a medicine that "suits me", the right to make mistakes in one's choices without this causing the negotiation to beak down.

I'm taking medicine again, not big doses, but still. I got worse after I stopped taking the medicines all at once. "You mustn't do that", the doctor said, but I said I would anyway because I was feeling so good. (…) OK, so it was wrong. I made a mistake, but the doctor agreed to let me make a mistake. Now I can agree that she was right and she can agree that I want to experiment a little with my medicine. Try out what suits me. (Lars)

The stories report innumerable occasions where the doctor has pre-scribed a change of medicine or the dosage. The psychiatrists proceed by trial and error to find a medicine or combination of medicines and a dosage level that they regard as optimal. But what may be optimal for the doctor is not always optimal for the patient. There are times when the psychiatrist's desire to reduce the symptoms and thereby give the patient some peace, but also to reduce them for the sake of people in the patient's surroundings, including staff, conflicts with the patient's desire for a better life, i.e. to be given a say in what medicine to take. When negotiations break down, the relationship does not disappear but continues on a different level. War has been called a continuation of diplomacy by other means.

When you were in hospital, did you feel that you were allowed to have a say in anything?
I can't say anything about that because I don't really remember. But after that time, I tried to get hem to change my medicine, but they didn't want to do it. And so I stopped taking medicine altogether and got sick again. And so it's back to the hospital again, and out again with medicines and they don't work, and so I stop taking them and get sick again because they don't want to give me anything else. And I went on like that for six years. Out and in. (Maria)

The alternative to negotiation is an escalation of psychiatry's and the patient's actions and counteractions. To avoid repeated negotia-tions the patient can be "put on" injected medication, sometimes under some form of informal coercion. The absence of negotiation or its breakdown, which usually has to do with the patient's wish to reduce the dosage or change the medication, can result in various counter-measures on the part of the patient.

Interview subjects have described how they experimented on their on with varying the dosage. Some have cut back in secret, a step ahead of the doctor, while others have varied the dose depending on how they feel at the moment and keep a reserve of different medicines on hand. And some patients, have we have seen, have chosen to stop taking medicine altogether.

Side-effects

Just about every respondent in this study reports experiencing side-effects. At times it seems that side-effects are the medicine's only effect. When this topic is raised in the interview, it is often in connection with the staff's lack of interest in discussing side-effects:

> Cisordinol was the worst possible pill for me. It gave me so much anxiety, so much anxiety. And I didn't get any response from the doctor. "Won't do anything about it", [the doctor] said; "We neither can nor want to do anything about it." But then doctor [name] took over and now we got... My father had read about some new kinds of medicines, and so finally I was allowed to switch to Leponex, and it's worked for me so far. But I've heard about others who've also been on Cisordinol and it gave them anxiety. (Sven)

The exclusively pharmaceutical solution may, from the patient's perspective, be worse than the problem it was intended to remedy.

A person who is confronted with often frightening, incomprehensible and deeply disturbing experiences tries to remedy the situation in some way. These ways, both when they are successful and when they fail, are regarded by the person's surroundings as a sign that he/she is ill. Neuroleptics, the most common means by which psychiatry tries to remedy the patient's attempt at a solution, fails and becomes in turn still another problem for the patient to contend with. Psychiatry's remedial attempts have nothing to do with the patient's initial problems; rather, it focuses on the person's failed attempts to solve those problems. Psychiatry's own failed remedies lead to new problems that have to be solved, while the focus of the intervention is shifted from the patient's initial problem but does not disappear from the person's life (Haley 1982, Watzlawik, Weakland & Fish 1987).

Sören was hospitalised after having devised over a period of several years a way of managing his anxiety which he sees as being related to his increasingly acute psycho-social situation. This is a situation in which he feels trapped between a father who is on a downgrade and his own social insecurity and loneliness:

How long were you in hospital?
Pretty close to a year, almost to the day. Toward the end I was often let out on a free pass. Neuroleptics take away the feeling that I'm stuck. But at what a price! I've never felt so lousy. I swelled up. Your limbs feel detached from your body. The side-effects give you tingling sensations that were so unpleasant. You can't scratch them and make them go away. They're inside your legs. You're overcome by a kind of restlessness that you can't get out of your system. It was sheer torture. Maybe it's OK for others and for certain situations, but don't pump in such huge amounts, when you've never had it before, even if you're acting strange...

I could think the thought, OK, if I'm nuts, I'm nuts, but it will resolve itself. I'm not abnormal inside, it's just superficial, it's psycho-social and can just as well work itself out by psycho-social means. Why do they have to fill me up with all these medicines. But I couldn't say it. (Sören)

Thus, medicines sometimes supersede the patients' own ways of managing their problems. Sören's way of managing his severe psycho-social situation was through a form of meditation that he devised on his own and which consists of staring at a fixed point for long periods of time. Sören admits that this way of trying to solve his problem was not very good, but points out that it nevertheless enabled him to live with the problem. However, with his coming into contact with psychiatry, his actions are not regarded as a way of managing, but as a symptom to be counteracted and for which he is put on medication. If or when the medicine overcomes the symptoms/the person's way of managing, the person may be even more at the mercy of the problems that caused him/her to adopt that way of managing in the first place.

Things get to be hell when the medicine starts working. I lose contact with just about everything. My sense of security crumbles. I can stand and stare at a point and it's my only security in the whole world. It's the only thing I have. It's my anchor line and it is the only way I can put up with all that other stuff I don't want to have anything to do with in the world around me. And the line is cut off! I suffer the worst anxiety attacks. It's like you've completely lost your footing. Not to know anything at all. I wander around in the flat and can't fix on a point anymore. (Sören)

Although the medicines' side-effects are described in many of the stories as severe, quite a few of the respondents report that what they experienced as traumatic was that there was no discussion about medication at all. The patient's efforts to communicate are interpreted in these instances as lying within the realm of pathology. For Sören being medicated for the first time while a patient in the outpatient clinic resulted in the breakdown of his own ways of managing his problems. Shortly thereafter he was admitted to the psychiatric hospital:

They did the rounds once a week, trailed by a group in white… and there you're lying. I had started to talk a little bit, but they stood in front of me and talked about me using a lot of jargon: "We'll put him on that medicine and see what happens…" I began to have a really negative experience with neuroleptics. I became desperate. I was used to deciding for myself, but now I couldn't anymore. I was so desperate that I was hitting my head against the end of the bed, sometimes demonstratively, but they didn't change the medication. Showing desperation can be a way to communicate, too: "I feel awful, can't you help me!" (Sören)

Conflicting points of view

The way medicine is discussed in the interviews is often ambiguous: as a necessary evil, the necessity of which is questioned by the respondents. With recovery, it seems that medicine ceases to be an overriding issue in the person's life. The reduction of symptoms is one side of the story, but what the respondents emphasise most of all is the importance of a social life. To no longer feel subjected to the medicine and to feel able to live *your own* life. The majority of the interview subjects were ambivalent to the psycho-pharmaceuticals with which they had been, and sometimes still were being, treated. They were ambivalent, not only to the medicines that did not help them (actually, this is where they were least ambivalent), but to those that had helped them, and just because they had helped:

> I was very sceptical to medicines the first time, and they said we'll give you as little as possible. So they've always listened to me when I said that I want less and less medicine. I think it's pretty dismal that I've been on medication now for 12-13 years, that's not good… I'm a bit afraid about that. That's a lot of years. (Tina)

After being on medication for a longer period, many began to question whether it would be possible to cope without the medicine, after all. Even when the medicine helps, the question is always there: Could I make do without it, on my own?

Another way of relating to medication, which seems, however, to presuppose having control over the medicine, is to "feel healthy with medicines".

> So when they signed me out I was on 500 mg, 400 mg in the evening and 100 in the morning and that's almost a year ago, and now I have 250 mg in the evening. I'm going to cut down a bit more but I don't see any value in being wholly free from medicine. That's not saying it wouldn't be nice, but it has no value of its own. It's not necessary because I don't need to feel I'm healthy without the medicines. I feel healthy with medicines. It's a question of what we mean by medicines in this case. I regard my life as being perfectly satisfactory now when I'm on the medicines as when I wasn't on them. I just don't see that there's any big difference. It's true I have to think about things like sleep and I have to think about the medicines every day. So, yes, it can be a hassle. But still, there's nothing that says I have to be off medication as soon as possible, that that's when I'm really healthy. I don't see it that way. Otherwise it's very common to associate being free from medication with being healthy, but there are people who are on medication but don't tell anyone. (Jan)

Self-expression

Many of our interview subjects write, play music and/or paint and see a connection between these past-times and their recovery. Although several had begun using these forms of expression while they were under psychiatric care, they seem to work even for those who engage in artistic endeavour wholly on their own. For a few of the persons we interviewed, creative expression has even become a source of income: they have sold their artworks on the open market.

> Much of my therapy is sitting down writing. I write what was prose at the beginning, but now looks to me like poems. A lot has to do with my realising that comprehensibility is at the cost of not saying everything; instead I refine it.
>
> A lot has to do with the process of writing, formulating, reformulating, refining, and that way working through out. Eventually, it gets to be something that I think holds up. (Bengt)
>
> I wrote and wrote, and I began to paint. And I began to discover music, something that… wasn't there for me before. I was a fanatic about it, maybe, but it was like becoming myself. I had found a little corner in the world where I could exist without getting killed. That's how extreme it was, like. [Music, painting, writing], there's no doubt they've been a means of self-therapy; without it I wouldn't be sitting here today. Without it I wouldn't have had the energy to make it through your ordinary psychiatry, to succeed in the struggle to come to therapy. It has to do with being creative. With expressing yourself. With transforming an inner life into external forms of expression and that way both unloading it and, you know, reflecting yourself in your self by listening to what you've accomplished, looking at or reading what you've accomplished. Maybe even coming so far as to being appreciated by others… That's what gives you dignity. (Lars)

Talk

Conversing with other people is an important tool in the recovery process. Such conversations can be divided into three groups, where the first two groups take place within a therapeutic framework:

- psychotherapeutic treatment, often long-term (as much as ten years for some of the people we interviewed)
- structured talk sessions, often of short duration and supportive in nature

- ordinary conversations; with friends, acquaintances and treatment staff who have no formal therapeutic training, that take place outside a structured therapeutic framework

In their life stories the respondents point at especially two features of conversations that have contributed to their recovery. These conversations have been about "both this and that", about the problems and suffering the person has experienced, but also about everyday events that have nothing to do with suffering; about interests that the therapist and patient have in common. This applies of course to everyday conversations, but even the two forms of structured talk contain similar elements. Switching between these two levels during the therapy sessions seems to be closely connected with another characteristic of conversations that have contributed to recovery; namely, the lack of emphasis on therapeutic techniques and instead an emphasis on the characteristics of one's partner in the conversation. Both these features of beneficial conversations are exemplified in the following excerpt from one of the interviews:

... this is a very special person. He's more known abroad than in [name of country]. He's very controversial, but internationally he's a celebrity... What helped me in all this? It's hard to say because it didn't happen on a verbal plane actually. But it happened of course during our sessions. Sometimes we talked about his work, like about seminars on his research, and then suddenly we got to talking about my life.

What do you think has helped you?

You could compare it to an atomic explosion, like [the therapist] used to say. He understood very well what I had to say and I could... He had confidence in me, and his fantastic charisma had the effect of giving me the courage to take a look at my own life and talk about it. I think he was the first person I've met in my whole life who listened to me and treated me with respect ... I had never experienced that before, and I was nearly 40. (Elin)

As is the case with the circumstances surrounding medication, what is important in psychotherapy is having a personal relationship with the therapist. This is more important than technique, or rather, it is inseparable from technique. In the above example the respondent becomes a patient, co-worker and adept of the therapist all at the same time.[4] This quality of "both the one and the other", both in the relationship and with respect to the person's identity, seems to constitute an essential element that recurs in most of the life stories.

Actions

The individual's own actions and the actions of others are discussed in Chapters 8 and 9. We shall nevertheless briefly comment here on their great importance for initiating and maintaining a recovery process. The actions of other people gain special importance when they are contrary to one's expectations, expectations about oneself and the other person.

An important characteristic of many of these actions is their ordinariness. This is an illusory quality in that the actions take place in a context where ordinariness is an exception. But just because they are so commonplace makes the actions invisible:

> One morning I was arrested. The police came and knocked over my door and then they stood there kicking me; I still have a nick in my shin. They took me into custody in [city 1], photographed... then I was locked in a cell to wait for transport back to [city 2]. After that me and another prisoner sat handcuffed in a police wagon and were driven first to [city 3]. In [city 1] I didn't get anything to eat. The police treated me like shit. But in [city 3] a nice policeman gave me lunch. I was so grateful. Plus I remember that he brought me some comic books. That was worth gold. (Irene)

Whether everyday actions will be experienced as just everyday acts or as an unusual intervention depends on the context. The life stories collected in this study indicate that when people have a low expectation of how others will respond to them, everyday actions lose their everyday character; but not within the framework of traditional psychiatry. Here the respondent draws her own conclusion:

> Fair-minded people have helped to balance things out. Like when the policeman gave me food and some comic books, against the police brutality in [city 1]. Your so grateful when someone treats you decently. You remember it. I was so awfully grateful. They give you back your

human value somehow. A feeling of being... If everyone treats you like shit, you become a piece of shit. If someone treats you right, well maybe you are good for something. (Irene)

Scenes

There are mainly three scenes upon which the stories told in this study take place: psychiatric institutions, the organised arenas of everyday life (Hansson 1993) and public arenas. What is remarkable is that it seems that almost any place can suffice as a waystation in a recovery process. Although certain scenes are apparently conducive to the re-covery process, it seems that almost any scene can offer some scope for breaking with chronicity. Perhaps this is why patients have recovered in different eras offering wholly different conditions for re-covery. There is no straightforward cause-effect correlation between a particular factor, a particular environment and recovery. Although certain environments provide a wider range of opportunities, the opportunities are not in themselves necessities. Moreover, new oppor-tunities can always arise.

The scenes where psychiatry is practised are accorded central im-portance in all of the stories, either as unresponsive environments (which thereby are an obstacle to recovery) or as environments that create opportunities (which thereby become a scene for the recovery process).

Inpatient facilities

A hospital ward can be a place where recovery is promoted if it offers the patient an opportunity to rest up and to meet others. Several of our respondents experienced round-the-clock hospitalisation or a stay in some other residential institution as a chance to take a "time-out". The institutions had a positive effect if they did not impact unduly on the person's life and instead offered a chance to rest up, to take a limited time-out from responsibilities when daily life was experienced as too stressful, room to just be:

> The most important thing about the children's home was that they left me in peace... I had stayed there three years before and I remember it was

heavenly, so I knew what to expect. The staff hasn't changed, but there are other children of course, but I know I'm going to have my own room. I choose my own room. I have a few of my things with me. (…) I began to make my room into a whole new world. I discovered in myself an enormous creativity that I had never made use of before, but I apparently had it in me all the time. It just poured out of me. I borrowed a typewriter from the office and began to write poems and short stories. (Lars)

The institution's main positive function in these cases is to leave the patient "in peace". Patients often describe their participation in the ward's treatment programme as a concession to the system in the hope that they would be left alone the rest of the time. Providing treatment justifies the staff's professional status, but in some patients' eyes it is more of a nuisance than a help. In the few instances when the hospital ward is mentioned in the interviews as a place that has contributed to recovery, it is in connection with the patient's having met a special person.

It seems that even in the most inhospitable scenes, patients can discover openings for recovery; but also, in practice this constitutes a criticism of the scene and of its rules and routines.

Hospital wards are often inhospitable settings. Their function is to receive, treat and accommodate persons who are considered incapable of living in society. Repeated hospital admissions are also taken as confirmation of the person's difficulties, of his/her chronic condition.

But by breaking with the given conditions of the scene (its routines and rules), fertile ground may be produced for recovery. Susanne, for example, has found "an oasis" in a little corner of the ward where an occupational therapist had set up an office:

Mostly I was there on my own because not many of the other patients were not interested in that kind of thing. She didn't have a room of her own, but… She had a space in the corridor… those long corridors. It was a space at one end of the corridor where they had some handicraft stuff on a couple of shelves – and twice a week she sat there. Was available… So she had a whole different way of getting in touch with the patients than what the nurses had. She had a lot more time… that was important, you know. Just the fact that she chose to devote several hours at a time twice a

week and just be there... So it was up to folks to come and sit down, talk and have a cup of tea or you could do something else.
So she was a person who was available?
Yes, the nurses were always too busy... They did the rounds and... They made up these agreements that were such a bother, and so you were supposed to "cough up" something about something or other; that's what it felt like anyway. If I asked to talk to a nurse, then it had to be about something. So what was really nice about her... that she... that it was a bit more fun being around her.

Susanne describes the place on the ward that helped her recovery as a space that contrasted with the rest of the ward. Here there is time. Here there is an opportunity to converse, to "just" drink a cup of tea with another person. Here there are no demands for change, but instead an invitation to try out a few things. And here there is a person, a professional who is different from the other professionals. She has no preserve of her own, instead she sits out in the corridor exposed to the patients' wish to choose or reject her. She could represent an opportunity, but she was not a necessity. Thus she broke with the ward's rituals for how the meetings between patient and staff are to occur.

> You didn't have to produce anything to be there. She was very clever. Even if you felt anxious to perform and felt you should do something, you didn't have to. She succeeded in creating a little oasis where you could come and be and do something only if you wanted to. She was an important person for me. She was. I'm so glad she was there to coax me so that I got started with that stuff again... (Susanne)

What is a help to Susanne on the ward is finding a place that is basically different from the rest of the ward, an "oasis" in a desert landscape. It is place where she need not perform to be accepted.

> I end up on the admissions ward. There they take away a free pass they had promised me, so I succeed in escaping and taking a taxi home. When I get home I'm devastated. I'm there to get help... Later, on the same ward I tell them that I'm going to sign myself out, and that's when they get me a bed on a quieter ward so that I can rest up. A good thing they do on that ward is let me paint in my room. The ward also has a piano, so I play it.

That was good for me. And I got my meals and vitamines. It was more or less quiet on the ward and that's what I needed. (Ruth)

Meals, vitamins, rest, painting and access to a piano... It would seem that it is only when the ward becomes something other than what it was designed for that it succeeds in contributing to the recovery process.

Outpatient facilities

Out-patient clinics and private therapy facilities are never specifically mentioned except in connection with the routines that regulate contact between patients and staff and the personality that the therapist displays.

If you look at the room we're sitting in. [The interview was conducted in the therapist's office at the facility to which Lars went for treatment]. This is not what a therapist's office looks like at a clinic. That says something about the atmosphere of this place. An atmosphere that's dignified. You can't go to a damn clinic, for there you're just one case among many getting your 45 minutes and that's it. Here, it has to do with a process, there are no set time limits.

She wasn't one of these "accredited"... She didn't have a nameplate on her door with her name on it and her title, if we're going to talk about symbols. No, she just sat there in her "artist's frock", as she called it and was a bit bohemian (...). OK she had some books on borderline personality and pathological narcissism by Otto Kernberg and most probably knew everything about it, but that's not what she had in her mind when she talked with me. And if you look at what she wrote in my patient record about me, she didn't use words like "pat." [patient] when referring to me, she wrote "Lars": You can see that she has listened to and been affected by what I said, maybe even touched. That was my experience anyway. Empathy, I felt, not antipathy, like you often find in psychiatry. "Oh, no! Well, we're just going to medicate him, put him in cold storage, then discharge him, but he'll soon be back..." You're just a registration number on a patient journal where they have to write down an anamnes, mental status, and that's that; mental condition, current situation. You're put on record, and so you're dispatched. For the moment. (Lars)

231

The essential factor in the contacts that take place on these scenes seems to be the other person. The presence of the other person broadens the scope of the scene. Sometimes the other person provides a place within the place. The other is also important in that he/she conveys a sense of really seeing and hearing the patient, or perhaps the person behind the patient. We return in a later context to what words like "being seen or noticed" and "being heard" can mean in practice.

Both in- and outpatient facilities are used in a similar way by severely mentally disturbed persons. Both seem able to function as places where patients can recharge their batteries and test themselves in relationships with just one or a few other persons. In both cases the official purpose of these scenes differ from how the service users put these resources to use. In none of the interviews was there any mention of a treatment programme or plan; rather the ward was first and foremost an opportunity to withdraw from the pressures of everyday life (for an extended period of time or for recurrent hourly sessions) and to act in relation to another person. This use of psychiatry's resources is somewhat reminiscent of what Strauss (1989a) calls "woodshedding". It is also reminiscent of the stage in the recovery process which Davidson and Strauss (1991) define as discovering parts of one's own self that have not been attacked by the illness and making an inventory of one's own capabilities. The relationship with staff members, whether clinic or hospital, who have helped a person serves as a foundation and a point of reference from which that person can once again begin to make use of his/her capabilities.

Organised daily life

Living outside closed residential institutions is rather a recent phenomenon for persons who have been diagnosed as suffering from severe mental disorders. The reduction in the number of hospital beds parallels the increase in the number of intermediate care facilities that are concerned with housing, work and recreation.

Intermediate care

Intermediate care facilities devised by the social services and psychiatry are concerned with central aspects of daily life that formerly lay within the total institution's area of responsibility: housing, work and recreation. In contrast to the psychiatric hospitals, these intermediate care facilities are spread out in the community. They are also open to local residents to a greater or lesser extent.

Intermediate forms of care are a relatively new element in the assortment of care programmes designed for people with mental problems. Several of our interview subjects have described from their own experiences what role these facilities have played in their lives.

> When they discharge me, they send me back home. No friends. Nothing to do. Still pretty much broken down. If [the day centre] existed then it would have been perfect. I would have had some chance of rehabilitation after leaving the hospital. But there wasn't anything like that. Just emptiness all around, so I try to go back into hospital again. I do anything, as long as something happens. I'll just have to go on associating with loonies and eventually they'll discharge me again. If [the day centre] had existed, this wouldn't have happened. (Ruth)

The lack of intermediate care facilities reflects an either/or way of thinking in psychiatry. Sick people must be hospitalised. If they are cured, they can be discharged and therefore do not need continued support. Intermediate care plays various roles in the recovery process. In the beginning, a facility like a day care centre can be a place to go to and spend time in – a chance to get out of the house and go somewhere where there are no overwhelming demands made on you. Later, it may turn into a place that is not "real enough", a place where adaptation to the visitors' difficulties becomes an obstacle to recovery, a painful reminder that the real world exists outside its walls. Ruth continues her account of the place which she believes that, had it existed earlier in her life, would have saved her from further hospitalisation:

> I go to [the day care centre] so that I won't feel so lonely. I don't have a job. I'm a pensioner now. Up to now I've coped on my own. [The day

centre] is a temporary solution for me, so that I won't isolate myself. I've made good use of [the day centre], it's been useful.

But actually, I wish I could spend more time out in the community. There are times when I suffer because the courses they give are a little bit like nursery school; I mean I've had a real art education. But then I've taken the courses just for the fun of it, not so seriously. But sometimes, you want a bit of seriousness, if you can handle it. (…)

I've said only good things about [the day centre] and with good reason, but I don't want to idealise it. It has a good atmosphere. But sometimes I feel I'd like to do something for real. And that's a good sign. Because actually [the day centre] is supposed to be an opening to working life. It feels a bit boxed in, which is both good and bad. The atmosphere can be quite intimate and sometimes that feels good. But not always. It's a relatively small place where you get to know one another and dare to be yourself. That's good. You can talk about your problems, you don't have to hide the fact that you've had a psychosis. (Ruth)

Intermediate care facilities aim at normalisation. They resemble ordinary settings in daily life and are designed for people who formerly had been defined as being beyond the boundaries of normality. This duality seems to characterise the range of activities provided in these settings and determines the experiences of those who use them. They are described as places where one can feel well or ill. They are places where one can both give and receive; they are arenas where people can reflect upon themselves in relation to others who know about their problems; they are arenas that are free from the mixture of permitted/ forbidden that characterises much of psychiatry. (See Basaglia 1968) Eric gives a description of this duality and contrasts it with a far less ambiguous place with which he has come into contact, a place where he is more clearly a patient:

I've helped to fix up the place. Laid carpets, painted it. It's mostly a place to meet others. If you're living at home it's good to have somewhere to go. You can meet other people, and most of all other people who also have had problems. For me, it's good, but I know a chap who gets nervous when he's here. He felt that it only got him thinking about his illness. But for me it works all right. You have a place to spend a few hours in the afternoon before going home.

On Thursdays they always have something going on in the evening; a barbecue, music, a lot of stuff. It costs 10 kronor (about one USD), which is really cheap. So, sure, this place has helped me. Much better than going to [the out-patient clinic]. There they have this lounge set. We all just sit there and look at each other, from 8 in the morning to noon. It really sucks. I only go there to get my medicine.

Down here it's another place altogether. It's like a little café. You can sit outside in the summertime... and everyone is really nice. At the clinic it's more like they're staff. Here they're more like friends. Up there you feel like there is the nurse, and now it's the nurse aid... well, they're not all like that up there, but I don't feel like being there.

In what way are they more "like friends" here?

Here we all talk with each other. Upstairs no one talks. They can sit and read a newspaper and then just leave. So down here you don't feel as if you're sick; you feel more as if you're a part of it ... an employee.

Is that a good thing?

There's more joy in it. When we were fixing the place up everyone was so happy when we saw it getting nicer and nicer. Then we had an art exhibition and hung all our paintings... Here the staff have a more positive attitude.

The woman I see over there, we say a few words to each other. I get an injection and then its "bye bye" and I go back home. That's it. There's nothing wrong with her. It's just that we don't have any contact. (Erik)

It seems that intermediate care can contribute to the recovery process mostly when it offers a place where people can just be and where they can practice meeting other people in a social context. Intermediate care can provide a place where people can test who they are and reject the one-dimensional role of a patient, a schizophrenic or otherwise mentally ill person; and to do so first and foremost through actual behaviour and real interpersonal relationships. Depending on what roads the recovery process takes, these places become either arenas upon which the person will have to continue to rely, or they become the starting point for venturing out into new arenas. Often the rules and regulations for many of these intermediate facilities are sufficiently flexible to allow people to simply "drop in". The relationships formed between service users and personnel can continue even if the user is no longer associated with the services on a regular basis. "I'm proud I've come this far", says Anne, after relating how she is able to complete more and more tasks at the day care centre. In her case, her being able to use the opportunity to establish an increasingly complex identity seems to take her further along the road to recovery:

> It helps to make time pass. And you have someplace to go. The mornings are the worst when you live at home. I wake up early and now that I start so early here I don't have to wait so long, even though I often get here too early. When I finish at 10, I want more to do, so maybe I'm going to start studying in an adult education programme. (Anne)

The user movement

In several of the life stories, the respondents talk about the user movement's own organisations in the two countries of the study (National Association for Mental Health and Wellbeing in Sweden and Mental Health Norway). The fact that the user movement is mentioned and in specific contexts is perhaps related to how that particular respondent was recruited for the study. In these instances, what has benefited the recovery process is the person's having been elected either as an ombudsman or as a co-worker in the movement. One has been chosen by others and can therefore be of some help.

> But then I guess that what made it all meaningful was that, after a few years, I joined the user movement. It's helped me an awful lot. Now I can get my teeth into something that touches me deeply, and maybe, too, I can help others who are in a bad way. It is very important too because I've seen that the health service can't cope, so someone has to go in and help. (Jan)

Thus the user movement is both an arena and an agency. But one's involvement in such movements can be very demanding:

> My idea at first was to be hired on a salary allowance, but I soon realised the advantages of being an elected representative. You could say that an elected representative works with a variety of questions within [the user organisation]. But I've cut down a bit now, because for a while there I was doing an 80-hour week. (Ester)

One's involvement can be so demanding that instead of contributing to recovery, it may threaten it:

> After awhile I became psychotic again. You could say that it was self-inflicted. I had been working too hard in [the user organisation], became too involved and didn't rest up and so things just got out of kilter. I had too much to do and wore myself out. So now I have to start all over with the medicines again and I'm still on [type of medication]. But this time I guess I've learned not to work myself to death anymore.

People who represent a user organisation are in an ambiguous dual situation. On the one hand, they come into contact with other organisations (public authorities, other user organisations and even private firms which the organisation has hired or is hired by) and participate on an equal footing. On the other hand, their position in the organisation rests on their having been patients themselves. Using Fuchs Ebaugh's term, they are an "ex"; but also, as long as they are involved in the user organisation, they remain an ex, with great difficulty to develop an identity beyond the role of an ex

Public scenes

Other places mentioned in the stories include those that are open to the general public; public arenas such as courses in adult education, cultural events, workout gyms and the like. Even places for exercising one's dog can have an impact. All of these are places where one can test one's sense of self and perhaps be affirmed; they confirm that a person is able to be among people and interact with them, not as a patient or former patient, but as a person, one among others.

> *So at that time you had been hospitalised continuously for two years?*
> Yes, hmmm. So the years after that have been a long process of learning to stand on my own two feet and continuing with therapy and finding myself. One of the things I also got out of being on the ward: there was this woman there – she wasn't an occupational therapist, she had a kind of diffuse position as a social pedagogue – anyway, she got us to go in for training at [the gym] and I kept it up. And that was the first step I took towards approaching other people. I signed up as a volunteer, a volunteer

functionary. I was a hostess there. It was very tiring but this was a very important period in my life. Because this way, I entered that kind of environment from an entirely different direction than I would have done earlier. (...) But I took a small step on my own and signed up as a hostess. I went to the office at [the gym] and asked if I could do a little work – without any salary – just to have something to do. Afterwards, I felt I was able fill my days with something more than just being sick and living from day-to-day and going to therapy. (Susanne)

So here Susanne lived a double life. She was a patient on a hospital ward (for the past two years at that time) and she worked in the office at a gym. It may be that at certain times one kind of life is a pre-requisite for another kind of life to be possible (Strauss et al., 1992b). Susanne uses the ward as a place of refuge where no one bothers her; she says that what helped her on the ward was a staff member who had a "diffuse position", who brought her along to an activity outside the ward. With her mental health worker she learns a main rule of social intercourse and to be more self-reliant. At the gym, among ordinary people, she tests her own self by engaging in social intercourse. As the life stories show, the surrounding world appears to contain a wealth of resources and opportunities that could be used in a recovery process. Given the chance to rejoin that world, this time better equipped to manage everyday stresses, the person can make use of its dynamics where the one opportunity opens the door to the next.

[The psychologist] encourages me and suggested that I study art theory at the university. Just having a goal helps a lot. It has helped. I was obliged to take an upper secondary school degree in languages, and I managed it. And being at the university was a lot of fun. I travel. I go to parties. They let me use their studio. So there's more to it than just studying, which is mostly a lonely job. That has helped me. (Ruth)

At home

As a consequence of deinstitutionalisation and the expansion of the social insurance system to cover people who have never entered the job market, a relatively new scene appears in the stories: the person's own home. Long-term hospitalisation has usually resulted in a total break with social life outside the institution. For this reason many patients no longer have a home to return to. A survey conducted by the Swedish National Board of Health and Welfare shows that half of the patients who had been hospitalised in psychiatric institutions in 1991 did not have their own place to live. Among patients being treated in rest homes in 1991, 75% were without an own place to live. (Official Reports of the Swedish Government 1992:37) Homelessness and its probable relationship to the reduction of hospital beds has been much discussed. Whether these findings are related or not has not yet been determined, at least not in Sweden and Norway. What is evident, however, is that many homeless people are suffering from mental ill health and that thousands of people are virtually homeless. (Halldin 2000, Official Reports of the Swedish Government 2000:14, Ågren, Beijer & Finne 2000)

Having one's own place to live is thus by no means a certainty. For many people who spent long periods of times in psychiatric institutions, access to a place to live depended on the relatively well developed welfare system that was in effect in the two countries at the time the interviews were conducted.

Nevertheless, if an own place to live is not, in the short historical perspective, a certainty for all people, it is for our interview subjects; it is so much a certainty that the fact that it has not always been so is only mentioned in passing:

> So I had an examination where they photographed my brain, but there was nothing wrong with it and I told the doctor that I was a voluntary patient and that I could leave whenever I wanted, but that I wasn't going to leave because I had no place to go, so I'm satisfied with the bed I had. And so the doctor says: "You're not leaving? Why don't you try to find a place you could go to?" So I got ahold of a little cottage in [place-name] and moved there. And I said to myself: "Never again the hospital. Now I'm finished with all those thoughts." (Erik)

Getting one's own place to live becomes for Erik and several others of our respondents a platform for continuing their recovery process; a place where they can be left in peace; a place where they can have a sense of integrity. Nonetheless, being left in peace can also be similar to being abandoned. Earlier in his life Erik has experienced homelessness and abandonment:

> After a month, after I had been sectioned, I ended up in a bachelor hotel. Alone. They promised they would come to visit. But I was left all alone. Not a single person did I have to talk to. I just sat in the room and that's when those thoughts came back again. I was desperate. (Erik)

> When they discharged me, they sent me back home. No friends. Nothing to do. Still pretty much broken down. (Ruth)

In both cases, feelings of abandonment result in "readmission". On the other hand, however, the price for not being abandoned may be finding one's home transformed into a kind of institutionalised housing. For people with severe mental problems, a place to live can be an ambiguous concept in that it is less a place of one's own as it is a housing arrangement; a place to live, but also to be cared for, trained, supported; a scene to which other people can claim the right of access.

> At that time I was in contact with the night-team almost every night. They came to my home and we talked until they [the hallucinations] went away. We talked about everyday things. The night-team was really swell. First they told me that I had to be readmitted, but I said that I just wanted to talk. And so we talked, sometimes about problems, sometimes just about things in general. (Anne)

> And now it's [a psychiatric nurse] who comes to my place. She visits me twice a month and it doesn't cost me anything. If she came more often I would have to pay. And I think that after-care has been very good to me. I've had the help I need, but you have to contact them yourself. They don't run after you. I needed someone who could give me injections. And someone to talk to once in a while. And so it was just for someone to come to my place, you know. (Tina)

One's own home can thus be both an agency and a scene for recovery. But to be so, the home should also be part of a broader social life; a place where one can close the door to others (Forsberg & Starrin 1996) or invite others to come in for a visit; a place to leave in order to go to work, or to meet other people or to find amusement.

A medicalised view

Several of the scenes upon which the stories evolve and the agency utilised on these scenes are medicalised. Many of the key scenes take place in psychiatric institutions – mental hospitals, psychiatric wards and out-patient clinics. But medical personnel also visit scenes outside the domains of psychiatry, imprinting them with a medical way of thinking. And then there is medication which is independent of the scene where it is dispensed. Mental health staff play a central role in all of the life stories in this study. Psychiatrists are decision makers. They are important in many ways despite, or perhaps because of, their often cited inaccessibility.

The language of medicine and its frames of reference recur in the interviews. The respondents have learned to use this language through their association with psychiatry. Several report that they have read psychiatric literature in an attempt to understand what has happened to them.

Medication is a topic in all of the life stories. Certain social insurance benefits, such as sickness pension and other forms of monetary allowances, are tied to medical assessments.

The social insurance system is more or less taken for granted and when mentioned in the interviews it is often as a background to other events in the person's life. Judging from these stories, less time is devoted to discussing and deciding on possible forms of financial support and social interventions than to medication. Moreover, these forms of support play only a minor role in the respondents' worldview and construction of their life stories. Medication, on the other hand, implies hopes of being cured, even though those hopes are often crushed. Social interventions generate no such hopes.

But at the same time, there is a discrepancy between how doctors and users talk about the effects of medicine. The relationship between medicine, user and recovery can be described in four ways:

- Medicine can be seen as a prerequisite to enable the user to begin to manage his/her social and psychological problems and thereby begin the journey to recovery.

- Medicine can be seen as one factor among many that can contribute to the recovery process.
- Medicine can be seen as the direct cause of recovery. In such a context, the establishment of a good relationship between doctor and patient is merely a means to strengthen the patients' so-called compliance, by which is meant their willingness to take the medicine as prescribed.
- Medicine may be wholly without meaning or even play a negative role in the recovery process

It is the first two possibilities that are described in the stories as being the most common.

The stories describe a number of scenes upon which important events in the recovery process have occurred. It is not possible to determine if these scenes are related to different phases in the recovery process, if they have occurred in any special order; the exception is the psychiatric hospital which, as we have seen, can under certain conditions function as a starting point or a base from which the work of recovery can begin. Places that have once been of importance for recovery can recur at a later time in life or may never recur again.

From a recovery perspective, the central aspect in the scenes and the agencies that we have discussed here is their ability to permit and promote ways of being that transcend the traditionally rigid division between sick/healthy, discharged/abandoned, hospital admission/total care and care provider/care recipient.

The life stories show, however, that it is not the place itself that is crucial for the recovery process; all places can become a scene of and for recovery. The difference between these places is that some of them provide means for facilitating recovery, whereas these ways and means work more in the background in other places; when put into practice they constitute a strong criticism of the rules of the institution.

Characteristic of the material conditions discussed in this chapter in their complexity; they are depicted in the stories as complex scenes where the person can exist and develop and as intricate and useful ways and means. In fact, the material conditions are just as complex as the people whom our respondents describe themselves as being.

242

---

[1] An exception is the therapeutic community movement whose origins derive from the early days of psychiatry. Here the institution itself is the foremost instrument of treatment (this also applies to the anti-institutional movement, but here it is the surrounding environment that is ascribed this function) (see Basaglia 1968, 1983, 1987, Castel 1976, Jones 1968, Scull 1979, Swain 1977).

[2] Medicines used in psychiatry have different names. Psychopharmaceuticals are medicines that affect the mental processes. Neuroleptics is the common name for a class of medicines that are used to treat symptoms of psychosis (the term anti-psychotic medication is incorrect in that the medicine does not remove the psychosis, rather it reduces certain of its symptoms). Besides these, there is a wide range of other medicines used to treat other types of mental problems.

[3] See Castel 1973, 1981 and Lerman 1984.

[4] This is not an exception in psychoanalysis. Freud was known to hold lectures for his patients. (See Roazen 1995)

8

In search of a lost self
Finding oneself

To speak of the invention of the self
is not to suggest that we are, in some way,
the victims of a collective fiction or delusion.
That which is invented is not an illusion; it
constitutes our truth.
Nikolas Rose, Inventing our selves

There is an extensive body of literature describing the effects that chronic illnesses have on identity. Bury (1982) refers to chronic illnesses as
a "biographical disruption" (see also Radley 1994, Strauss et al. 1984,
Charmaz 1983). In addition to the illness, the individual has to contend
with extensive changes in his or her life, in social interaction which
generates and maintains a sense of identity. Chronic illnesses can be
divided into those with which the individual identifies and those
which, despite their chronic course and obvious effects, nevertheless
remain separate from the individual's identity. Estroff (1985) has made
an interesting distinction between these two classes of chronic illnesses
in the effects they have on identity; she categorises chronic illnesses in
Western society as "I *am*-" and "I *have*-illnesses".

The picture becomes even more complicated when we consider
mental disorders: the very disorder is described as an assault on the
individual's sense of self[1]. The identity of a person who has a mental

disorder is thus subjected to a two-flank assault; besides the illness itself, there are the effects following in the wake of the illness, as is the case with anyone who has long struggled with an intractable problem.

Psychiatry, however, has concerned itself primarily with "the illness". It has devoted relatively little interest to how a person's identity is affected by having to live the life of a "chronic". Although there are studies pointing at the iatrogenic effects of life in total institutions (Barton 1959, Goffman 1961, Wing & Brown 1970, Estroff 1985), these research results have played a minor role in the psychiatric body of knowledge. Neither are the theories on the effects of stigmatisation (Goffman 1968, Scheff 1984) accorded much attention in the world of psychiatry. People with severe psychiatric problems are often reduced to their diagnoses; to a collection of deficiencies and disturbances. Their problems are regarded as expressions of the illness that have little to do with normal social interaction. By definition, normal social interaction can have only little or diffuse impact on persons who are periodically mentally disturbed in that the illness attacks the sense of self and persons so afflicted have great difficulty in relating to their surroundings.

The annihilated self

Severe mental disorders differ from other illnesses that have the chronic label. Schizophrenia, the other psychotic disorders and personality disturbances touch the individual's very self, the person's identity. Barrett (1996) writes:

> The "schizophrenic" becomes the antithesis of the idealized person, or, more characteristically, is thought of as part person, part non-person. (p. 179)

The dissolution of the person has perhaps been best described by Kraepelin (1971, from the 1919 edition):

> ...there are apparently two principal groups of disorders which characterise the malady. On the one hand we observe a *weakening of those emotional activities* which permanently form the mainsprings of volition.

In connection with this, *mental activity and instinct for occupation become mute*. The result of this part of the morbid process is *emotional dullness, failure of mental activities, loss of mastery over volition, of endeavor, and of ability for independent action. The essence of personality is thereby destroyed*, the best and most precious parts of its being, as Griessinger once expressed it, torn from her. With *the annihilation of personal will*, the possibility of further development is lost, which is dependent wholly on the activity of volition. What remains is principally what has been previously learned in the domain of knowledge and practical work. But this also sooner or later goes to ruin unless the failing inner mainspring is replaced by outer stimulus which rouses continual practice and so obviates the slow disappearance of ability. Whether and how far the malady directly injures the mental faculties apart from their gradual disappearances through disuse of mental function needs further inquiry. (...)

The second group of disorders which gave dementia praecox its peculiar stamp has been examined in detail especially by Stransky. It consists in *the loss of the inner unity of the activities of intellect, emotion, and volition* in themselves and among one another. Stransky speaks of an annihilation of the "intrapsychic coordination" (...). This annihilation presents itself to us in the disorder of association described by Bleuler, in *incoherence of the train of thought, in the sharp change of moods as well as in desultoriness and derailments in practical work*. But further, the near connection between thinking and feeling, between deliberation and emotional activity on the one hand, and practical work on the other is more or less lost. *Emotions do not correspond to ideas*. The patient laughs and weeps without recognizable cause, without any relation to their circumstances and their experiences, smile while they narrate the tale of their attempts at suicide. (...)

The work of the patients is not as in healthy people the expression of their view of life and temperament, it is not guided by the elaboration of perceptions, by deliberation and moods, but by *the incalculable result of chance external influences*, and impulses, cross impulses, and contrary impulses arising similarly by chance internally. (Italic mine, p. 75)

What is being described in this long excerpt is the almost total annihilation of the individual, a description we often find in psychiatric literature pertaining to the diagnosis schizophrenia. This way of describing people with severe mental disorders is still widely used today.

246

Hatfield and Lefley (1993), for example, divide schizophrenia into two main categories: disturbances in the sense of self and disturbances in emotions, relationships and behaviour. These are further divided into several sub-categories: disturbed perception as a primary factor, the loss of the sense of the self, disorders of attention, disturbances in emotions, fear and anxiety, depression, guilt, mania, apathy, blunting and inappropriate affect, and disturbances in relationships and behaviours.

What characterises a person who "is" schizophrenic or is "a schizophrenic" are specific malfunctions. Hatfield and Lefley (1993) write:

> People with schizophrenia are seen as unsocial, eccentric, suspicious and solitary. They have poor empathy with other people, are rigid in behavior, communicate in unusual styles and prefer to be alone. (p. 62)

A publication by the Swedish Psychiatric Association (1996) lists the most important symptoms of the schizophrenia diagnosis as being:

> (...) delusions, disturbed thought processes, self-absorption, emotional disturbances, perceptual disturbances (hallucinations) and cognitive disturbances, that is, disturbances in the ability to receive, process and give information. (p. 11)

This annihilation of the individual is, logically, irreversible. Because the person's sensory impressions do not accord with "reality", social or psychological interventions can have no effect, at least not in the way intended by those providing the help. And even if the cognitive and emotional ability to more or less correctly perceive the signals sent out by the environment were still intact, severely mentally ill people lack the ability to process these signals and express their emotions, thoughts and experiences in an "appropriate" way. And lastly, efforts to help schizophrenic patients are obstructed by the patients' impaired volition which no longer serves as a rational tool under the individual's control. Instead schizophrenics perceive signals that are either non-existent or apprehended incorrectly, signals which more or less haphazardly, randomly and irrationally determine the person's emotional state and "will". The prerequisites for communication, for influencing the person through psychological or social interventions, no longer exist. All this is why severe mental disorders are labelled as chronic.

However, this conception of severe mental disorders has been questioned in recent years, partly through the efforts of service users and former service users to articulate their experiences. Hatfield and Lefley (1993) write:

> Accounts of patients with schizophrenia raise many questions about how reliably we interpret what they are experiencing. While traditionally we have thought these patients to be in affect and lacking in interest in relating to others, our patient accounts suggest that there are many exceptions to this generally held belief. (p. 66)

History of the self

Both in the accounts of patients and in the accounts and theories of psychiatry, we find the notion that within every human being there is a central, fixed and integrative entity (Rose 1996). Thus persons who have recovered share with psychiatry a common cultural conception of the human being. It is important to recognise this common cultural heritage now when there is increasing doubt that the self can be conceived as a uniform/homogeneous, autonomous and fixed entity (Burkitt 1991, Danziger 1990, Gergen 1989, 1991, Rose 1996, Sampson 1989). In psychiatry, however, the self is seldom put in a historical context.

According to Danziger (1997) the idea that every human being possesses an own identity was first formulated by Locke at the end of the 17th century. The Industrial Revolution in Great Britain broke down what used to be the bases for establishing social identity, i.e. class, family ties, religion and profession. Empiricism threw further doubt on a concept that has had a central place in human identity: the eternal soul. Human beings were no longer made manifest through their actions. They, or rather the self, had now become the self-directed owner of its own actions and experiences. No longer a prisoner of fate. The self observed other selves as well as itself to attain its own ends in the best possible way.

In his earlier writings, Adam Smith reflected on the self and its role, and it is these reflections that later became the foundation for his economic theory. An important tenet of this theory is that when one observes oneself, one becomes two individuals: there is the person who is being observed, and there is the person who is doing the observing and who passes judgement.

> The self, thus set free, can now also be improved. Self-esteem is not simply a given, it has to be won through a carefully thought out presentation of oneself in everyday situations. (Goffman 1959)

Instead of the indivisible eternal soul, we now have the increasingly fragmented and circumstantial self:

> While the original division was between the self as observer and as observed, in the nineteenth century, with the increasing emphasis on the topic of self-control, the division between ideal self and real self assumed more prominence. From this position it was not a tremendous step to assert that there could be not just two selves in the same person, but many. (Danziger 1997, p. 147)

The fragmented self has a history of its own ranging from pathology to normality. From the notion of a self as a central, uniform and largely fixed entity to the notion of a self that is continuously adapting to new situations and thus lacks a central standpoint whereby a person's actions become explicable. Nevertheless, when the concept of self was reintroduced into American psychology, it was in order to "do justice to the unity and coherence of the human personality" (Danziger 1997, p. 148). This return of the notion of the self as a central unifying entity fixed over time and place led to a number of hypotheses about the human personality. One such hypothesis has to do with the individual's striving for consistency, for example between words and deeds. Another hypothesis has to do with concepts like "the true self". Today these hypotheses are integral parts of how we envision the self.

The persons interviewed in this study concur with contemporary psychology's concept of self. It may even be said that their life stories often contain a change in their way of relating to themselves – a changeover from having been controlled by destiny, a chronic, to persons who have conquered fate and have started to take charge of their own lives, together with, but also in opposition to, other people. This transformation parallels the historical development from a belief in the eternal soul and immutable destiny to envisioning the self as its own (co-)creator. Bruner (1987) quotes Amelie Rorty who describes how narrative forms have had a similar development over time:

> ...the folktale *figure* "who is neither formed by nor owns experience", to *persons* defined by roles and responsibilities in a society for which they get rights in return (as, say, in Jane Austin's novels), to *selves* who must compete for their roles in order to earn their rights (as in Trollope), and finally to *individuals* who transcend and resist society and must create or "rip off" their rights (as, say, in Beckett). (p. 19-20)

In like manner the persons we interviewed in the present study fit in with Hydén's observation (1995b) that:

> ...patients who recover from illness through treatment have at their disposal cultural resources that enable them to show how their usual 'Self' has changed and, not the least, that this change is in contrast to their former state. These resources seem to range from being able to *realize* the true Self (Maslow 1976), to *restore* or *reconstruct* the Self (Kohut 1977, Williams 1984), to *regenerate* a Self (Hawkins 1990), to *create* a new self (Schafer 1992) or to find *a newborn* Self (Hawkins 1993). (p. 76; italics in the original)

These theoreticians and the respondents in this study both share the same cultural environment. They use the same concepts, have a similar set of mental images and articulate similar theories about mental disorders and the main features of recovery. One such central concept appearing in several of the stories is "an own self" and the loss and subsequent regaining of that self. It is not, however, the whole of the self that is lost; some parts remain – a self that is aware of the loss and goes in search of itself, or at least, part of itself.

The loss of an own self

The loss of the self and the search for the "own self" is, in narrative terms, the central "plot" of most of the interviews. Revolving around this central plot are various stories of practice; these may be concerned with underlying problems (alienation process), the experience of suffering or the recovery process.

The loss of the self is described in several of the recovery accounts as resulting from a conscious striving to be someone one is not:

> There was a man who I kind of looked up to, who interested me a lot... For some reason I wanted to be like him. And so I went around... for a whole year I went around and tried to keep an eye on how I walked and stuff like that. That's what I was doing and I got so stuck in doing it that in the end I thought I was him. So... that's why... I think maybe that's how I lost myself. (Sven)

For many of the respondents, the self was lost through trying to be someone else, either someone in one's immediate surroundings or a more remote idol:

> Of course it was a fantasy world, built on music stars, my own omnipotence and belief that I could be something really fantastic in those fields... But so what! It was my way of existing. (Lars)

In several instances the loss of an "own" self occurred early in life, long before others began to identify the person as being deviant or ill:

> Even as a child I had invented at least two personalities to protect me from the painful experiences I was having. (...) I didn't want to talk to anyone about all this because I believed and hoped that it would disappear if I could just get away from home. (Elin)

> My task was to dissimulate. To act healthy, or more healthy than I was. It was one of the basic principles drummed into me as a kid. Not to show that I exist, ever. (Lars)

The transformation of the self can also take concrete form and be directed against the body. Nils describes his struggle for existance, tracing the roots of this struggle to his childhood:

Some of it has to do with losing yourself, with being too sensitive, with experiencing yourself as unreal. To shut down so that... the delusions and fantasies I had back then. Such suspiciousness, it can devastate anyone. (...) Either you had close yourself up inside or act hysterically and like some kind of unreal... like there was nothing in between. And then, too, it has to do with existing, not existing. Being or not being. That's what's it all about; like when someone tells me I don't measure up; criticises me or so; all of a sudden I'm not allowed to be the person I am. Something like that sticks with you for the rest of your life; once you get the feeling you don't exist, then you're dead, you know. (Nils)

To measure up, to avoid devastating critique, Nils decided to make himself over:

I tried to find what were external causes inside myself instead; in myself as flesh-and-blood. First I began with my teeth. I looked like a walrus, I thought, back then. Today I wish I had my old teeth back. I found a dentist who extracted four healthy teeth, and retracted my teeth so much that when I was supposed to sing, I couldn't...

Then they operated on my tongue because it was... it had gotten too big. They had pushed my teeth in so far into my mouth cavity that there was no room anymore for my tongue. (...) I thought it would help me be a better performer if I got my teeth retracted, and that I would have more luck with girls, and I would sing better. I remember standing on the stage when all of a sudden it struck me that there was just emptiness. It's hard to describe the feeling, that you have no right to exist. It's a bit like when you lose contact with yourself and... I remember it as a total disaster, I couldn't sing with my tongue like that, so I got in touch with another dentist and they contacted someone at the hospital. And so I went in for an operation. A professor was supposed to operate on me and I come in and I'm, like, paralysed. I'm totally driven by... "For Christ sake operate on my tongue so we can put an end to this once and for all; so that I can start singing again, so that I can get on with my life". So I went there and in comes this assistant surgeon, and here's me, 25 years old. Now, afterwards, I don't know why I didn't object and insist that Professor [name] was supposed to do the operation, he's the one who examined me, he's the plastic surgeon. (...) I wanted it done. So I got it done. The underside of my tongue grew back the wrong way, the muscle became enlarged, as big as a pingpong ball cut in half. Today I don't know where I got the energy to survive the decades that came after; because after this first operation, I had three more major operations, the last one Professor [name] did for free because he understood my predicament and so he cut away everything, all the scar tissue.

I associate all this with what I learned as a child about being silent. Because I became silent again. My tongue hurt so much and what was supposed to be the solution to my life, that I was going to have a beautiful smile, and make it with girls, I was going to be a real performer, a great singer, I would get answers to the question of why I had got along so poorly in company. I didn't get any answers at all. Just the opposite, I became more and more silent. (Nils)

This attempt to find a solution, however extreme it might seem to others, is logical from Nils' own perspective; and the subsequent failure is even more extreme. Take away this inner perspective, and what remain are symptoms of severe mental disturbance. The loss of the sense of self triggers the process that brings the person into contact with psychiatry and results in a diagnosis.

But often, what has been identified as the symptom is not the loss itself, but rather the person's efforts and subsequent failure to manage his/her life after experiencing such a loss: a self in search of itself. Several of the stories contain descriptions of a schism, not only between what is experienced as the own self and a different foreign self, but also within the own self. A schism between a part within the person that is in search of a second part which, if united, would make a whole.

This common feature of many of the life stories – the feeling of being inferior – gives rise to two main ways of managing the situation – hiding the inferior self or exposing it by attention-seeking behaviour. Although some people might use both ways during different periods in their lives, most use primarily the one or the other.

Hiding the inferior self

In the absence of a self that measures up, in one's own eyes and in the eyes of others, some people create an alternative self, a surrogate self, one that conforms better with the person's own expectations or with what he/she believes are the expectations of others. But success in using this strategy bears with it the seeds of a breakdown later in life.

The better the alternative self works and the more it is confirmed, the more depleted becomes its creator. What is being confirmed and has success is not the own self, but the alternate self that was created to hide the own self's shortcomings. The alternative self is given nourishment and a life of its own. The tools are no longer under the control of their inventor. With less and less scope to interact with others, the own self atrophies. The distance between the own self's shrivelled existence and the expansive power of the alternative self may, at some critical point, lead to a breakdown; a breakdown brought about because the person can no longer contain the contradictions within.

> But what became a problem was that the role closed off so many other sides of myself. I was playing a role for other people and was so scared they would find out who I really was and how stupid I was and how frightened I was… So I never allowed myself to be anyone other than someone who was strong and tough and capable and nice to be around and… (Susanne)

Seeking attention

Some people, when they experience that they are not accepted for who they are, begin to behave in an eccentric manner so as to draw attention to themselves and to the vulnerability of their situation. They become someone else in order to be seen as they are. This way of behaving seems to bear the seeds of its own failure, as well. People seldom realise that a person's eccentric behaviour may be an attempt to draw attention to a problematic life situation, to a self that is under threat. Usually they regard such behaviour as expressing the person's real identity. The person's identity becomes reduced to a set of behaviours, to the alternative self. Thus the person is presented with a new identity and a new social context that confirms that identity through mechanisms of inclusion and exclusion. Drug abuse brings a person into contact with drug abusers and other social outcasts and leads to a process of exclusion from other social groups:

> No one cared. You realise now the kind of signals you were sending out. Really powerful signals, but no one noticed them. (Irene)

However, the way of behaving is doomed to fail even from this perspective because it seems that the new identity is unable to offer a satisfactory substitute for the person's own identity. In either case, the person is forced to set out on a search for his/her own self.

The continuity of the self

Regardless of which strategy the person chooses, the life stories show evidence of an inner continuity between who the person was before the breakdown and onset of illness, during the recurrent periods of hospitalisation and throughout the recovery process. This continuity stands in sharp contrast to how psychiatric literature describes "the schizophrenic's" fundamental break with the rest of humanity. This state has perhaps been most clearly expressed by Karl Jasper:

> If we try to get some closer understanding of these primary experiences of delusion, we soon find we cannot really appreciate these quite alien modes of experience. They remain largely incomprehensible, unreal and beyond understanding. (Quoted in Barrett 1996, p. 22)

Continuity is maintained through the search by one part of the self for its complementary part. We can find a similar idea of continuity in the work of Davidson and Strauss (1992) who focus in their research on the sense of self during the recovery process:

> And once there is a sense of self that can be seen as responsible for managing the illness, it then also becomes possible for the person to take a more active and determined part in his/her social and vocational rehabilitation, developing, copying mechanisms and learning to exercise self-control over symptoms. (p. 140)

The self, a sense of identity, sometimes has to be won despite opposition from the person's surroundings (including psychiatry); a belief that one is, or at least could become, something more than just a patient, something other than a chronic whose perhaps only hope lies in simply accepting his/her limitations. However, in this study we found that accepting one's limitations could be a platform for transcending them. Ruth, for example, describes the gulf between the environment's expectations of normality and her own dreams for her life:

> I left the hospital and began to work, but I had a few ambitions to be an artist... and maybe I'm being fresh when I say the medicines drove them away. Now I'm supposed to adapt to a normal life. So I'm working in a tobacco shop and it's so damn boring. (...) I'm 20 years old and want to do something with my life, not work in a tobacco shop all my life.

It is first several years later that Ruth returns to art:

> I found my way back to painting. I see it as my only chance... painting. That's what I always wanted to do. It feels like a gift after all I've been through.

Since then she has had several exhibitions of her art and has taught water colouring and art history.

Further on in the text we will return to the idea of the recovered self. The question here is what is there within the person that could promote recovery? What can the person do to set out on and make progress along a road to recovery?

Personal qualities

Contrary to the concepts found in psychiatry – a language that emphasises the vulnerability, weakness, fragility and shortcomings of people with severe mental disorders – many of the respondents in the present study point at other kinds of personal qualities besides vulnerability: "I had a kind of driving force within me." (Richard)

Amidst all the problems and a great need for support, there are also personal strengths and personal qualities particular to the individual.

Possessing a driving force is mentioned by several of the respondents as one of these qualities:

> I'm that kind of person, I think. Otherwise I probably would have died already at birth if I hadn't had that attitude. I think there's a powerful driving force within me. I don't know what to call it, the capacity to endure, to put up a good fight. (Jan)

Other characteristics mentioned in the recovery stories are being a fighter and being daring, tough, stubborn, creative; that one has inner resources, good genes, ambition, and that one has the ability to get going under one's own steam. These personal strengths, which are emphasised in the recovery accounts, indicate that the recovery process is hardly a spontaneous self-going process; rather, it is a very demanding undertaking and the person must mobilise all his/her inner resources to make any progress at all.

> I've always been stubborn, already as a child. I am stubborn. There were times when I was so depressed I was ready to give up, but I keep fighting and put up with the suffering. You could say that it's part of being an artist. Your have great heights and declines. In my case, it has to do with never having enough money to get by on.
>
> I've had to struggle to have an artist role and not always just a patient role. Unfortunately, I have to have both of these roles because I've been a part of it for so long and so much in psychiatric care... I try to think in terms of an artist role as being more healthy and that it can be very liberating, but I know that I still need some support. And I get it at the day centre. (Ruth)

Strengths and resources that enable one to endure, to struggle on despite the onslaught of the illness and despite the environment's lack of understanding seem to be central personality traits in people recovering from psychosis. Ruth is clear in pointing out that her own qualities are the basis for her resistance to being reduced to a psychiatric category, to a set of problems. But she does not deny that she has problems, although she sees them as being linked to the enormous financial difficulties she has had to contend with for most of her life. She defines herself in terms of a dual role: both service user and artist. Not either/or, but both. And she relates her possibilities to benefit by her innate abilities to the external support she finds in the form of professionals and the activities offered at the day care centre.

Ways of managing

Recovery is a demanding process that requires the individual's total commitment. And even though the disorder cannot be separated from either the person's life before becoming a psychiatric patient and being diagnosed, or from the recovery process and the successive regaining of autonomy, it is still possible to detect a common thread running through the person's way of relating to his/her life: the person is, for the most part, active; active when he/she copes with the first feelings of inadequacy; active in relation to the first symptoms; active sometimes even when seemingly most passive; active in finding ways to manage the symptoms and difficulties that life as an identified chronic entails; active in relation to the illness and to the surrounding world.

The own self interacts with the alien parts of the self. Even when it cannot exert control over these parts, the own self works out a way to live with them. It does what it has to do to survive with them and influence them in the desired direction. That is to say, these parts of the self develop ways to purposefully influence both these split-off parts of the self and the environment in order to exert influence over the alien self. This means in turn that the person still has the ability to exercise judgement in the face of a confusing and frightening situation and in relation to the own self, including the alien self. It indicates the continued existence of volition and the ability to turn that volition into deeds, either by one's own efforts or with the help of others.

These strengths, which are the remnants of an own self or sense of self that exists alongside but in conflict with the disorder, are expressed as more or less purposeful, more or less successful actions with the aim of facing up to, resisting and managing that other self, the alien self.

Increasing attention is being given in psychiatry today to patients' so-called coping strategies. But to call them coping strategies is often misleading. To adopt a strategy means that one first acquires an overview of a particular situation, analyses the relevant circumstances and thereafter formulates a long-term plan that takes into account the opponent's possible countermoves. Although there are examples of strategic thinking among the persons we have interviewed, mostly they use simple, short-term and ad hoc measures in their attempts to manage their problems. Coincidences occur where a particular action or thought seems to counteract the emergence of a particular symptom or weaken its effect, coincidences which the person becomes aware of and makes use of. It has to do with finding ways of managing, of using tricks and ruses, of trying, of failing, with learning from the mistakes and with not giving up, or of giving up and then coming back again. That these ways of trying to cope are often innovative supports the idea that an uncorrupted self still exists beyond the disorder. But because the outcome of these ways of trying to cope are sometimes destructive, their creative aspects and the person's active part in them often go unnoticed by outsiders.

The ways of trying to cope that are described in the recovery stories in this study can be classified according to whether they are directed towards the symptoms, the environment or life as a whole. They can also be classified according to different sets of attitudes; the pattern commonly occurring in the literature on coping strategies is present even here: to either increase or decrease one's level of activity.

Several of the recovery accounts also contain examples of how the person purposely tries to avoid certain environments (scenes, co-agents) that have a negative effect or seeks out environments that have a positive effect. And lastly, we find examples of a way of dealing with the problem that could be termed "distancing through dialogue".

One step at a time

Recovery is a time-consuming taxing undertaking. It is an uneven and complex process that progresses by fits and starts, where sudden leaps forward are succeeded by periods of lull followed by forward movement again, one step at a time. In such manner, the progress made is gradually consolidated and reversals are forestalled.

I think I've come up with something. Somehow I've been able to create a bit of distance to my problems by telling myself that "OK, start with thinking it can turn out all right. And if goes to pot anyway, I just have to believe that things will work out eventually. It's a good idea to think like that. And that's how it is, I tell myself: "OK, you have a problem and this is the problem. OK. I don't have a solution. But I bet I'll find a solution afterwards." And it's good for me to think like that. And the kinds of things I've been talking about now, they distance me from the problem, I think.

How did you come up with this particular philosophy in life?

Well. I remember that ever since I got ill I've tried to improve myself, be more flexible in order to move ahead. Yes, I remember that from when I was in really bad shape. It was so bad I couldn't think a single thought, I can tell you. I laid on the bed and I couldn't formulate a single thought in my head, for myself, like. I can do that now, don't you think? Back then I couldn't do it. I remember just lying on the bed. I was almost at my wits end. I got out of bed and walked around the room. I called out loud: "I can't even think of a single thought." That was the only way I could get through to myself, to say the thought out loud. I couldn't say it inside my head. That's how uptight I was. I was all tied up in knots, like, inside. It was... nothing was moving in there at all. And not because it was dead, but because something was locked up tight, so tight that it was completely impossible to move around inside it all. Afterwards, I thought: "I'm going to have to work at this a little at a time. Try to loosen things up a little bit inside, do it in small steps, and maybe some day you'll make it." I wanted to loosen up the knots, if I only did a little every day. And that's what I did. Things have loosened up. And I only did a little at a time, like. But I've succeeded in untying the knots. (Sven)

That was being too greedy... So now I take it in small portions. I've learned that more haste, less speed is the better way, to give myself partial goals that are attainable. That way, you get positive feedback that it's working, and you don't knock yourself out. That's my strategy, my coping strategy I mean. Partial goals, reasonable goals, attainable goals, so that's one way I've learned to come to the point. I'm determined to get well, it's a kind of mantra for me. I ignore the pain of maybe I'll have a relapse. It's become a way of relating to the whole thing. (David)

There are different ways of implementing a one-step-at-a-time approach.

Diminished or heightened activity

Several of the respondents have learned with time to observe how they react in different situations. On the basis of this self-knowledge they have had to invent an optimal balance between, on the one hand, the life they want and, on the other, the "insight" that the road to that life is paved with dangers that obstruct an immediate realisation of that life – a balance between the intellect's optimism and the experiential world's pessimism. The balance can consist of learning not to do too much, of doing only so much as one can cope with. But in several of the life stories it seems that a balance is achieved by cautious pendulum swings between periods of activity and of seeming inactivity (the question is whether an "intentionally passive attitude" really is passive considering that it is the result of an active choice).

To be able to mange social situations, Richard's need to rest up between such occasions is perhaps greater than most people's:

> I spend a lot of time by myself because I have this huge need to just relax and recharge my batteries. When I'm with other people I get so excited that I need to calm myself down. If I go out in the evening I like to come home early because it takes me several hours to wind down so that I can go to bed. (Richard)

David describes how he completed a full university education while having psychotic experiences:

> Yes, I stuck with it and took my degree while I was completely psychotic and like…
> *But how did the rest of your life work out, when you were… You said that were able to zoom in on… but were you able to keep things in order in other areas of your life; did your daily life work out all right?*
> Yes, it did, but I was like a robot. I shaved every day, for example, which I don't do now! But it's more that I just didn't want to do it…
> *And you cooked for yourself…fix your clothes and stuff?*
> Yes, my clothes and everything, daily life worked OK…

Daily life worked out?
But it worked because I made it a habit. It wasn't anything you think about or did anything special about it, like, cooked a good dinner or... It was entirely "basic". Things went by routine, I mean... (David)

Daily life worked out because it followed a planned routine so that as few unexpected and problematic situations as possible could arise. On the other hand, ritualising daily life, i.e. reducing the level of activity that daily life requires, was a condition for coping with university studies which require a high level of activity. In the long-run, achieving this balance was an important step towards the desired life, towards recovery.

Thus, it is a question of a balance between higher and lower levels of activity in different areas of life where one level is a precondition for the other.

Distancing through dialogue

Another way that occurred for managing concrete problems and symptoms is distancing. Creating distance helps to counteract the risk of being swamped by one's problems, of losing sight of one's options. To achieve distance people use various ways to get into a dialogue about their problems, a dialogue they have alone with themselves or with other people. The dialogue a person has with him-/herself about, and sometimes accompanied by, threatening symptoms may be very literal indeed:

When I finally quit using Esucos (type of medication), when I stopped looking for happiness in a pill, and when I had learned to deal with my anxiety... I felt, it sounds so simple, but when I was up at the cottage all by myself and in the end could pretty well fend off much of the anxiety... But it always came back when I went to bed. It's been like that for lots of years and I got so tired of it. I didn't know how to handle it. Finally, I screamed: "OK. Come on, anxiety, damn you. Come on and let's get it over with!" Rage: "Come on damn you, let's fight it out, you and me?" I gave my anxiety a good tongue-lashing. Fought the fight with my anxiety. "I bloody well refuse to live this second-class life with you anymore, damn anxiety, always hanging over my shoulders!" Sometimes a miracle would happen and I'd get out of having an anxiety attack. And with time they began to thin out. Sometimes it would occur to me: "I haven't had any anxiety for two whole days!" (Irene)

Meeting one's anxiety head on seems at times to reduce its power and eventually disarms it. The dialogue with oneself can also be conducted with the help of external aids. Writing down one's experiences is a way of giving structure to the problems and of distancing oneself from them so as to better manage certain situations:

I got myself a big notebook and wrote down everything in it. About everyone I met and what I saw and how they reacted. (Erik)

External aids can also be a link between the person and his/her self:

There was a time when my life was dreadful, just horrible, and I have a tendency to magnify crises, you know; the feeling gets overwhelming and everything seems black as night. So I went and recorded stuff on my type-recorder. I sat there and said out loud to myself: "My life sucks these days. I don't have any money, and everything's so dreadful. I don't what to do, I'm flat broke"... and stuff like that. I sat there and described exactly how I felt. And then I replayed the tape and heard what I had said. It's exactly like a girl had come to visit, and then I saw things much clearer, and then I said: "Well, Maria, things aren't so bad. You could sell your car if you can't afford it. And you can stop getting the newspaper, and you can do this and you can do that."

I'm very good at solving other people's problems, you know. If someone comes to me, I know very well what they should do... It was like someone else had come to me and I then knew exactly what I had to do. So the next morning I sold my car and stopped getting the newspaper and I arranged everything. It wasn't me any longer, you see; and I could listen to that other person without any feelings and use my head instead.
So it's a technique you can use?
Yes, it can be a technique. And it's a good one. Because when I recorded the tape, I put into it all my feelings and everything, you see; and just said how bad things were. And then when I listened to the tape, I didn't have any feelings about it anymore. So it was kind of fun, for suddenly I fixed everything. (Maria)

The external aid, a tape-recorder in this case, opens up a passable detour. Taking a round-about-way through language is evidence of a far-reaching creativity in a world where the simplest daily chores may seem insurmountable problems.

The dialogue with others seems to be about getting "a second opinion" from someone one has learned to trust. In situations where a person has difficult deciding how to relate to his/her symptoms and the more all-encompassing life situations, the other can be a supportive self that the person has chosen on his/her.

> I have trouble saying no and [name of the contact person] told me to savour the words first and think about what I really want to say. If someone calls me up and wants a favour from me, then I say: "Wait a moment. I'll call you back in a little while." Then I call [the contact person] and we talk about it. He asks me what I think and what I want to do. So I think about it a bit and after a while I call up the other person. And so I've got help along the way. (Anne)
> *But how come you didn't "flip out" like you said?*
> I think it's because I had such a good friend, so I could talk about it a little. I could talk about what I was going around thinking and why I was so afraid. And she only said: "No, it's not like that" and "Just take it easy" and "No one thinks that about you". (Tina)

Changing one's environment

Other ways of managing difficult situations have to do with problems that are much more comprehensive than are the symptoms themselves. They are often concerned with how the environment responds to the person's manifested problems. Several of respondents describe occasions when they avoided a certain environment or certain people because they regarded these as having a negative effect.

> I moved to X-town with my husband in [year]. I felt that I didn't have anything to lose. The mental hospital was divided into an east wing and a west wing, and I had been in the east wing for ten years. If you were on the west wing you were incurable; that's where the chronics were. And it was called the asylum, too. I heard that they planned to move me to the west wing and that's when I realised that they had given up on me a long

time ago. I realised that if this went on a while more I would be incurable, I would be a chronic, I'd be brain damaged; and then I thought to myself, I have nothing to lose, so I took my stuff and moved out. (Elin)

It is also a question of establishing contact with people who have a positive influence:

... since [that year] things have looked up. First of all I began to realise that [name of the contact person] was on my side, and so I kept in touch with him. (Roland)

All these ways of managing symptoms and life situations indicate the presence of an active and intentional self, a self who tries to find solutions to extremely distressing and sometimes incomprehensible experiences. Many of these ways of managing problems are indications that the person is still in touch with reality. Viewed from the person's own perspective, and in context, much of this seemingly bizarre behaviour becomes comprehensible practice. There is, however, reason to discuss how certain symptoms are described in the interviews as coping strategies, yet are treated as symptoms by others who never take the trouble to consider what explanations the persons themselves give of their own actions.

Symptoms as managing and managing as symptoms

There are situations in which the ways service users manage their difficulties are confused with their symptoms. In the recovery stories, it is possible to distinguish between two ways in which symptoms and ways of managing are interrelated. The first is that symptoms may be a way to achieve something, a secondary gain. The second is that what might at first appear to be a symptom may very well be an attempt to manage a problematic situation. In certain cases, what psychiatry has classified as a classic symptom of severe mental disorder could have an entirely different meaning when seen from the patient's perspective.

Anne has been plagued for many years by voices and visual hallucinations. She sought help from psychiatry for these complaints. The hallucinations could be so intense that at times she had to be hospitalised against her will. At the time of the interview, she had not had any hallucinations for over two years. Anne has achieved some distance to her tormentors and we can discuss that period in her life from a different perspective. She is not tormented by them any more. These are the circumstances around the following dialogue:

> *How did you manage him (the "Reaper", a hallucinatory figure that Anne referred to earlier in the interview)?*
> In the beginning I used to bang my head against the wall. I did it in the hospital, too, so they belted me down and gave me an injection and then disappeared. And that's how it was for a long time. After that more voices appeared, men's voices. They mumbled and I couldn't hear what they said. And then they disappeared and "Reaper" went away too. How he disappeared, I don't know. I haven't heard him for a year now. This has been a wonderful year.
> *What made him disappear in the end, do you think?*
> I just didn't bother about it anymore. I didn't make up any fantasies. They said it was me, myself who... I was the only one who heard or saw him... and I thought about that a lot. That it was only me fantasising. It's me making a fool of myself and trying to get attention. To get people to pay attention to me because I felt so lonely. So I say: "I hear voices. Help me!" That gets me a lot of attention from the staff, and like... And I've gotten it too. I haven't been all alone. (...)
> *Do I understand you correctly: it was worth hearing the frightening voice, and being belted down and all that in order to avoid being lonely?*
> Yes, it was. I think I made myself mentally ill. Suicide thoughts, it's all mental, but it's a cry for help, too. That you so badly need someone to talk to you. To find a kind of togetherness that way. To have friends... Of course, it's not so easy to make friends, but... But maybe it was the only thing I could do. That's what I tell myself.

Anne describes a complex experience where she is subjected to hallucinations but can bring them on herself, too. And she is aware of two reasons for doing this. First of all, having hallucinations is an accepted way of getting attention from the service staff. Attention and companionship. Second, hallucinations are in themselves a form of companionship, an exceedingly distressful companion but sometimes less so than the alternative – social isolation.

The from-the-inside perspective of the life stories throws new light on ways of behaving which, when viewed from the outside, can only be regarded as symptoms of mental illness. Seen from the individual's perspective, however, these behaviours are comprehensible, acceptable, if not always successful, features in the person's life context (see Hatfield & Lefley 1993, p. 133).

As the interview continues, Anne explains that she preferred to bring on these horrifying symptoms because her feelings of loneliness were much worse. Talking about her life without "the Reaper", she says

> I thought: "I've lost a friend. A cruel one…". It was very sad.
> *Better a cruel friend than no friend at all?*
> Yes. I could bring him with me into town, wherever I wanted to go.
> *Could you decide over him?*
> Yes, when he was going to turn up in my head, that's when I thought, now I want him to turn up. We talked with each other too, sometimes. It worked pretty well. I didn't talk with my mouth, only with my head, so to speak. We talked about the weather. About my youth, cause I found it so awful, the years between 12 and 18. We talked about all that, and I magnified things. We talked about my mom and dad, and my sister and her children. He talked back just like there was someone there and we talked things over. He gave me advice. Bad advice. (Anne)

Drug abuse is one of the indications for a psychiatric diagnosis. But for the persons in our study who talked about their drug abuse, it was partly an attempt to cope with a much greater problem.

Irene describes her initial abuse of drugs as a form of "self medication". She describes different types of drugs, their uses and side-effects, and gives a rather balanced firsthand account of a way of trying to cope that could easily be reduced to only a symptom. Drug abuse can be a symptom, but not necessarily, and not only of mental disorders, but also of an existential life situation with which a person is being forced to contend.

> You didn't know what to do with yourself in [names a city]. They had a camping place and back then I had a friend whose older brother and his

gang were the town's first hippies. He was into that stuff. I got involved with that gang, too. It suited me perfectly. They had pills and they had dope. And there was beer and everything was just fine. I tried to get rid of the pain and anxiety by using the stuff as medicine. And it got to be a lot. I remember how we mixed the pills and drank and smoked. (…) Today I can see that it was a kind of self-medication. Back then I could have popped anything, just as long as it had some effect. That's what it was like for many years. It didn't matter to me what it was. Just as long as it took away… just as long as I didn't have to think. That's what I felt for a long long time: "I don't have the energy to think. I don't have the energy to feel." It felt so good, you took a little dope, and – suddenly a world of colours and content and feeling. (…)

Drugs to counteract the emptiness – did it work?
Both yes and no. During the high, of course. And yet, sometimes you felt like you were more empty than ever. Somehow. Of course you knew it was false, a chemical kick you bought either as beer or as a pipe or as pills. You knew that. But somehow, it worked better than not having any-thing, because you kept doing it…

What gave me the greatest kick actually was LSD. That made me feel on top of the world. An incredible feeling of well-being. You feel so good from head to toe. If you take the right dose. That's what I liked the best. When I was between 14 and 15 years old, I must have taken at least 50 to 100 LSD trips. I took a whole lot. The first time I was at [name of clinic], they gave me an EEG because I had trouble keeping my balance and they thought it had to do with LSD. I was terribly clumsy and they thought it was because of the LSD.

Sometimes, when you smoked, what happened was that you got even more engrossed in yourself and although you could, like, feel calm, you felt like you were inside a shell. You could sit there real spaced out and the world stayed outside. You were your own island. But that didn't worry me so much just then. But the feeling that you were all alone could get really very strong. (Irene)

Like the medications prescribed by psychiatry, there seem to be two aspects to alcohol and narcotics, as presented in the life stories: one has to do with the chemical substances themselves and their effects or highs; the other has to do with social interaction in connection with drug abuse. The chemical effects seem to be directed mostly against feelings of anxiety; the social interaction against feelings of loneliness.

Ruth, more so than Irene, is concerned with the companionship drug circles offer.

> I want to tell you something that I don't think the doctor would approve of; about that business with drugs I was doing. I think it was both a good and bad thing. It shook me up. At the same time it wasn't good, but I did drugs for only a little while. I was never a certified drug addict. But it had an effect; I never had any anxiety attacks when I was doing drugs. And also, I had a chance to experience, after being so lonely in the hospital and being isolated among all those nutcases, a very close companionship that I've never felt before. If it had gone on for a while longer, I would have seen a lot of its downsides, but because it went on for such a short while, there was something good about it all, even though withdrawal certainly wasn't easy. (Ruth)

Behaving in a way that seems incomprehensible to others alienates the person from so-called normal people and it is for that very reason that the behaviour is regarded as indicative of mental illness. But even such behaviour is explicable from the person's own perspective, explicable as an attempt to cope with a problem that, for the person concerned, seems worse than the problematic attempt at a solution.

> He was like a cartoon figure. Just a circle with two big ears and legs from the head down, like a stick drawing. That's what he looks like.
> *You saw him?*
> Yes. He showed himself to me. Maybe not the first month or so, but after a while. It was so scary. I was so frightened. It crept up on me. It began in the back of my head and then circled all around until it covered my whole head, like a bed sheet. It covered my whole brain. And that's when he appeared. It was horrid.
> *What did you do then?*
> I get so scared so I bang my head against the wall to get rid of him. And he does go away because it hurts him. It's so strange!... After that it's better. (Anne)

It is worth noting that these ways of managing, which may appear to be symptoms, are not wholly unsuccessful, at least not in the beginning. They give a measure of relief, which is why the respondents resorted to them.

Resistance as managing (from the institution's perspective)

Several of the life stories depict the respondents' efforts to maintain some degree of what they refer to as integrity and dignity in relation to the routines typical of the total institution. Seen in this light, Tina's and Lars' behaviour seems like a revolt when they describe what they regard as efforts to protect themselves:

> I was assigned a room and when the nurses came in to talk with me, they just opened the door and walked right in. It made me furious and so I told them: "Go out again and knock on the door and ask if you can come in. Otherwise I want a lock on this door. So I can lock it." Because it wasn't right, you know. It violated my integrity, when they just walked right in like that. (Tina)

Not only did Lars protest when the rules of normal social behaviour were broken, he also worked out a way to cope with how he was being treated in hospital:

> They sat there in their white coats, looking all the world like professors. So of course you get pissed off and you start saying crazy things. I recorded some of those conversations. I had a hidden microphone... I kept a little of my dignity, even if I did it in a provocative way... (Lars)

From the perspective of the institution, such behaviour may appear to be symptoms and resistance to treatment. Castel (1976) saw acceptance of the institution's leadership as the definitive proof that the patient had been cured. One's values may depend on one's perspective

Making decisions

Several of the life stories describe situations where the person makes conscious decisions that affect the recovery process. Several of the ways of managing described in the life stories are based, at least in part, on conscious deliberation, which makes them decisions. These decisions are discussed in the present context because they are explicitly expressed as decisions in the interviews and because they have an overall effect on the person's life.

Erik describes a situation which, in the language of psychiatry, means that he is suffering from delusions (he sees signs in the sky and hears a ticking sound in response to his questions to the higher powers that send him signals). He is being treated for schizophrenia and his current situation is that, through the many years of affliction and psychiatric treatment, he has lost his means of livelihood and his former social network. Also, he is deeply concerned about his ageing mother and her constant worry about him. Furthermore, he participates in an outpatient programme where he has formed a relationship with a contact person whom he values highly and his medication has been successively reduced, which seems to be working out fairly well. In this situation he decides to try to simply ignore his delusions. He does not want his mother to worry about him. He is fed up with people regarding him as sick. He has grown tired of his insecure social situation and of having to spend time in hospital.

> I just told myself: I'm not going to get involved in this stuff anymore. I'm just not going to think about it anymore. I'm not going to sit around at home and draw pictures and stuff. I'm not going to sit around and fantasise about someone else giving me the answers. And if I get any answers, the hell with it. It can go on ticking for all I care. And you know, it just stopped, all of a sudden. I've haven't heard anymore ticking since then. (…)
>
> I make a decision to stop brooding. Ignore it if I see any signs and take my medicine and something happens, that's how I explain it to the doctor. (…)
>
> *What made you take that decision at that particular time?*
>
> Because I said to myself – no more hospitals for this thing. So now I've got to get me some friends. I mustn't go around talking about all this stuff anymore.

This situation is loaded with critical and contradictory circumstances: a long-term psychotic patient makes a rational decision to ignore his delusions. He does it out of consideration for others – his ageing mother whom he wants to protect and a contact person whom he regards as an important relationship. He even takes into account the material circumstances of his life and works to change them (intermediate care, an own flat which he applies for and eventually gets). As a result of his having made this decision and its social consequences, his symptoms diminish and his medication can be reduced.

For Susanne it was a question of regaining control over her life. She regains control, both in relation to her own life, the feeling that she is able to direct it, and in relation to other people whom she experiences as having too much power over her:

You increased the tempo as you saw fit... you got things under control, it seems?
Yes, that's right, I did. It's just as you say, I got it under control and I felt that it was at my own initiative, I was the one who had made the decision. This was very very important for me. Because everything else I had been doing was decided by other people or by an inner imperative about what you are supposed to do in life.
Actually this is the first thing having to do with other people that I decided for myself that I wanted to do. (...) So, I can see that during that time I drove up the tempo a bit at a time and got involved a little bit with this and a little bit with that and used the gym as a springboard, a kind of fumbling period of trial and error... Just generally how should you act with other people? How do you talk to them... how do you communicate... without losing yourself, and without riding roughshod over the other? That was the big project of my life back then... (Susanne)

It may be that David, in the following excerpt, has formulated a general principle for how decisions, power and control are related to recovery:

I got the feeling that there were more and more opportunities available to me, that I was somehow getting healthier... that I was getting my life under control, that more and more opportunities were opening up for me and I could do things and had a little surplus.

272

The self finds itself

Recovery is often described as a process and not as a point in time when suddenly everything changes. Seen from this perspective, recovery is life itself. It is the successive regaining of control over one's life, of feeling secure in interpersonal relationships. For the self that is being described exists in relation to other people, whether or not this relationship is expressed as loneliness and isolation or are profound and enduring ones.

> I had a little problem functioning in groups; I kind of withdrew and let other people do the talking. But one-to-one it worked pretty good. But lately it's been getting better, I'm a little more on the ball and have more self-confidence and I've also joined a singles club, to sort of, you know ... I have a lot of time on my hands that I don't know what to do with... I have a bit of a bad conscience about calling my friends as often as I do, and it's kind of hurtful to feel that I need them more than they need me; that's not so good. So I've been trying to be a little more strategic about it and for a while I joined a user organisation, and last summer I worked at the hospital and it's really gone quite well. I'm beginning to have a little more self-confidence and getting some acknowledgement from others. It's beginning to come together now, but it happened after my health improved and I began to be able to recognise the early signs. (David)

Measuring up in one's own eyes

At the time of the interview, the respondents have all recovered to a greater or lesser extent. But regardless of how far along they have come in their recovery process, most of them talk about recovery in relation to how they perceive themselves and thus in relation to their symptoms/ problems. In each case recovering has made them feel more satisfied with themselves. Erik, for example, besides attending the local day care centre, lives in his own flat and has begun trial employment. He has begun to re-establish contact with the world outside the psychiatric hospital. He is taking what he considers a low dose of medication and has only sporadic contact with psychiatric services. Nevertheless, he still talks about having delusions. During the interview he refers to himself as divided. "It has nothing to do with me", he says in reference to his delusions. But these experiences now play a limited role in Erik's life. The delusions do not seem to be a threat to his self-image.

> I can still see flashes. I saw a sign when I was sitting on the balcony... there are still signs all around me, but the thing is I don't give a damn anymore... Bugger that! I don't think about it. I was looking at the sky, a clear blue sky, a week ago, and it was written "ITR". On a clear blue sky there comes a cloud and it's written "ITR". I just sat there and looked at it and thought: "Go on and have your fun, damn you, because I'm well now. I'm out of it." (Erik)

Sören, on the other hand, has had no contact with psychiatry for several years. He is not on medication, lives in his own flat without community support, but has intentionally not sought contact with the ordinary job market. He visits a local day care centre sporadically, but also engages in social activities of his own making. During the interview, Sören describes how he became reunited with himself at a time when he had reduced his medication, had made the arrangements for getting a flat of his own and had begun to socialise with people outside of psychiatry.

> I remember once when I was walking on [name of a street] in [a certain year] and I'm feeling: "Now I am myself. I'm back!" That was fun, even though I've had some problems since then as well, but everyone does. I had begun painting and it was a gas. I went to evening classes at the adult education centre. After that, I've just kept on with it and it's awesome having your own exhibition. (Sören)

Nils is another who expresses joy in the interview. He has talked about his life, his experiences and his recovery, and just doing that has contributed to his recovery.

> I think it's the joy of experiencing who I really am. To have found... maybe saying the joy of finding your way back home seems sentimental, but the joy of knowing this is me and of having the chance to talk about... the central nerve in my life just now is telling about it. Not for it's own sake,

but because I refuse to be silent again. I refuse to be shut out – shut out and silent. (Nils)

During the interview Sven summarises his experiences and formulates how he sees them – from having wanted to be someone else to trying to find his way back to himself:

And my uncle said something very true and something that I've also thought myself. It's something he said to me once when I was talking about the illness: "Yes, but Sven, maybe later you'll be able to find your way back to yourself". And that was a good thing to say, at least for me, because it was so true. because, before I got sick, I was myself, you know what I mean. I was. And while I tried to loosen up inside, like I tried to coax myself back into myself. Maybe that sounds kind of funny, but I've, like, tried to find a way to get back into myself. It's hard to explain how you do that, but you know what I mean. (…)

And I've found the way back to myself a little bit. You remember I talked about wanting to be someone else and that's just where it comes in… I wanted to get back into myself because I nearly climbed out of my own skin, somehow, because afterwards I began to really think that I was someone else. I behaved and talked and thought just like him, this person I thought was really tops… (Sven)

Not either/or, but both

The self has been reunited with itself and is able to present itself in front of others. It was not a disaster. "I am the illness" has gradually become "I have" and even "I have had" a problem. The biographical disruption (Bury 1982), which the experience of having lost one's self results in, has been transformed into a new life history that can be incorporated into an *ongoing biography*.

However, the break between "before" and "after" (before the onset of the disorder and recovery and after the onset of the disorder and the recovery process) should not prevent us from noticing that in the majority of the life stories some degree of continuity is still maintained. The element of continuity is reflected in the story plot (a heroic person in search of him-/herself), but also in the stories of practice.

In several of the stories the first symptoms appear to be the person's efforts to find a solution to a life problem or identity problem. These attempts are sometimes successful, but in most cases they have led to a crisis, a breakdown.

Through these stories of practice we get a glimpse of persons who, in the midst of the deepest suffering, cannot be reduced to that suffering, whether it be illness, functional disability or whatever. The suffering and symptoms are real. None of the persons we interviewed deny their existence. They exist; sometimes they are understood and can be explained, sometimes not. But they exist for the most part in the context of the person's efforts to manage a difficult and bewildering situation.

That some ways of trying to cope seem bizarre and are doomed to fail make them no less an expression of the person's continued existence as a complex being. From this perspective, "symptoms" must be perceived in their experiential context. What from the outside can be interpreted as "negative symptoms" may actually be expressions of the person's active efforts to cope with a problematic situation. (See Corin & Lauzon 1992)

Throughout the whole course of events being described in the interviews, there are repeated examples of the respondents' ways of relating to themselves and to other people. Both the breakdown and the subsequent recovery are depicted as a relational interaction, one that is most certainly highly complex, but still recognisable to other human beings; recognisable to oneself. The other is not a stranger.

Lastly, there is reason to once again point out that the respondents in this study are firmly rooted in the same cultural heritage as that of psychiatry. This applies not only to the content of their delusions and hallucinations, but also to the central conceptions that guide them during the onset of the illness and through the recovery process; for example, the desirability of having a good enough integrated, coherent, stable self.

---

[1] In psychological theories the first person pronoun "I", like the term "self", has a particular meaning separate from everyday usage. The references to "I" and "self" in the interviews, unless otherwise indicated, denote their everyday usage.

9

Others
Co-actors and counter-actors

The actions speaks louder
than the words.
Keb' Moe'– on CD, "Just like you"

The impossible relationship?

In the psychotic world, such as it is described in much of the literature
in psychiatry, there is very little room for other people. The symptoms
and mental breakdown disrupt the basis for the person's ability to
direct his/her words and actions toward other people and comprehend
their words and actions in turn, at least as the others intended them.
Cullberg (1999) writes:

> … the patient's way of thinking, interpreting and experiencing are
> dictated from very regressive, primitive levels of the personality; he has
> regressed in his thinking to the level of a two-year-old. Events lose their
> ordinary meaning and the patient interprets them in his own highly
> personal way. Concepts like love, death, friendship, deceit and morality
> are as irrelevant to him as they are to the little child. (p. 268)

Against this background, it is not surprising that the Swedish
Psychiatric Association (1996) write:

> Besides producing a disturbed sense of reality, the illness also adversely
> affects the individual's relationships with family and friends, work
> capacity and possibility to lead a normal social life. (p. 11)

277

If we accept Bleuler's characterisation of schizophrenia and its basic symptoms of autism, distorted associations, ambivalence and emotional affect, and accept what he described as the second level of symptoms, which comprises hallucinations, delusions, disturbed behaviour and compulsive behaviour, then it is not surprising that the social relationships of persons so afflicted are either no longer functioning or have become so distorted that they can hardly be called relationships.

The conclusion drawn in a number of studies is that the social networks of people diagnosed as psychotic are more limited and of a different kind than those of the general population or of patients with a diagnosed neurosis. The psychotic person's social network comprises few individuals outside the family circle and professional caregivers. (See e.g. Pattison, Defransciso, Wood, Frazier & Crowder 1975) Beels (1978, 1979, 1981) has analysed the early career of people with a schizophrenia diagnosis as a network crisis. Not only is the patient's very identity questioned, but also that of the person's family and of the self-image the family tries to project. However, Salokangas (1996) is critical of the idea that the onset of schizophrenia always results in a network crisis for patients, their families and friends. Although the patient's social network tends to shrink in connection with the events surrounding the initial hospitalisation, it expands again after a time, except for those patients who no longer had any contact with their families when the breakdown occurred.

Ewertzon and Forsell (1999) find the current view on the social networks of patients diagnosed as psychotic to be problematic. Most of the knowledge on this subject is based on studies of American conditions. Ewertzon and Forssell show that in Sweden the social networks of first-time patients do not automatically decrease during the first year of hospitalisation. Nor is there a marked decrease in the social network of the family as a whole during this period.

With time, however, the life conditions of people with a severe mental disorder limit their possibility to maintain and expand their social networks. Nevertheless, there are certain categories of people who remain a part of the patient's network:

1. Family members, many of whom continue to give the patient material support when society's safety net is insufficient, but who, at the same time, are often described in the psychiatric literature as an emotional threat
2. Other people with mental problems of their own and in whose company the patient's problems may be aggravated unless their social encounters occur in some form of professionally led self-help group
3. Professionals, primarily from the health care sector but today also from the social services

The stories of the persons in this study depict periods of deeply felt loneliness but also of actual isolation.

According to most of those we interviewed, loneliness, expressed as feeling isolated even when there are many people around, was the original problem which their first unsuccessful attempts to find a solution were intended to remedy. In several instances it was these attempts at a remedy that brought them into contact with psychiatry in the first place.

For several of our interview persons, loneliness tends to lead to social isolation during periods when the symptoms are especially acute. The symptoms themselves, various side-effects of the illness and an insecure financial situation render more difficult contact with others outside the circle of family, caregivers and fellow sufferers. In the stories rock bottom is hit when the person stands alone and is isolated both from his/her own self and from others. But this is never quite the case.

People who have recovered, without exception, see relationships with others, both people and pets, as being of central importance in the recovery process. These others may serve as vicarious bearers of hope, the hope of one day living a different life than that of a chronic. Sometimes the others provide material support. They may also be recipients of the person's own demonstrations of caring, as when he/she gives the other a gift. The others may symbolise continuity and wholeness in the patient's life. Lastly, it is in relationships with others that the person tests the viability of his/her recovery.

The various others mentioned in the life stories play somewhat specialised roles in the recovery process. For purposes of analysis, we have divided these others into four categories: family, professional, "ordinary" people and pets.

Family

Family members play two distinct and diametrically opposed roles in the recovery stories: as the direct cause of the individual's current problems, and as a significant contributor to the recovery process. In some of the stories family members were given both roles.

We asked no questions during the interviews about the subjects' backgrounds nor what they thought had caused their problems. Nevertheless, as mentioned earlier, the respondents presented a number of hypotheses regarding the cause of their problems. They tried to place the recovery process in some sort of explanatory context. One such context was childhood and the decisive impact of parents on the child's growing years. Persons who had been treated with psychotherapy were more inclined to refer to their childhood in the interview.

Irene and Lars are two respondents who describe their mothers as having played an important role in bringing on their current problems. Fathers are seldom mentioned; and when mentioned, they are assigned a generally positive but peripheral but role:

> It all ended when they got divorced. My mum had been having an affair for several years. (…) So after two weeks, there you were in [name of town] with your mum and youngest brother. Down there you had to manage on your own. My brother stuck it out for about half a year then moved back with my dad. I wasn't allowed to. A lot of prestige was tied up in my staying there. They weren't really interested in me, just in what people would say.
>
> After only half a year they bought a house in [a neighbouring resort town] and so she and [name of mother's new partner] wanted to go visit, but I wasn't really welcome. So every weekend I had to take the train to granny and granddad who lived in another town. If they weren't home, I had to spend the weekend with different employees in my mum's firm while they went off on their own. Every holiday I went to my dad's place. (Irene)

I lived for three years in the most horrible torture, day and night, it never stopped. When I was 13 and just entering puberty, I must have been extra impressionable then. Having to see my mum naked all day long. Even if I wasn't so aware of what it meant back then. To be forced to lie beside her in her bed, naked, and rub her breasts and all those other rituals we had to do and which created like an incestuous tension, which I felt… I think it was… I'm just speculating now because I can't know what that little child was thinking… but I found it intolerable and I knew about the institution because I had spent some time there three years' earlier when my mum and dad were getting a divorce. So I knew it existed. I knew that there was hope of rescue. (…) I had a little contact my dad who was living by himself then. Instead of going to school I went to his place when he came home for lunch and he gave me some money to buy yoghurt or something and I was with him instead of going to school, and my mum didn't know about it. So I cheated on her in the maximum way. (…) Dad tried to help, too. I think he contacted the social services or the child welfare authorities or something or other, and told them that this couldn't go on, but they didn't do anything, not until I walked into their office and said: "You've got to put me in the institution. And I'm never going back to my mum." (Lars)

Irene and Lars describe different degrees of abandonment during childhood, a circumstance in their lives which they see as being directly related to their mental problems. It can be worth noting that both Lars and Irene had other persons in their family who played a positive role in their lives. In both cases, the grandparents are important because they stood up for their grandchildren in opposition to their own daughters. Constellations are formed consisting of grandparents and absent fathers who have become estranged through a combination of divorce, death and drug abuse. There are several such constellations in the life stories.

Are your grandmother and grandfather among the "benefactors" [a word Irene used earlier in the interview]?
Yes, they died late, in [year]. I have since read about so called "significant others", something you have to have if you're not going to go completely off your rocker. That's what they were for me, even though it was at a distance. They stood up for me. Grandmother got more and more angry

with my mum. She cried on the phone at the end and said that she should have adopted me herself. I told her that she was already old when I started getting into trouble and they wouldn't have let her. "We should have taken you away from your mother and that bastard [the mother's new partner]. I'll never forgive your mother." You need those ... (Irene)

I had my grandmother and I also had mental pictures and impressions from the short time I went to school. Apparently it gave me enough, an inner life force. So somehow there was the seed of a life force that said "Take up your sword! You have a right to your own life!" My mother couldn't take everything away from me. Even if it was hidden from me, it triggered my making the decision that I couldn't stay there anymore because there's something that's going to keep me from surviving it.
Can you give an example of what your grandmother did to give you that idea?
She was my father's mother and, first of all she liked me a lot. I've always felt that way, and she has always shown me I was her favourite grandchild. She has a lot of grandchildren. I have always felt that she really liked me a whole lot, even though she was immature in her own way and never understood the psychological mechanisms behind social relationships and things like that. But anyway, for me she has always been a normal person who takes care of her house, who can take responsibility, who stands pat, who is stable; she can put up with stuff and doesn't break down in the face of internal or external threats.
How do you know that you were her favourite grandchild?
You feel it. It's not something written down on paper... It's just something I know. She has special affection for me. She always has. She still calls me "Lasse-my-pet", even now. She is pretty old but she's clear in her head and has helped me a lot, although she doesn't really understand the seriousness of my problems. Like when people say they have problems with their nerves or are a little depressed. That's how she thinks, but she knows somewhere what a terrible time I've had. (Lars)

The presence of good, if remote, figures and their importance for the person's ability to manage difficult life situations has been described in the literature in connection with so called super kids (Werner 1995) and with KASAM[1] (Antonovsky 1991). One of the factors that enhance our ability to manage difficulties later in life is having had a good relationship with a primary caregiver during infancy.

It must be pointed out, however, that persons recovering from severe mental disorders cannot be described as "super kids". Nor are they likely to have a high KASAM score. They have not been able to manage the difficulties they encountered in life; instead they have experienced such deep crises that they have been classified as mentally ill and were hospitalised. This makes their recovery even more remarkable.

Some parents play a more complex role when it comes to understanding the causes of the problems and how these problems are later managed in the recovery process. These family members stand by the person, in good times and bad. The relationship may be riddled with conflict at times, but through their resilience these family members embody the hope of better times and continuity in the person's life.

There are several aspects to continuity. In the stories reported here several family members emerge as guarantors of continuity of time and place. Jan gives an illustration of these two aspects of continuity when he describes the role his mother has played in his recovery:

> If I have to look for what I call a lifeline, it's my mother and our confrontations. She has never given up, despite my screaming at her. Despite the traumatic experiences we had earlier in our lives, she never gave up. I guess that's been the most important thing. She has always been there for me, no matter what I did, she has always stood by me. That's why I'm so grateful to my mother. I don't what would have happened if I hadn't had her. She's very important. And then, I've had some friends. But I think my mum has meant the most. She has always been there for me, no matter how I behaved, no matter what I shouted at her, or what I did, she's always shown me her best side. There's no question about it, she has meant the most. And from what I can see, everyone has a good opinion of her. Yeah, sure, I've had a pretty wide network, but most important of all has been my mum. (Jan)

The person being described here is in no way a wholly good human being. On the contrary, Jan implies that he and his mother have had some tough times together. They have had their share of conflicts (and perhaps still do). But it may be that it is for this very reason that the role his mother has played in his life has been so important. She has stood by him the whole time, from childhood to the present. She has been there for him through the good times, and through the bad. She has been both the good mother and the bad mother. And has stayed. She is someone to visit, someone to borrow money from, someone who calls him up from time to time.

She represents a collection of events in Jan's life which, had she not been there, would have been split up among other people, such as others in the family, mental health workers, friends and workmates, and among other places, such as the home, hospital wards, outpatient clinics, workplaces, and so forth. Thus, she embodies and can harbour the contradictory totality of Jan's life experience.

The role played by family members in the recovery process can perhaps be most easily contrasted with the role of the institution, a place where the patient meets a series of professionals, each with a different role, and who take over from one another according to their own rules (own time schedules, vacation periods, time off for study) and without any direct connection to the patients' particular needs. Generally speaking, professionals work in institutions where the care of patients is divided between a day staff and a night staff. There are other professionals who work more long-term with patients either at inpatient or outpatient facilities.

I was lucky in several respects. One of the things that was so lucky for me was that back then they had this little unit, the admissions ward. It had five beds and you couldn't stay there for long because it was only for pre-liminary examinations. In principle you could only stay one night. But for some reason I spent a whole week there. It was because there was no demand for beds. That's when I got into very close contact with the staff. I never had to run out into the corridor and feel desolation; when I went out into the corridor, there were always staff right outside. There was an office behind glass. As soon as I opened my door, they could see that I went out. Right away I could get into communication with the staff. They let me into their space.

What was so lucky for you?

It was that little unit… and having the staff close by.

284

Did they do anything special?
No. It was just so open. I could always talk to them. I don't remember any of our conversations, but I remember that they let me borrow a typewriter. Closeness, that the unit was so small, that I didn't have a bad time with desolation, because desolation is the big problem, actually; just that total loneliness; it didn't get worse in that unit. Thank God they didn't send me somewhere else, because that could have reinforced the desolation. (Bengt)

Another feature characterising family members is that they take responsibility, sometimes serving as a connecting link to psychiatric care. In several of the life stories, it is parents and siblings who arrange for the person to come under psychiatric care:

... I felt that this can't go on anymore and my wife and I went to the hospital and we met the doctor who was on call then and my wife asked the doctor if there wasn't some other way of handling this than what we were doing. He looked at us for a long minute and then said, well yes, actually there are therapists who work differently but there are not so many of them, and then he tells us about this man [name of a therapist]. (Nils)

In such manner, some family members become an important boundary-setter and a helping hand when a person is in danger of losing his/her bearings, or has already done so.

Pets

Pets are mentioned often enough in the recovery stories to warrant being taken into account as a contributing factor in the recovery process. In each case the pet in question is a dog. The foremost feature of dogs as pets is that they help to break through the patient's isolation and that they are living creatures upon which the patient can shower affection and care. Dogs help to break through isolation because they offer companionship in themselves, but are also a less demanding form of companionship than human beings. The companionship they offer can be a substitute for human company, but it can also be a way to find human companionship.

Irene gives an example of how her dog became the only meaningful companion she had during a difficult period in her life:

Last spring I made my life's best investment by far; I bought an Irish sheepdog. A big wonderful dog. (…)
It sounds like most of what has happened after you left the psychiatric hospital you arranged on your own?
Yes, no one helped me. I had no friends, no one I could confide in, no one I could talk to; instead, all those years afterwards you had to do everything on your own. It really hurts, that no one cares about… but I can't say that I was all alone because I had my dog. She meant so much to me. She has been my loyal companion. She was the one I sat down and talked with. We took long walks together. It was mostly for her sake that I tried to stay sober.

Erik got himself a dog when he had come quite far along in his recovery process. For him as well, his dog fills the function of breaking through his isolation, but in a different way than for Irene:

Together with him I get out more. We take walks outside a lot. He loves to swim. When my mother goes out to the cottage on weekends, I go down to the lake and swim and cook on the grill. And I have my friend with me. At home we can cuddle. You're talking to him like you're crazy or something, but that's how it is. The more you talk to him, the smarter he gets. He knows exactly when I'm setting a boundary. My dog has given me a lot this past year. Before that I was so lonely.

Dogs as pets also help to normalise a person's life in that they are a way of making social contacts. Dog owners meet other people when out walking their dog; not as a patient or former patient, but as a person who is no different from anyone else. A pet dog serves as a topic of conversation that has nothing to do with illness, suffering or psychiatric treatment.

Erik is quite clear about how his dog is regarded at the day centre he attends compared with the clinic where he goes for psychiatric treatment:

The contact person at the work centre always asks about my dog. They never do that at the clinic. They don't give a fuck about my dog. They don't realise how much he means to me. He means all the world to me.

Because dogs need care and are dependent on their owners, but also because they show such affection for their carers, they provide scope for the patient's capacity to take care of someone else (not only the one who is taken care of), the capacity to give. In this way, owning a dog also demands structuring daily life in some way:

Another thing that this is all about is that I was living with my parents for a while, in [year] I think it was, I guess it was for two summers; well in any case my ex-wife and the boy come out with a little puppy for me. So I moved back home by myself because I had a dog. Having a dog kept me occupied and then moving back to my own flat gave me something to do. Even if it was only for a short time, I think that owning a dog was important. It was like a sign to myself that I should move back to my own place. That was a kind of outside help. And that's why I could take still another step after I started taking a medicine that helped. (Jan)

Professionals – the components of professionalism

Professionals play a central and positive role in all of the life stories we collected in this study. But compared with the large number of professionals our respondents have met through the years, few are mentioned as having contributed to the recovery process.

The opposite of professional is amateur. In etymological terms amateur means one who loves. One who does something for the pleasure of it. Professionals are salaried employees who have at least some specialist training. It is their job, and therefore demands can be made on the professional that cannot be made on the amateur. In order for professionals to be regarded as professional, they must follow certain rules that constitute an expression of their basic knowledge and the basis of their professionalism. These rules are grounded in a body of knowledge that distinguishes the professional from the amateur, but they are also rules that create a distance between the professional and the patient.

Parsons (1951) lists four demands that the professional caregiver is expected to fulfil:

- "The obligation to do everything [the therapist] can do within reason to 'help' his patient" (p. 457)
- "... a special permissiveness to express wishes and fantasies which would ordinarily not be permitted expression in normal social relationships..." (p. 458)
- "...the therapist is expected to control his countertransference impulses and that such control is in general a condition of successful therapy" (p. 458)
- "... the conditional manipulation of sanctions by the therapist" (p. 458)

Therapists are thus allowed to place themselves above the rules for normal social intercourse because they are, and continue throughout the therapy to be, aware of themselves and of their altruistic goals, and because they can separate their own needs from those of the client/ patient. It is possible to tell the therapist about one's most forbidden thoughts and feelings, without risking incurring the kind of response that ordinary people would give. Instead the therapist will deliberately, by drawing upon his/her unique qualities, guide the patient, simply by not reacting in the way others would react. The therapist's power and position is in conformance with the patient's role. The patient is released from various obligations in the society (such as work, social interaction, taking sick leave) in exchange for agreeing to be treated.

A professional client-therapist relationship differs markedly from the normal rules of social intercourse. It is this difference that is behind the patient's being able to break the rules connected with intimacy, such as nudity, physical touching, expression of primitive drives, expression of forbidden thoughts and actions. This lays the ground-work for treatment and recovery. In the same work, Parsons points out that this is true not only for the psychotherapeutic relationship but also for the whole field of medicine:

Indeed, the effective utilization of these aspects of the physician's role is a prominent part of what has long been called "the art of medicine". (p. 459)

To achieve this neutrality, says Parsons, therapists must fulfil certain obligations. They shall not talk about themselves and their personal lives. Nor shall they enter into reciprocal relationships with their patients:

> In general, that is, the therapist does not reciprocate the expectations which are expressed, explicitly or implicitly, in the patient's deviant wishes and fantasies. The most fundamental wishes, we may assume, involve reciprocal interaction between the individual and others. (p. 458)

Parsons writes later in the study about the patient's "attempt to 'seduce' [the therapist] into reciprocation". (p. 458) The attempt to establish a reciprocal relationship is merely a way to obstruct the therapist from doing his job and to avoid undertaking the necessary work with oneself that the patient must go through in order to recovery.

Infringement of these rules is regarded as a sign that the therapist is unprofessional, lacks the prerequisite knowledge and personal maturity and is incompetent to help the patient with his/her problems. Such infringements are a serious threat to the efficacy of the treatment and go a long way to explain failures in therapy.

Parsons takes his model of professionalism in health care from the psychotherapeutic tradition, but also from Freud, who, as Parsons points out, was in turn part of a tradition that stretches far back in time. The main task for doctors in the Middle Ages was to remove all obstacles that could prevent the illness from running its natural course. If the illness were allowed to run its course, it would fade away of its own accord. The notion that illnesses have a natural course has survived other notions of that period. A common thread in the thinking of theoreticians about mental hospitals at the end of the 1700s and later among the early psychoanalysts was to create a setting where pathological processes could have free rein, secluded from environmental influences. Early modern medicine was based on observation. And to be observable, illness processes have to develop unhampered in an influence-free environment – in a hospital or laboratory setting. In like manner the neutrality of the psychotherapist and of the therapeutic setting is intended to allow the pathological processes operating within the patient to come to the surface unfettered and undisturbed in order to be analysed. The analytical setting was devised by Freud, partly as a reaction to hypnosis, which he did not regard as a form of treatment but of manipulation. With correct treatment instead of manipulation, long-lasting results can be achieved. Psychoanalysis was thought to produce results, not by manipulating the patient, but by coming to grips with the underlying disorder. (Swain 1994).

Implicit in this line of reasoning is the idea that it is possible to provide the same type of care for all patients. The professionalism of the therapist guarantees it. Central to this conception of professionalism is the assertion that the person who has been professionally trained (and accredited by the state) ceases to be a unique individual during work hours and can be anyone who has the same training. It is the technique that is essential, everything else is an irrelevant influence and not treatment and placebos; it is whatever "one pleases" and therefore belongs to the category unscientific, which signifies that something may have an effect but is not treatment.

Severely disturbed patients are said to be disturbed in their capacity to establish social relationships. For this reason only a few accredited professional groups can claim that they possess the means and methods for reaching such patients and exerting a deliberate influence over them. The only acceptable ways of reaching the patient are through chemistry and/or through the highly ritualised therapy session where the rules directing the sessions are the instruments by which the therapist tries to reach whatever might still be intact of the personality.

Professionals who facilitate recovery

The professionals mentioned in the recovery stories comprise a broader group than those that normally figure in such contexts. In addition to doctors and therapists, the stories also mention nurses, mental health workers, social workers, hospital aids, employment counsellors and supported housing counsellors. If professionalism as defined by Parsons is represented primarily by the first two categories, these professionals influence in turn the other groups of caregivers by virtue of their training, supervision and the power of the leading ideas within their professional culture.

The professionals who are described in the recovery stories as having contributed to the recovery process constitute a paradox. The basis for their claim to professionalism is a technique that has developed through the scientific study of the nature of severe mental disorders. But this technique seems to play a subordinate role in recovery (which calls into question the scientific claims upon which their respective techniques are based).

It could be said that professionals who contribute to recovery in these life stories do so partly because they display the same qualities found among ordinary people, among amateurs or non-professionals. In addition to the qualities that Frank and Gunderson (1987) mentioned – openness, warmth, empathy, active engagement, optimism – other terms occurring in the literature are "being heard", "being seen", "feeling respected", "being the focus of attention", "the other's willingness to devote their time" (see e.g. Olofsson 2000). These are rather abstract terms and give us little help to grasp the underlying reality to which they refer. They can easily become all-inclusive or blanket concepts. Such blanket concepts do not emanate from the context of practice and are therefore abstract, despite their apparent commonplaceness. It is not easy to know what they mean in practice. In fact, they teach us very little about theory and practice. Olofson (2000) expresses this problem when she writes:

> The question is how do professionals and patients together learn to understand and confirm each other's perspectives. The answer is rather naïve, but quite simply, through talking and listening to each other. (p. 59)

The naïve answer is hardly enough. Analysing stories of practice allows us to penetrate the practice behind these abstract concepts to see how therapists actually go about giving of themselves, what they do when they listen and see in ways that are conducive to recovery.

The collection of stories in this study contains descriptions of which professionals have contributed to the persons' recovery. These descriptions call into question the traditional formalised conception of professionalism. The stories mainly describe actions of the professional that constitute infringements of the formal rules of professionalism, actions that broaden the framework for professionalism. But it also seems that it is not these new boundaries for professionalism as it relates to patients that is of primary importance. Just as important is the actual infringement of the rules. In the choice between patient and institution, the professionals come down on the side of the patient. In doing so they take a great risk. They have ignored the tenets of their professional knowledge and broken rules that constitute their professionalism. Without this base, who are they? Amateurs?

To break the rules is not only a threat to the professional's identity (as a professional), it may also incur the risk of exposure, and therewith formal and informal reprisals; to be classed by other professionals as "unbounded" (Topor 1996a), which thereby equates them with the patients.

Also of importance for persons who have recovered seems to be the knowledge that the professional does not break rules for all of his/her patients. What will have an effect is highly individual. This is not about inventing a new technique. If it were it would be a new rule and not an infringement and the professional's actions would not bring the risk of reprisal. If an infringement becomes a new rule, it is not an infringement. It becomes instead a new institution and as such creates the need for new infringements.

By breaking rules the professional emerges as a person. It is likely that the infringements reported in the stories were not conscious actions based on strategic planning and on having found the appropriate references in the literature pertaining to the theoretical and practical elements of the therapist's school of therapy. Rather, it seems that the professional is drawn into the interaction with the patient and is unable to resist being "socially responsive" (Asplund 1987b). A genuine interest in the other person breaks down the disciplined responsiveness of professionalism. (Asplund 1987b, see also Nilsson 1997)

The patient appears to be quite aware of the rule infringements when they occur. He/she may even feel moved by the infringement and become aware that something important is happening out there which could happen inside him/her as well. The persons who spoke about these incidences have all had years of practical learning about rules, about what applies and what does not apply. Breaking the rules generates a sense reciprocity or mutuality; the patient and the professional become "accomplices in crime", dependent on each other and on the relationship they have entered into with one another. The recovery stories point out several areas where such infringements have occurred.

Professionals who base their work on maintaining distance apply a number of basic principles in their professions. The main one is, as we have seen, that professionals should not reveal themselves as persons. By stringently regulating the time and place for the therapy sessions, therapists acquire a tool for their work which also serves as an external support and identification badge for their claim to professionalism.

Time

In psychiatry patients' contacts with treatment programmes and staff are generally regulated in fixed units of time:

- There are telephone hours, office hours and visiting hours regulate when patients can come into contact with the mental health services.
- The therapy sessions take place according to fixed time schedules for the patients already in the system in order to regulate their accessibility to the therapist. How long should each session last? Where and how often should they occur?
- Therapeutic methods and the institution's organisation and division into sectors regulate the terms and duration of the contact. Short-term therapies are by definition limited in time, as are therapies based on a system of buy-and-sell services. An ongoing contact can be broken off for reasons that are unrelated to how the patient feels when the stipulated length of time for the therapy has been reached.

- The duration of the contact may also depend on how the person is assessed by the organisation or organisations that are responsible for the patient's care.

Patients are shifted between hospital wards, between in- and out-patient facilities and between the psychiatric services and the social services according to the institution's own rhythms and routines. The lack of continuity is often a practical arrangement, although during their journey through the institutions patients often come into contact with persons they have met and places that they have visited before.

The examples of infringements of both the regulatory system of institutions and the rules of professionalism touch upon all these aspects. In its simplest form, the infringements have to do with the professionals giving the process the time it needs, with keeping the patient when they are not obliged to and despite legitimate opportunities to terminate the therapy.

Anne tells about an occasion when she first met the mental health worker who became her contact person on the ward where she was being treated and later after her discharge.

Why did you choose him that morning?
He's nice. He's the kind of person I've been missing, was what I was thinking.
How is a person who is nice to you?
I had had a bad night and was belted down, and so he came in that morning and was supposed to keep watch over me, as they say. But he untied me. I was feeling calm and we went for coffee and we sat and talked and I felt that we really got close to one another. He sat there and drank coffee with me. He wasn't in a hurry, he didn't have to go off somewhere. He had time to listen. I needed that then. There was no rush. And when I was finished, after we had eaten and I had taken my tray back, he was still sitting there when I came back to the table. And we talked a little bit more. That's my kind of person. That's how I want people to be. It was so cosy. We were honest with one another. I asked if I could have his phone number and if he would like to be my contact person. He thought I meant my contact person at the hospital and so he was, but afterwards I asked if he could continue with me. I didn't know

how he would get paid, but it's worked now for 11 years. He's paid by the municipality. (Anne)

It is worth noting that this is a psychotic patient who makes note of the mental health worker's conduct, judges it as adequate for her needs and makes the suggestion that he become her contact person. In Anne's story the health worker stands by her, not merely as her guard, but more as a partner in the relationship. She notices this. It is not part of the routine. Anne knows. She has been belted down countless times. Words like "nice" and "cosy" are introduced and given a frame of reference in the actions of the health worker: he has chosen her. He puts her above hospital routine. The fact that the contact has continued for 11 years at the time of the interview points at an aspect of time that is mentioned in several of the stories: to know that one has enough time, that the institution's organisation will not be allowed to interrupt an ongoing contact. This assurance, that one will be given enough time, has for some persons become a basis for starting a recovery process:

> That's important, I mean… Being calm, not being pressured, just letting things come of their own accord… He told me afterwards that it wasn't necessary to pressure me and ask me a lot of questions, because I could get going under my own steam… I had this great need to talk and get things off my chest. But I think that time was the most important thing. He was there and was there and was there, regardless of what I did. If I tried and failed, he was still there for me. (Susanne)

The therapist who met with Susanne gave her power over aspects of the therapy: confidence in her desire and ability to make progress.

> And so I think that there probably are patients you have to set limits for and put a frame around them, but one thing that was very important for me, now when I think about my therapy, was that he always said that we had plenty of time. And he had pictures of things – that he showed me – like when he said: "Our therapy is like a book. And you are the one who decides how long that book is going to be. You are the one who ends the book." (Susanne)

The therapist's words are also a recognition of Susanne's ability to decide about her own life within the framework of her need for help. She is not reduced to her shortcomings.

> I thought about getting to that point... but at the same time I struggled to get further... but I didn't have much hope... there were times when I was really down... and it was just like he said, that it was his job too, to keep hope alive for me. And if you can't keep the faith yourself, I'll help you anyway.
> *Did you believe him when he said that?*
> Yes, I believed he meant it, but I didn't believe it was true. But I did believe he meant what he said...
> *So he was kind of like your anchor?*
> He was... He was all I had... So of course when he talked about things like that... I wanted him to say it... It was important to me that he said it. But I had, like, planned my life to be a long-term patient, I ... (slight smile) I did that... (Susanne)

At the same time Susanne's therapist compromises himself in a way that is not allowed. Professionals change jobs, institutions are shut down, reorganised, change treatment methods. Operating funds run out. To extend the length of the therapy beyond the time regulated by the institution is one way to put the patient's needs before the concerns of the institution, to decide in favour of the person behind the patient.

Several of the interview subjects mention that their relationship with their therapist continued even after the therapist had changed place of employment. Susanne continues her narrative:

> It's important to have – not a lot – but at least one good helper along the way. Someone who is resilient. Who is always there. And what I feel has been the most important of all that my therapist has done for me is to have put up with me all those years. He stood it for eight years. He didn't use that little trick that many therapists use when they change jobs – as a way to get rid of their patients. He took me along to all four jobs. (...)
> If he changed his job, he took me with him along with the rest of his stuff. All that time he made sure that he had time for me and that I was the one who decided how much time I needed. That made me feel very secure.
> *You didn't have to hurry...*

That's right, I was allowed to be in the process. And that's something that has really impressed me, both then and afterwards, but maybe mostly afterwards when I can see how valuable it was.

The therapist had somehow arranged at his new place of work that his colleagues would accept his working with a patient who came from outside their jurisdiction.

In Nils' case his contact with the therapist survived a move of over 100 miles from where the therapy contact was originally initiated:

> In [year] when he moved to [name of city] and I had to get through this huge, long, exhausting therapy before we were finished. I mean finished in quotation marks, for it's never really finished.
>
> So he had just taken a job in [name of city], it had to do with his not being able to keep his private practice any longer and he had to make new arrangements for himself. For me that was an awful let-down. He abandoned me just like my mother did. (…)
>
> I wrote him a 20-page letter where I poured out my anger… Every time, when I was a kid and as an adult, whenever I expressed my anger I was abandoned; but then I went to see him in [name of city], and I got the feeling that he wasn't going to abandon me. Maybe that's a little part of the answer; the memory of his sticking by me, of not abandoning me, that he was a person who listened, who stuck around. (Nils)

In several cases, the contact continued even after the therapy was officially terminated.

> Yes, ever since then I've had contact with her – like two or four times a year. We've also written to each other a few times, but not as my therapist. She was my therapist for a couple of years, psychiatric. (…)
>
> About half a year or a year ago after he had started with a new job, another therapist and I agreed that we would… he wouldn't be my therapist any more but we would still keep in touch. And that's what we've done… we've talked with another once a month… on the phone. And then we met at Christmas time. I think that was just great. (Ester)

Continued contact after the conclusion of a therapy, when there are no treatment plans or financial agreement to regulate the contact, creates an opening for redefining the relationship between the former patient and the former caregiver.

Time, documentation, financial compensation

Many of the rule infringements we have discussed so far have to do with the duration of the therapeutic relationship. But many of the stories of practice collected in the study touch upon still another aspect of how time is regulated, or how time is managed during the therapy sessions themselves. That professionals make themselves available during their free time, outside the regulated time frame and without payment, constitutes a breach of the boundary separating professionalism from amatuerism, a transgression against the very foundation of professionalism. If the encounter between patient and therapist occurs without any financial compensation within the ordinary framework, then why does it occur? What drives the professional to do it? An own need? An idea of the patient's needs?

The last time it was [name of a nurse who makes house calls] who phoned and I didn't manage to answer a question properly. I just stood there with my self-confidence at rock bottom – it was so low that she realised over the phone that I was in bad shape. So she started coming here three or four times a month, on her own time; she just came. And I said: "You're not allowed to do this. You have to be paid for your time here!" But she said that she just wanted to get to know me better. (Tina)

A similar thing happened once with [therapist's name] during her vacation when she was still living in [name of town]. The treatment home was closed for the summer holidays, and so she did me a favour and came and helped me assemble a loom. We met at the treatment home and worked for several days tying the thousands of threads. And then she taught me to weave a very complicated pattern. Since then I've done a lot of weaving. And here you have [therapist's name], someone who is renowned world over for her fantastic contributions, and here she is weaving with me. It feels great.
The Goddess climbs down. She was a goddess to me in the beginning. Now she's a grandmother, like any other regular grandmother, with faults and... Certainly I know that she has exceptional knowledge on this

subject, but that's not what I think about any more when I'm in therapy. (Lars)

To give of one's own time seems in practice to be a deconstruction of the therapist role but also of the patient role.

Jan met a doctor who not only broke the rules regulating the times for therapy but also infringed upon other major aspects of the customary relationship between doctor and patient. Jan sees a direct link between such infringements and his recovery:

> What also helped me during that period was the contact I had at the hospital with a visiting doctor from America. It's as if we were buddies. I could go out there and talk with him for an hour or so without anyone putting it on my record or charging a fee. At the time I was coming off medication, and I could talk to him about everything that was going on, or about anything at all. It was like supportive therapy after I was discharged. It gave me a boost. It just turned out that way. I guess he enjoyed having a visitor, so there was some mutual exchange. Also, he was important to me, most of all, like I said, because he didn't have anything to do with my records. It felt like it didn't really have anything to do with psychiatric care. As soon as you opened your mouth in care you got a few more lines added to your record. But it wasn't like that with him. (Jan)

Here, the infringements of the rules regulating time concern when the sessions were to take place ("I could go out there...") and their duration ("... an hour or so..."). And it seems that here the doctor does not appropriate all control over the content of the talk, which does not necessarily focus on the patient's problems ("...could talk to him about everything that was going on, or about anything at all").

The doctor does not ask for payment for his work. Nor does he write everything down in the patient's records, which Jan appreciates and associates with his recovery ("Also, he was important to me, above all, like I said, because he didn't have anything to do with my records."). That these infringements have the character of help becomes clear in the following excerpt: "It felt like it didn't really have anything to do with psychiatric care." This said about a professional psychiatrist whom the patient describes as having been important for his recovery.

Mutuality – the therapist as person

It could be argued that in the kind of relationship being described in some of the stories, the patient ceases to be only a patient and the therapist only a therapist. Instead, a relationship develops based on "mutuality" to use Jan's own term ("I guess he enjoyed having a visitor, so there was some mutual exchange.")

The idea of mutuality, that is to say mutuality in practice and not merely as rhetoric, means that the patient has something to offer. For patients mutuality means having something to give, something that might be of value to another person; one is not always in the position of being a recipient:

> From the time I was discharged in the fall of [year] until the fall of [three years later], I've had relaxation therapy with a psychologist I met at the children's psychiatric clinic, and I really liked that. So I travelled once a week from [hometown] to [city where the doctor practised] and had relaxation therapy with him.
>
> He was a person I liked a lot and I felt that he was someone who had a special liking for me as well. He drove me home after therapy and we had a meal together. He was a bohemian type and I got a chance to shoot the breeze and play a double-bass fiddle and eat health food. The atmosphere was really nice and I gave him some music cassettes I had recorded and he thought that was a lot of fun. (Lars)

In psychiatry the predominate image of professionalism sees the patient as a recipient – of treatment, care, medicine, talk. On the short-term, this probably is not a serious threat to the person's identity. But on the long-term, it could be a threat to the person's identity and position in social life. Reducing the person to only a recipient breaks down the reciprocity typical of most relationships and which has been described by Marcel Mauss, among others, in his study of gift-giving in so called primitive societies. Mauss (1968) focused on the central role that reciprocal gift-giving plays in social life and for personal identity. The reciprocal exchange of gifts, "Potlach", is the cement that binds tribes, clans, superiors and subordinates, families, individuals. It is a ritual that includes certain mutual obligations.

> The totality of the act is more than the obligation to repay a gift with a gift; it has two additional essential components as well: the obligation to give gifts and the obligation to accept the gift. (p. 27, translated from the French.)

On the importance of gift-giving for social life, Mauss wrote:

> To fail (neglect) to give, or to neglect to invite, is, like the refusal to accept, tantamount to a declaration of war. It is to reject friendship and social intercourse. (p. 28)

This is what the role of a sick person and the kind of professionalism advocated by Parsons are all about. Sick people are released from their social obligations, they need give nothing other than their submission to treatment. The cure re-establishes the social order. But for those who have not been cured a new problem arises: what was at first a temporary condition becomes permanent

In reference to the importance of gifts for the person's identity, Mauss drew the following conclusion from his study:

> A gift that has not yet been repaid with a gift in return degrades the recipient, especially if he has no intention of repaying the gift. (p. 85)

Bearing in mind Mauss' argumentation, it is interesting to analyse the rule infringements that the respondents talk about in these life stories. Infringements tend to establish mutuality in the relationship. Mutuality between patient and professional can be established at different stages in the relationship. Sometimes it exists at the very start, sometimes it is successively built up as the persons get to know each other. However, mutuality between professionals and patients seems to be rare and when it occurs is taken note of by the respondents. But they report mutuality as being not only uncommon, but also important for their recovery. From Mauss' perspective the professional's rule infringements could be said to re-establish the patient as a person, as someone who participates in social life on the same terms as everyone else, a person who counts for something.

Mutuality appears in two different guises. It can, on the one hand, be a conclusion that the respondents draw from their experiences of the professional's rule infringements. If the professional has broken certain rules and routines, and has done so only for this one person in particular (and not for others) and took risks in doing so, then the therapist must have benefited in some way from the encounter. This first aspect of mutuality has to do with an exchange on a person-to-person level.

Bengt's story gives an example of such an exchange. At the same time he provides a clue as to what made him feel that he "was listened to".

> That's when I had a meeting with the employment counsellor. We started to talk about the job, but pretty soon I was sitting there and describing my experiences. And this person was interested, she listened, and she didn't just listen but asked questions too, so after I had told her something, there was usually something in what I said that she asked me about. That's what made me feel she was interested in what I had to say. And I looked forward to our meetings. I was able to think: "I mustn't kill myself, for I have to meet her because we are going to continue our talks. Life really sucks and I want to kill myself, but on Tuesday I'm supposed to meet this person and on Thursday that person. I'll just have to stick it out and see what happens." It was this counsellor who made me feel more and more appreciated. In principle, it was because she listened and could make interesting comments. Ask questions that helped me develop what I had said. My being so verbal is an advantage. (…)
> *Were the counsellor's questions different from other people's questions?*
> I don't remember how she expressed herself, but when I was sitting there and talking, she used to interrupt me: "Listen up, about what you just told me, what was that like?" A little bit like you're doing now, trying to find a way in. And so I felt she was really interested. And just my feeling that she wasn't indifferent to me, that she was interested. Actually, we were supposed to talk about jobs, but we didn't. And so it took the time it took. We didn't just sit there for the little time of my appointment; well yes the time I was supposed to be there, but then it took the time it took, a little bit anyway. Feeling that was awfully important to me. She got to hear a lot,

but she put up with listening and being interested and thought that there was something there that she got back herself. That's almost certainly why she put up with it and let it go on. It was the feeling of having made contact instead of what is so frightening: desolation. Feeling abandoned and all alone. That's the nitty-gritty of psychosis: that maybe I'm the only one alive.

Ruth throws light on another way to achieve mutuality described in several of the stories: when professionals equate themselves in some respects with the patient on a personal level:

He's good because he puts himself out. Sometimes he tells me his thoughts about his own life. He did that when there was some reason for it. To me it felt like being in his confidence. He didn't tell me things in detail, but it was like he saw me as an equal by telling about his own experiences, and I thought that was just fine. It worked really well.
What kind of things did he tell about?
One thing was that he liked to paint, so right there we had a lot to talk about. What it felt like to go on a trip with other amateur painters, if people stood behind you and stared over your shoulder, how that could be so irritating… That's just a little example.

Mutuality can, on the other hand, also be built on the exchange of personal property between therapist and patient. Treatment and care in exchange for music, paintings, poems. The exchange of items is free of charge, but could entail an expense for the professional if he/she buys something from the patient. The item is something the patient has produced, a part of him-/herself. If a certain item could delight someone else, maybe that delight could also apply to the person who made it.

In both cases – the exchange of personal experiences or property – the therapist transcends the professional framework, in the latter case as a customer, in the former as something new which the respondents make a great effort to describe.

In an excerpt quoted earlier, Jan gives a definition of the relationship that developed between himself and the doctor who "helped [him]", who "was important". Jan concludes that what he has described, what helped him towards recovery, "felt like it didn't have anything to do with psychiatric care". The doctor's rule infringements had nothing to do with the routines of treatment. He describes his relationship with the professional as "like we were buddies", an as-if friend. With these words, Jan describes a relationship that nullifies professionalism. "Being buddies" is the opposite of being a professional. At the same time, for most people who have been in contact with psychiatry for a long time, their earlier friendships have usually been broken. Note that Jan does not say that he and the doctor became "buddies". He uses an expression that occurs in several of the interviews (see also Topor 1996): "we were like buddies", or as-if friends, where the words "as if" give a special connotation to the word buddy or friend.

The concept of an "as if" friend contains a wealth of meaning for understanding the relationship between a person with severe mental suffering and a professional who has ventured to break the rules. The idea of an "as if" friend can perhaps be understood as a first attempt to define a "new" kind of professionalism. New is in quotation marks because this kind of professionalism has certainly occurred before, but it has seldom been formulated in positive terms in that it conflicts with the predominant interpretation of the code of professionalism.

> Physicians as described in Parson's sociology are in turn responsible more to professional codes than to individual patients. According to modernist universalism, the greatest responsibility to all patients is achieved when the professional places adherence to the profession before the particular demands of any individual patient. (Frank 1995, p. 15)

Lars sees a problems in his relationship to a psychologist with whom he was in contact during his teens. As a teenager Lars had already acquired considerable experience of therapists. The interview takes place when Lars is older and has become even more knowledgeable about professionals.

> There was a lot of laughter therapy. It was supposed to be relaxation therapy, but usually I just lay there laughing, and that was good; it was OK for me to do that. There was nothing else for it and he laughed too in

his infectious way. He was precisely on the same level as me, exactly where I was as a 14-year-old and a few years on.

He was very unprofessional I'd have to say. Although he of course had read the books and had his diploma.

Anne also uses the words "as if" to define the relationship that developed between herself and the mental health worker who had been her contact person:

We visit each other at home. Or we go out and have a meal together or go to the cinema or listen to music. That's great. We like the same music, or rather I've started to like his music. Sometimes he comes over to my place and brings his children. We go sledding. That's really fun. It's as if we are a family.

Although Erik does not describe it in detail, his relationship with his contact person at the day centre he visits occasionally gives further concretion to this new kind of professionalism that, according to several of the respondents, have contributed to their recovery:

[The contact person] has helped me with my mother. But on the ward they didn't do anything. Most of the help I've had was here at the day centre. A lot of what I've told you, I've also told [the contact person]. And she listens. She doesn't interrupt and say that it's all just fantasy. (...)
What is it that is good about [the contact person]?
She's nice, she's kind. After I had worked for a month she gave me a rose. I dried it and keep it at home. Small things like that. Last month when I didn't have any money left, she let me borrow 100 kronor [about 10 USD] until the end of the month.
She phones me up and asks how I'm doing. She phones my mother and tells her how things are going for me at the job. That's made my mother feel a whole lot better. She says she's so happy that I'm well again. I've explained to her that I still see things around me, but that I don't care about it anymore. That's what feels so good, that even my mother has accepted it.

Besides the examples we have presented so far, there are mainly two kinds of rules that the therapists in question have broken: the rule to meet only on the ward or at the clinic and the rule to maintain distance to the therapist's own person. Infringements of the rules regulating time and place often occur together. Meetings have taken place away from the therapist's place of work, in the patient's home (which has become accepted in the last decade as official "home visits"), but also in public places when the encounter cannot be explained as a form of social training, and in the professional's own home.

Looking back at his first contact with the world of the institution, Lars describes an infringement of the rules regulating place. He talks about the emotional impact when a professional breaks the rules and does it for a particular person. For his part, he felt that he was not just any person, that he was chosen, that he possesses certain qualities (not merely an illness) that another person has been able to see.

> At the children's home they let me go home with [people on the staff] and have a snack with them. They asked me to paint a picture and then they bought it from me. When I was supposed to move from the children's home, one of the staff wrote me a nice little letter and wished me all the luck in the world. Lots of small stuff like that. And you felt... Of course, I was one of many, but even though there were a lot of children there I felt special in some way. I felt they liked me because I was... despite what I was. I was up to mark. I could even let others hug me. Body contact. For me that always used to be abuse... (Lars)

Person

By breaking the rules of time and place, the professional also reveals hidden sides to his personality and his own life. Lars describes such a situation:

> I saw [the therapist] at the post office when I wasn't feeling so good. He was standing there like any ordinary person. And that did something for me. Knowing that he was like any other ordinary person. He's not just my psychotherapist who I look up to. He's also an ordinary person and doesn't have to be anything else than just an ordinary person.

This observation leads Lars to draw a broader conclusion:

I don't have to be the perfect patient. I don't have to be the worst patient or the best. I'm just a person who's had the privilege of getting qualified care. And that gave me an enormous lust for life that I carried around with me all that weekend… Life gives you these small injections sometimes.

It seems that when professionals who have a certain relationship with a service user show themselves to be people with problems and abilities, they become a bridge that the person could use to crossover; a bridge between the oftentimes paralysing effect of mental suffering and regaining the personal abilities that have long been denied. For Lars, this means that he does not have to be "a perfect patient". By showing his own complexity, the professional creates an opening for the patient to relinquish the one-dimensional role of patient and accept his/her own complexity. Not just healthy or sick, but both, at one and the same time.

Irene describes her meeting with a counsellor who eventually came to mean a lot to her in reaching a turning point toward recovery:

But I was lucky. I was given a contact person, a counsellor who knew my brother. He was a social worker. He had been to sea. He wasn't at all like the social workers I had met in the social services. No, this was a dependable, a chubby kind of guy, about 30 or so. He had been part of the leftist movement and he surely must have smoked a joint or two in his younger days. He had a completely different attitude about everything. I never understood how he ended up here in this mental hospital. I don't know why, but he was so darn nice to me. He boosted my confidence from the very first moment: "You can do it!" "You'll make out just fine!" He was always saying things like that.

There are several places this brief passage that show identification through the acknowledging of complexity. The counsellor is provided with a history of "surely" having used drugs earlier in life, which was also Irene's big problem at this juncture in her life. A bit further on in the interview she exclaims: "I never understood how he ended up here in this mental hospital!" In both cases the professional and the patient begin to resemble one another a little bit. The professional is not someone who is always happy and successful; he has his little flaws, too, which are not so very different from the patient's. And because of this, it is not impossible for patients to imagine that perhaps they too might be a bit like the therapist in turn. A loser, but sometimes a winner too – both, simultaneously. At the time of the interview with Irene she has been working as a social worker for several years after having successfully completed university studies.

Hatred and recovery

The interviews describe a number of incidents when the professional has broken rules for the patient's sake. Irene describes such encounters with professionals and their importance for her recovery. But she mentions as well an entirely different aspect of relationships with certain professionals and family members which she say has also helped her: the hatred she has felt for all those who have harmed her:

> You know, you can really feel hate. I hated. I was wild with hate. I hated my mum. I hated my stepfather. I hated my social worker. I hated all the public authorities. If there had been a Red Army cell in [name of city], I would have blown up every single building where there was a public authority. Such hatred, it was all-consuming. It enrages me when people humiliate you like they did me. I felt: "Here I am, at the mercy of those bastards again!"

Irene succeeded in transforming her feelings of humiliation into hate, and her hate eventually became a driving force in her recovery:

> When you identify with your executioners, you begin to die. If you've been humiliated as much as I have and lose your capacity to hate, then you've had it. But as long as you can still hate… I've hated my way past my mum and my stepfather and all who have insulted me, raped me, humiliated me, and I've been able to keep the hate going strong… I think that has been the main driving force. The year I spent out at the cottage, I sat there and said to myself: "Now I'll show them. One day they're going to eat up what they did to me. One day I'll show them that I'm better than them." Really powerful. It sounds so primitive. And that's exactly what it was. When you're in that kind of situation… I had refused to take a disability pension retirement. They had taken my son away from me. They

had declared me an unfit mother. The doctors told me I was going to die. It was sheer will power on my part.

Irene is very clear about the role hatred has played in her recovery process. The clarity of her description casts light on the many incidents reported in the interviews when the respondents felt humiliated by their families and/or certain professionals. The question that Irene's recovery story raises is whether these people serve merely as a contrasting image or whether they could also function as a driving force for someone who has stepped out onto the road to recovery?

Hatred's role in recovery work is not discussed by any of our other respondents, but Patricia Deegan (1997a) talks about the impact outrage had on her own recovery:

> I know that anger, especially angry indignation, played a big role in that transition. When the psychiatrist told me the best I could hope for was to take my medications, avoid stress and learn to cope, I became enraged. (However, I was smart enough to keep my angry indignation to myself because rule number 1 is never to get enraged in a psychiatrist's office if you're labelled with chronic schizophrenia!) I also remember that just after the visit I made up my mind to become a doctor. I was so outraged at the things that had been done to me against my will in the hospital as well as the things I saw happen to other people, that I decided that I wanted to get a powerful degree and have enough credentials to run a healing place myself. I had a survivor mission that I felt passionately about. (p. 81)

The parallels between Irene's and Patricia Deegan's descriptions are unmistakable: both were outraged by the treatment they received as "a hopeless case", the point of which was that they must simply accept their situation and condition; they both transformed their hatred into a driving force; they both made it their goal to become a professional themselves in order to show the others that they were mistaken in their doomsday prognosis and that also severely distressed people must be treated with dignity.

The feelings of hatred that can grow in people with severe mental disorders as a consequence of the humiliations they have suffered complicate our understanding of the factors that contribute to the recovery process. It is not only the "good" professionals and other people who are mentioned in this context, although Irene's depiction and analysis are not formulated as clearly in any of the other interviews.

The nature of the infringements

None of the psychiatric workers mentioned in the stories break rules all the time. Nor have they broken rules for all their patients. The infringements are committed against a background of rules; in fact, they mostly follow the rules. But not always. Furthermore, when we bear in mind that the therapists being referred to in the stories are affiliated with different schools of therapy, it is quite likely that the sets of rules they each follow differ somewhat. This was evident in the research on therapy that focuses on so called non-specific factors. It is essential that the therapists believe in their particular model of therapy, whatever the model. Infringements of the model's rules, as we have seen in our material, are how the professional builds up the non-specific factors. In these infringements we see the source of the patient's experiences of being met with empathy, of being seen and heard.

All of the stories in the study contain examples of rule infringements. Does this mean that all infringements are therapeutic and promote the recovery process? It is hardly likely that we can find grounds in the material for drawing such a conclusion. Any number of therapists may have committed similar breaches without it having any positive effect. The infringements may not even have been noticed or regarded as worthy of being mentioned in the interviews.

And infringements may even have negative effects, although none were mentioned in the recovery stories. Rather, the line of demarcation goes between professionals who sometimes break rules and those who always put the rules before the patient. Using Burke's perspective, it could be argued that all aspects of a drama must be present before something can happen. The person in question must be present as well as other people who are involved in a common action that creates meaning, and one or more arenas where the person's competence and self-esteem have room to grow and be expressed.

Ordinary people as means and end

There are other people besides family and professionals who have played an important role in the respondents' stories of their recovery. In fact, their specific value lies in their being neither family nor professionals. Their relationship to the patient is not based on blood ties nor on conditions of employment. They represent the world toward which the recovering person strives. Normality. As representative of the normal, they are a scale by which recovering persons can measure themselves.

Measuring up in the eyes of others

The recovery process is described as the search for parts of a lost self. An important aspect of the search for the self and of putting to the test the person that one is in the process of becoming is finding the courage to be oneself in front of others:

> So I went along with the interview and got the job. I was so glad to get that job, even if I was scared, too, and wasn't all sure that I wanted it. I felt like… was a little bit normal again. That I could do the interview and get the job without putting on an act. (Susanne)

A straightforward honest encounter with someone with whom one has no previous ties is an opportunity to be confirmed as someone who measures up. When the encounter works well, it brings the person a step closer to recovery. When the "other" does not have a professional relationship to the person, a new relationship can be formed that allows the person to step outside the patient role, to live among other "normal" people; to be "normal" oneself.

> *Do people treat you differently now?*
> Yes, now they say hello. Before, when I had to hobble around – I could hardly walk – no one said hello, except when my mother was with me. Now it's more cheery: "How nice to see you! I didn't recognise you!" They ask me if I'm sick, if I have cancer, or HIV… Now, when I look at myself in the mirror I see that I've lost weight, too. (Anne)

311

A final step that only a few of the respondents have taken is telling other people that one has a past history as a psychiatric patient, people the one feels accepted by.

> But... in the fall of 1990 I met the man I'm married to now... I met him through the gym and we became acquainted because I was involved with a committee. We started to talk together a lot and I thought he was very nice. I was so surprised to meet still another man... not just my therapist, who didn't try to push himself on me, or put something over on me, someone who had boundaries... and who wasn't just out to sleep with me. I couldn't believe it was true. Totally unexpected... And eventually I got the courage to open up to him a little about what I'd been struggling with and he took it very well. He was open and honest and said that he didn't have any personal experience of this kind of problem, but he managed to open up to me emotionally.
> *It sounds like he could stand hearing...*
> He did ... he wasn't frightened off by any of it. So all of that year, from the summer onwards, we got to be really good friends... we had these long telephone conversations and I talked my head off and really lived it up and felt... a couple of times I felt panic, you know... scared that maybe I'd said too much and so now he doesn't dare go on with this, he's going to try to get out of it.
> *Was he the first person you became close friends with?*
> Yes, absolutely, for a long time. He was the very first person I didn't overact with – who I was completely honest with – didn't try to be anyone but myself, and that was a daring thing to do, I'll tell you. But it was a good thing, too. And so... in some incredible way or another we could stand being together. We were both of us just as embarrassed and un-certain, so it's quite moving that we made it. But when I had the relationship as a base and felt: "Now I'm going to put everything I have into it" and stopped watching the scale... because I fully realised that I couldn't have a relationship with someone and do all that stuff about food. That would upset everything. So I put everything I had into it, just like when I was put in hospital or began going to therapy. I wanted it! And so I stopped all that stuff with that boring point system. I was honest with him about it... that it was pretty risky and that I could gain an awful lot of weight and was afraid he wouldn't like me any more... (Susanne)

Here the person is accepted not only in her new guise, but with the whole of her history. Perhaps it is at this point that she becomes able to transcend her old role and no longer define herself as a patient or former patient, as a person who will always be in a dependent position in relation to others.

The others

Other people (and pet dogs) seem able to play a crucial role in the recovery of persons with severe mental disorders. Contrary to the idea that a severely mentally disturbed person's social relationships are mostly characterised by the disorder, the life stories collected in this study provide examples of mutuality, permanence and deep interpersonal relationships. These relationships are not built solely on the person's need for help (although the need exists and is acknowledged), but also on the ability to give something in return.

A main characteristic of other people, and of encounters that promote the recovery process, is their complexity. In many cases the family is the embodiment of the person's complicated personal life history where periods of pain and suffering alternate with periods of hope and trust. The family represents continuity in a person's life history because it has been around from "the beginning". Furthermore, the family has often been present in the arenas that were created to deal with these problems. They have also stood by the person where there are no arenas. By continuing to "be there" for the person, they are living proof that complexity is "acceptable". There is someone who can put up with you. In several of the stories where the parents are described as having failed to be supportive, the grandparents have stood by in their stead. They are often at a distance, but have openly taken the person's part against their own children.

The professionals' complexity is related to their position as salaried employees. The basis for their relationship to the patient is a commission structured by certain rules and regulations. The person's legal rights are the point of departure, but in actual clinical practice the rules are formulated from certain assumptions contained in the theories upon which the professionals base their professionalism. The rules are imbedded in the institution where the professional works, but also in the ethical considerations and clinical techniques of the particular professional's theoretical school. The rules and how they are explained and applied convey a framework of meaning that may give structure to the patient's experience.

Bearing this in mind, every professional who is mentioned in the stories has having been important for the recovery process has broken some of the rules of their profession. The infringements are highly individual, although many of the professionals in question have broken the same kind of rules. They are individual because, although many commit them, they are seldom mentioned as being part of daily practice, as belong to the care culture, as something from which professionals could learn. The infringements arise in connection with and as a part of a relationship between two people.

The fact that the professional is willing to break a rule conveys to the patient that it is possible to question the one-dimensional relationship characterising health care: healthy-sick, staff-patient, giver-recipient. Breaking rules can create a condition of mutuality where the patient is both a recipient and a giver, which thereby changes the person's status as simply a long-term patient, someone whose basic humanity has become thoroughly disrupted.

Pets, dogs, seem to have played an important role in some of the recovery stories. They serve as training opportunities in the person's regaining a belief in an own ability to enter into mutual interpersonal relationships.

Other people, as we have seen earlier in Chapter 7, may be important reminders in times of deepest distress that the person has value. An important consideration here is that the relationship need not be permanent nor even long-term; it need not be based on blood ties, nor on the psychiatric worker's terms of employment. During the recovery process other people become both the means and the end. They are the means by which the individual can re-evaluate him-/ herself. To be among other people and not be treated as a psychiatric patient could be a step towards the bolstering self-confidence. Other people can be an end by the very fact that they "live a normal life". To live among these other people, sharing with them parts of one's personal history in all its complexity, and still be accepted is the final step towards ceasing to define oneself solely as a patient or former patient.

Still another factor in the recovery process that emerges in these life stories is that in some cases family members, pets and professionals who have broken the rules are said to have prevented the person from committing suicide, not by actually interrupting a suicide attempt, but by being there for the person. Thus they become a "vicarious bearer of hope". Even if one can find no reason for wanting to live, one can nevertheless continue to do so for the other person's sake and because the other person believes that one's situation can and will improve.

---

[1] Antonovsky (1991) defines KASAM as: "… a global position expressing the extent to which people have complete and enduring but dynamic trust that their internal and external worlds are predictable, and that there is a very good probability that things will turn out for the best." (p. 13) KASAM has three main components:

1. Intelligibility. This is a cognitive concept used to define the person's view of his/her surroundings as orderly and interconnected, i.e. predictable in contrast to random and inexplicable.
2. Manageability, which Antonovsky defines as "the extent to which we feel that we have the necessary resources to deal with the demands that arise from the stimuli that steadily bombard us." (p. 40)
3. Meaningfullness. This concept is more emotional than cognitive and refers to the person's ability to become engaged in the kinds of questions that help us to find meaning in life.

10

Managing the contradictions
The complexity of human life

To live outside the
law you must be honest.
Bob Dylan, "Absolutely Sweet Mary"
on CD "Blonde on Blonde"

Background
Research on recovery from severe mental disorders can be divided into two periods:

1. From the turn of the century and up until the 1980s, a number of follow-up studies were published showing that diagnosed schizophrenia did not necessarily follow a given chronic course of development. Not only did the course of the illness vary from person to person, but also quite a few patients recovered.
2. Since the 1980s a number of articles on policy have been published on the significance of the recovery concept for understanding and treating mental disorders and for developing rehabilitation programmes. Also during the 1980s research began to focus on the factors that contribute to recovery and the possible stages in the recovery process. In the 1990s still a new trend could be discerned: service users and user organisations appeared as important partners in research and in the formation of clinically oriented recovery programmes. Thus, the focus of research has shifted from investigating the occurrence of recovery to seeking

to discover which factors could facilitate recovery from severe mental disorders.

In general, research has had problems to establish a connection between the frequency and course of recovery and specific psychiatric interventions. There have been periods when the frequency of recovery was just as high before as after the introduction of modern psycho-pharmaceuticals. Nor can the high percentage of people who have recovered be explained by psychotherapeutic interventions alone. Combining various psychiatric interventions has been known to delay relapse, but has not resulted in a higher percentage of recovered patients. The frequency of recovery has also been shown to be higher in developing countries than in the industrial world, despite the enormous difference in medical resources between these two parts of the world.

Factors that are known to have an impact on the recovery process are medication, the person's own volition and determination, and support from the person's surroundings. However, it is difficult to ascertain in practical terms the content of these factors and how they interact.

This is the background to a study on the factors that contribute to recovery and how they work in actual practice. The study is based on interviews with 16 persons who have recovered from severe mental disorders. We found some variance among such factors as gender, age, diagnosis, treatment and institutional culture, but cannot otherwise say anything about the target group's representivity.

Were the interview subjects really so severely disturbed? Their condition had been assessed long before the start of the study. On at least one occasion in their career as mental patients, they were judged as suffering from severe mental disorders. They had been diagnosed and we can assume that they were treated for the diagnosed disorders. To have been diagnosed, treated and cared for as severely mentally disturbed people has been the common reality for the respondents in this study.

Had they actually recovered? At the time of the interview, all of the respondents satisfied the criteria for either total or social recovery. The recovery concept implies that the most difficult phase for persons who have recovered is behind them. Does this mean that they have recovered for all time? In psychiatry the concept of relapse highlights this problem.

How long time must have passed since the last "illness episode" before a new onset of illness can be regarded as a separate event and not a relapse? How long must a person have been recovered for the recovery to be acknowledged as such?

There is no guarantee that the persons who participated in this study will not experience mental problems again in the future, that they will not once again be hospitalised. But they had all been out of hospital for many years at the time of the interview. And it does not seem that in the intervening period their plight had been overlooked by the responsible public authorities; they had not been abandoned, they had not suffered a "relapse" without anyone noticing it.

But even if their recovery should prove temporary, there is still much that we can learn from their experiences. The main question is whether severe mental disorders follow a natural course that is impervious to human intervention, that is not affected by the persons themselves or by others in their surroundings. If people who suffer from severe mental problems can be helped and are able to help themselves, if there is a way to understand and affect the course of the disorder, then there is an obvious need for knowledge about what words, actions and other interventions are required and how they operate and interact. This is what the data in this study can shed light on, whether or not the recovery is permanent.

Complexity

The analysis of the stories of practice in context reveals an overarching category which I call complexity. Its most distinguishing feature is the idea of "both, simultaneously", not "either/or". This feature characterises both the individuals concerned, the people around them and the places and the means that facilitate recovery. It encompasses the possibility to be both mad and rational at the same time.

Thus complexity implies that our analytical categories contain contradictions. An important aspect of the stories of recovery practice is that the main emphasis is not to resolve the contradictions but to find a way to live with them, to be able to live with being oneself and experiencing less pain in the process; to manage the contradictions. To recover does not mean to become someone else. Rather, in the interviews the recovery process has been described as discovering a way to find one's self; of being able to manage problems, but in a different way than before. What helps a person to live with and through these contradictions without risking being reduced to either polarity, without risking being excluded from his/her social context? "Both, simultaneously" because even if the contradictions are bi-polar on a conceptual level, they are not mutually exclusive but intertwined.

It seems that the attempt to ignore the contradictions, to demolish one of the poles in the contradiction often creates more suffering than it alleviates. The individual and the circumstances of his/her life become one-dimensional, which in the long run is experienced as an act of violence to one's own person.

Managing contradictions is neither a method nor a treatment programme. The recovery process seems to depend on and consist of opportune coincidences that occur at times when the person is in a position to take advantage of the opening that is created to break with his/her one-dimensional identity as a mental patient and accommodate a more complex identity. It may be possible to increase the likelihood of such coincidences occurring, but they cannot be planned in detail. One way could be to remove the elements of segregation in how society and public institutions regard and treat people who deviate from the norm, and instead offer them a variety of opportunities, a "smörgåsbord" of interventions that reflect the plurality and diversity of human needs.

There are many contradictions that require managing. In the following, several of the more important and general ones are illuminated.

Developmental course and concepts

• *Breaks and continuity*

In essence, psychiatry builds its theories and practice upon the assumption that mental disorders constitute a fundamental break with the circumstances of ordinary human life:

- *Break with rationality*: People with severe mental disorders cease to be regarded as normal and comprehensible. They become something "other". They violate the norms for behaviour, for

interacting with other people and the conventional ways of thinking and feeling.

- *Break with ordinary interaction*: Professionals treat people with
  severe mental disorders differently than they treat others. "Chronically ill" people are equated with their problems, for this reason
  other people should act differently towards them. The implication
  is that family and friends would have much to learn from the special way professionals regard and treat someone who is mentally
  ill.
- *Break with ordinary community life*: The institutions for people
  with severe mental disorders have been built on social isolation.
  There is the actual geographic isolation typical of psychiatric
  facilities and intermediate care institutions. But people can also be
  isolated in narrow parallel societies that are organised within the
  broader society to meet special needs in a daily life context.

Exclusion and classification are mechanisms for breaking down the
complexity of individual lives into small unambiguous entities arranged
so as conform to the divisions within the caring organisations and thereby facilitate the smooth handling of large groups of people with special
problems.

The people in our study who have recovered describe their mental
problems as a radical departure from ordinary events in life. The occurrence of turning points in their life stories indicate that the hallucinations, the extreme anxiety, the delusions were completely different from
anything they had ever experienced before. The pain they associate with
their mental problems is different from the pain they used to associate
with real life. But at the same time, the respondents emphasise that their
life histories have a continuity that encompasses both "psychosis" and
"normality". This continuity is in contrast to the way they describe how
psychiatry has treated them, where interest in the person's history is
focused on the actual onset of the illness and not on the person's life in
its totality where mental problems are an integral part. Focusing on problems alone casts the totality of a person's life history in shadow, whereas
acknowledging a person's life history could help to confirm and maintain the true complexity of human identity.

The recovery process is described in the interviews as the regaining of control over one's own life. Important steps in this process are re-establishing personal relationships and regaining access to places outside the world of closed institutions – an own place to live, a place to work – and to public institutional arenas that are not associated with psychiatry and the social services. In such places the emerging complex self has the opportunity to be tested, confirmed and flourish in relationships with other people.

Here, prospective studies could generate important knowledge about the recovery process. The studies conducted to date indicate that growth and development are complex processes that proceed at an uneven pace. Progress is uneven depending on the extent of the person's problems and shifting care needs as the person moves through the care apparatus; it is complex in that the person can both function well in certain areas of life and less well in others, simultaneously.

- *Illness, total and social recovery*

The categories social and total recovery indicate varying degrees of recovery and as such imply the ranking of individuals, but also the very opposite of ranking. The newly awakened interest for the recovery phenomenon is a result of the closing down of psychiatric institutions, a policy initiated some 30 years ago in Europe and the USA. In practical terms, deinstitutionalisation is a critique against traditional psychiatry's conception of chronicity, mental degeneration and the necessity of removing from society individuals who deviate from the norm (if for no other reason than for their own care and protection), thereby establishing a norm for human conduct to gain acceptance in this society, a norm that excludes mental illness (Basaglia 1982).

The fact that thousands of people who do fit the norm of mental health, or at least of someone who has totally recovered, nevertheless live in society opens up new perspectives. If normality used to be formulated in terms of either/or: either sick or healthy, either hospitalised and bereft of responsibilities or a free agent, then the complex idea of "both the one and the other, simultaneously" in relation to mental health status and life situations and as described in the recovery stories means a broadening of the concept of normality; a broadening of our understanding of what a person can be and should be allowed to be.

The concepts of total and social recovery can be used to distinguish between "normal" and "less normal" people. But they can also open up for the perspective that life consists a continuum of situations and conditions in which people find themselves.

The requirement that there must be total absence of symptoms for the person to be assessed as wholly recovered was problematised by Manfred Bleuler. He noted that careful study would soon reveal that individual symptoms of schizophrenia can be found in almost anyone. Basaglia (1982) wrote:

> It has to do with understanding that a person's worth, whether healthy or unwell, goes beyond the value of health or illness; that the illness, like all other contradictions, can be used as an opportunity to regain one's self or to become estranged from one's self... (p. 9, translated from the Italian).

The person

• *Spontaneous cure – an exhaustive undertaking*

The spontaneous-cure hypothesis was introduced by psychiatry to explain the high percentage of patients who recover from severe mental disorders. Self-healing presupposes the existence of a natural process whereby the illness will eventually cease if allowed to run its course. Besides the problem of determining how not to treat an illness so as not to interrupt its presumed natural course, there is a paradox wherein the idea that people with severe mental disorders are chronically ill conflicts with the idea that severe chronically ill people can heal spontaneously.

The idea of spontaneous cure also implies its opposite: cases where patients recover because the causes of their illness were successfully treated. Treatment research has focused primarily on studying the outcome of a narrow range of treatments practised within psychiatry and a few schools of psychotherapy. There are two problems with this approach. First, it reduces the efforts of these professional groups to their respective technical tools. Research on the placebo effect and on so-called non-specific factors indicates that technique-centred studies have serious limitations. Second, by focusing on this approach research relinquishes the possibility to study the possible effects on the illness course brought about by the person's own efforts, by the efforts of the professional groups involved (such as mental health nurses, nurse aides and staff in supportive housing) and by others in the person's surroundings (such as other service users, family, friends and acquaintances) as well as the effects of other factors (such as the person's financial situation and housing arrangements). Instead, what remains for research is an abstract figure who has been reduced to a few controllable variables; thus is lost the possibility to study the impact of social life on people with severe mental disorders. The spontaneous-cure hypothesis was launched when it proved impossible to link recovery to specific forms of treatment practised by certain professions, but also because it was not considered necessary to study patients in their social context.

What emerges in the interviews is the existence of just such "non-specific factors". The life stories do not give us a basis for isolating specific professional interventions from their context; rather, the opposite. Contrary to the idea of an illness that follows its own course independent or treatment or other input, our interview subjects describe a struggle in which they have played an active part, a struggle in which a series of co-agents and counter-agents have participated. The notion of spontaneous cure risks making us blind to this struggle, and it makes it more difficult to grasp the forces that are at play in a recovery process.

The study of social life involves serious methodological problems. It is seldom possible in any meaningful way to reduce it to variables that can be manipulated and controlled as in laboratory tests. The question is whether the difficulty of establishing experimental conditions is to be allowed to determine what questions are researchable, and how this impinges on what happens in real life outside the research laboratory.

- *The disturbed self – the active self*

In contrast to the idea of a person whose life is thoroughly dominated and devastated by mental disorder is the image that the stories of recovery give us of a person who actively seeks to manage the confusion caused by these experiences. But this does mean that the image of the devastated person can be replaced with the opposite image of the patient

323

as the one who knows best what he/she and others should do to end the suffering – the image of the patient as being more normal than staff and co-agents.

Time after time the respondents point at the simultaneous occurrence of confusion and uncontrollable experiences on the one hand, and their own purposeful efforts to gain control over their lives and to manage these bizarre experiences on the other. The simultaneous existence of a self that is experienced as alien and of a self that is struggling to find itself is the basic contradiction which both the person himself and those around him are called upon to manage. A self in need of help.

- *Symptoms – solutions or ways of managing*
In psychiatry symptoms are the expression of the illness on the behavioural level. The symptoms are customarily interpreted as external phenomena emanating from processes and impairments having an as yet undiscovered biological or perhaps a psychological epicentre. But the life stories told by our interview subjects indicate that symptoms may also be attempts to manage one's life. They appear as attempts to solve problems, some more successful than others, where the less successful attempts become new problems that have to be managed, problems that sometimes serve to disguise the underlying problems. Cullberg (2000a) follows a similar line of reasoning when he writes:

> The function of the protective mechanism can be compared to the posture assumed by a person with a slipped disk. The sick person has discovered that he can relieve the pain somewhat if his movements are stiff and contorted. (p. 190)

The risk is that the environment will put greater effort into counteracting the unsuccessful ways of trying to cope and less on resolving the underlying problems. Symptoms such as voice hallucinations and addiction are extremely distressful ways of trying to cope, but they may be less distressful than the underlying suffering the person is trying to master. To concentrate on symptom suppression alone could have the effect of undermining the person's problematic attempts to avoid even greater distress.

Others

- *Disrupted relationships – the central role of relationships*

In contrast to the idea of a person whose personal relationships are characterised primarily by the disorder, or who may even be considered incapable of forming relationships, is the idea of a person who recognises that he/she has problems in relation to other people and talks about these problems as being one of the reasons behind the mental distress, a person who is fully aware of the importance of personal relationships and succeeds in forming them. Such a conception presupposes that there are inherent contradictions in people with severe mental disorders, or in Cullberg's (2000a) words:

> A crucial psychological experience is that parallel with the psychotic way of functioning we often find a non-psychotic part of the personality which we must try to work with, either directly or indirectly. (p. 166)

The central role that variation in personal relationships can play in the recovery process has seldom been researched. The stories of practice in the present study have given meaning to expressions like "to be noticed" and "to be listened to". Situations where being seen and heard occur during the recovery process often involve professionals. In such situations, two kinds of contradictions are being managed:

- *the professional as friend*
- *the good listener, the authoritarian figure, the bad professional as potential helpers*

Many of the atrocity scenarios about psychiatric care depict the staff as inhuman. They are deaf and blind to the person's needs. They are disrespectful. Their power over the patients is wielded like a weapon. The good professional is therefore often depicted as the complete opposite. The good professional is a person who shows respect and who listens and "sees" the patient. Descriptions of this kind tend to be one-dimensional and define a role that professionals cannot possibly fill. By investigating situations where people with severe mental disorders report that

325

they have been heard, noticed and respected, we can obtain a multi-dimensional picture of the kind of professional who is able to facilitate the recovery process.

Unlike the idea of achieving a cure, recovery implies a change in both the practice and identity of both patient and professional. A new characteristic, "like buddies", emerged in several of the interviews. The professional who is regarded as if he/she were like a buddy is a real-life person with shortcomings, needs and interests; someone who is a realistic identification object. Such professionals can build a bridge between the absolute poles typical of the language of psychiatry: either healthy or sick, either a staff member or a patient.

Buddy-like relationships arise in circumstances where the professional breaks rules by putting the patient's interests before the institution's. These infringements imply a criticism of the rules whose main purpose is to erect barriers between patients/the sick ones and professionals/the healthy ones. These infringements often consist of commonplace acts that acquire special import because they put events of everyday life back into situations where they had been shut out by the rules of the institution. It may very well be that at the very moment service users discover a "buddy-like" identity trait in the professional, they discover a new identity trait in themselves; they are no longer only patients, they are also like buddies themselves.

The life stories contain examples of reciprocal relationships that broke with the routine practice of the institution. By breaking the rules of the institution the professional incurs certain risks, risks that reflect the value that the professional places on the service user and which greatly surpasses the value service users place on themselves. Risks of this kind have high emotional value provided they are not elevated to a new rule that is meant to apply to everyone; rather, the uniqueness of the experience must be preserved. Thus the very fact that rule infringements are unjust in that they do not apply to everyone is what prevents them from becoming a new method, a new treatment programme. Some of these rule infringements are directed against institutional routines that have been devised to separate people from the totality of their lives and from the community at large. If discovered, professionals who question the institution's rules through their own practice could be accused of lacking limits of their own, which implies that in this respect they are no different than the severely disturbed patients in that they are incapable of setting limits. This is a way for the institution to avoid being subjected to close examination on the basis of the practice of others. Often rule infringements must occur in secret with the result that whatever new knowledge we might have learned from them remains hidden.

The life stories in this study are not about breaking rules as a matter of course, even if rules can change. To make it a rule to break the rules becomes instead a new rule that has to be broken. To replace the one extreme with the other means denying the complexity of the persons and human situations being described. Recovery is concerned rather with managing the contradictions between the rules and the infringements of the rules.

Besides the "buddy-like" relationships that are described in the interviews, there were instances where reciprocity was attained through the person's "voluntary subjection" to a strong personality. In this case, reciprocity develops in step with the other person's gradual relinquishing of his/her mythological status. The relationship allows the user to become an apprentice. By making use of the master's wisdom the apprentice gains insight needed to transcend the patient role. In the master-apprentice relationship the professional's way of working is not too unlike that of the African medicine man. The patient never has to discuss his/her problems explicitly; the charismatic therapist does not need the patient's help to grasp the truth of the patient's situation (Nathan 1994). The patient is given access to and comes to accept this truth, subjects him-/herself to it, is trained in it and may be transformed into a master in his/her own right.

The interviews also contain a few examples where still another type of professional emerged as a catalyst in the recovery process – the "bad professional". The case in point is that of a professional who repeatedly insulted and humiliated the patient. In this case the patient seemed to have been able, under conditions that we have no basis for determining, to transform the insults and humiliation to hatred and a desire for revenge; this in turn became a driving force in the patient's recovery process. The person was determined to prove the bad professional wrong by showing that he/she was better than the professional. It is not likely that an effect of this kind can occur on its own; the person needs the support of other professionals or other persons who are able to facilitate the recovery process in a more positive way.

There are three patterns characterising the kind of relationship between users and staff that seems to promote recovery. Some users switch to other key professionals as their needs change. Other users maintain contact with different helpful professionals simultaneously to address different needs. Still others have a staff member who has accompanied them for a long time and who continues to play a major role in their lives. Lastly, there are some examples of these three patterns occurring simultaneously.

- *Family as cause – family as solution*

Throughout the history of psychiatry dating back to the first half of the 1800s, the family has been cast in the role of prime cause of the "identified patient's" problems (Castel 1976). Their guilt has either been implicit in the genes (a degeneration process spanning over several generations) or explicit in the dynamics of a family life undermined by the parents' own unsolved psychological conflicts.

In recent years family groups have formed organisations and won growing respect in both psychiatry and the community. With their newly acquired power to influence, the family movement has succeeded in several instances to bring about a radical re-evaluation of their role in the problems, daily life and treatment of psychiatric patients. Where the family used to be regarded as a burden to the patient, today the patient is often seen as a burden to the family because psychiatry and the patient have failed in their attempts to solve the patient's problems. Families are described today as the patient's foremost support and psychiatry's closest ally. They are expected to co-operate in the treatment plan for the patient and even in the treatment itself. Whether as cause or solution, both images imply a one-dimensional view of The Family; either/or. In the life stories a more complex picture emerges where the existence of both problematic and happy occasions in the family's common history plays a central role in determining the family's possibility to contribute to the recovery process. The family can be regarded as both a contributing cause of the patient's problems and as a source of support in managing the problems. Continuity is the distinguishing mark of the family. By standing for continuity the helping family represents both a common if intricately woven thread running through the person's life and a promise of continued access to a social life outside the domains of psychiatry. In a social context the helping family can be the bearer of hope – others accept me; and of despair – they are the only ones I have left, and they have caused the problems and interfere with my recovery.

- ## *A comprehensive view, continuity and total institutions*
Formerly, admission to a psychiatric hospital was the only form of help available for people with certain kinds of mental disorders. The psychiatric hospital was envisioned as a kind of therapeutic community where the staff could form a comprehensive picture of individual patients by observing them in a range of settings over time. Continuity was guaranteed though the long periods of incarceration and the total control that the institution had over the inmates. Continuity and a comprehensive view were regarded, as they still are today, to be crucial therapeutic tools. But at the same time, the provision of care in the psychiatric hospital was associated with the risk of institutionalisation and was seen to promote chronicity.

After the end of the second world war the large residential institutions were replaced by a network of smaller institutions spread out in the local communities. This development caused considerable organisational problems.

Today, too, care institutions are expected to respond to the patients' need for continuity and a comprehensive view, whether the institutions are organised on the principle of geographic proximity (sectorised organisation) or in accordance with a diagnostic model (specialised organisation). But regardless of organisational form, their treatment programmes are compartmentalised. Divisions exist between wards, in- and out-patient facilities, between psychiatry and community social psychiatry, between units specialising on youths, adults or the elderly, between the social services, psychiatry and primary health care, between the national insurance office, the employment agency and other agents who have a responsibility for the patients' wellbeing. In this fragmented institutional world "co-operation" is a key word for re-establishing continuity and a comprehensive view. But in the recovery process continuity and a comprehensive view are not abstract concepts on the organisational level; they are concerned with real-life relationships in a narrow social network.

The life stories in this study show also that there is risk that the present network of institutions may develop into new total institutions. The regression toward the total institution is not so visible, but the effect is the same as in the old institutions because the new institutions are in may respects omnipresent. They are as impossible to get away from today as they ever were. On the face of it, the principles of continuity and a comprehensive view are important for recovery, but their reverse side is control; this is a fundamental contradiction that should be brought to light and managed.

What matters here is whether there are connecting links between the institution and the outside world, bridges that people with severe mental disorders use to reach the other side. What matters also is whether there is a real possibility for them to vary how much support they receive from the institution and how much insight the institution is to have in their lives until such time as the contact no longer exists or has developed into something else; perhaps even a kind of friendship.

- *Official life of institutions – secret life of institutions*

The closed wards of mental hospitals have been described in terms of total institutions, worlds where the inmates' daily life is controlled and planned in detail. In the therapeutic community the staff's efforts and the way of organising daily life are intended to cure the patient. The finding that extended stays in an institution causes chronicity and have a negative psychological effect through institutionalisation is not contested today. Nevertheless, Warner found in his review of recovery research (1985) that people have been able to recover even when psychiatry only had such institutions to offer. The life stories in this study, as in earlier studies (Topor 1993, 1996), point at the occurrence of a rich and varied secret life inside the total institution, a life that can be seen as constituting a radical criticism of the institution's rules.

In *The underlife of a public institution* (1973), Goffman wrote about the secret life of patients in mental hospitals. The book contains examples of how inmates find ways to improve their circumstances. The persons in our study also give examples of a secret life existing between patients and staff, a life that breaks the institution's rules designed to maintain the separation of patients and staff. These rule infringements tend to promote continuity in relationships between individual patients and one or several of the staff. It is in connection with rule infringements that our interview subjects describe situations where hospital staff were most helpful.

It seems that in closed institutions the staff's contribution to recovery occurs, not when they slavishly fulfil their duties, but when they break rules by allowing the patients to be excused from some of the institution's routines. Situations of this kind are described in the interviews, not as negligence but as accommodating the patient's need for a respite from the pressures of social life on the ward. Here the psychiatric ward functions as a place for "woodshedding" (Strauss 1989a), a place where patients can relatively undisturbed gather strength, make inventories of their personal resources and take the first tentative steps along a new path in their lives.

The underlife of the institution is in contradiction to the official justification for maintaining closed institutions. Nevertheless, it seems that it can play a certain therapeutic role in recovery, particularly when its rules are broken in practice.

• *Organised daily life – just daily life*

The dismantling of the large-scale psychiatric hospitals that was instigated in the last few decades has created a new institutional setting in the form of intermediate care facilities, institutions that bridge the gap between the closed hospital ward and the world at large, and, judging from our interview material, have the potential to develop the same contradictions that our respondents have described as having been important for their recovery.

These new arenas provide the means to discover, test and develop new and unalienated aspects of the self. Even people whose lives are characterised by extreme mental anguish have a right to exist in society;

they need not be patients all their lives if given the right kind of support in daily life. The right to be both healthy and unwell. Various forms of housing support, work and leisure-time activities are mentioned in several interviews as arenas for testing one's self.

Intermediate forms of care, as the name implies, can become an intermediate world where the actors have greater possibilities to make their own rules and create new roles for themselves. For example, today there are a number of co-operative enterprises employing service users. These co-operatives operate on the open market and offer opportunities for its members to interact with people outside the circles of care and family, and in other capacities than that of patient. User co-operatives can operate within psychiatric institutions to provide sanitation services or run a coffee shop, to give just two examples. Activities of this kind pose a challenge to conventional patient and staff roles. The patient is simultaneously an employee and the staff are customers for the users' services (Andersson 2001, Gallio 1991, Rotelli 1994).

There are other studies as well (Hansson 1993, Topor 1987) indicating that the special conditions of work at these institutions make it possible for staff to relate to users in a different way than what closed institutions and outpatient clinics once thought was desirable. What were once regarded as rule infringements by the old institutions are now acceptable practices in intermediate care institutions, which means that the complexity of each person has a better chance to be affirmed.

However, implicit in the intermediate care institution is the risk that it could easily become a world of its own, a parallel society or an oasis, if you will, in the midst of two threatening worlds. A utopia whose goal is to separate itself from the world of the institution and the community at large. In the life stories of recovery, these oases are depicted as being essential, but also that there has to be a road leading out to the surrounding society and even back to the few remaining total institutions.

- *Medicine as chemistry – medicine as personal relationship*

How does medication work and in what context is it given and taken? Even ineffective substances can work if they inspire hope and trust in the patient. This phenomenon has long been known as the "placebo effect". Many studies have been made and hypotheses formulated about what causes this effect. The substance's appearance, the patient's expectations, the therapist's expectations, the resilience of the therapeutic alliance, and the patient's reflexes conditioned by earlier treatment have all been studied. The hypothesised connection between a positive reaction to the placebo and specific personality traits of the person taking the placebo has proved to be unfounded (Boström 2000, Åsberg 2000). In traditional medicine the placebo effect is regarded as an irrelevant and disruptive factor (Lemoine 1996, Åsberg 2000).

In the present study we focus on the psychosocial context of medication, an aspect that is rarely discussed in studies of placebo. When it is discussed, it is with a different meaning, namely that the placebo effect is related in part to the prestige and authority of the medical profession and its practitioners. The interviews bring to light quite a different aspect: the patients' participation in their own medication; that is, making use of the user's knowledge and personal authority when prescribing and administering the medicine. As presented in the life stories, the patients' participation has little to do with "compliance". Compliance means that the patient accepts the doctor's authority. Participation means that the patient has some power over the treatment process, including the right to participate in the decision making. And this regaining of a sense of power is not lost if the consequences of a particular decision are negative. Having power implies the right to fail as well as succeed.

Compliance takes into account only the chemical effects of the medicine; what is important is that the substance gets inside the patient's body. Participation is not about chemical effects, it is about people having power over their own life.

The complexity of medication as treatment has to do with the medicines' chemical components and the context in which they are prescribed and administered. This context comprises various aspects, both psychological (colour, name, etc.) and social. The social aspect is concerned in part with medicine as a tool of power. To manage one's own medication means, to be viewed the medicalised psychiatric profession as a subject in one's own life, at the same time as the need for medicine is connected with the difficulties the person experiences as the subject in that life.

- *Social insurance system: liberation – a security trap*

All of the interview subjects mention socio-economic security as a self-evident condition for their recovery. Social security is so much taken for granted in the Nordic countries that it is seldom noticed. All of the interview subjects had some form of income, either through gainful employment or through the social insurance system. All had their own place to live, except for one who lived with his parents. For several of them obtaining housing and employment were advances they made within the framework of their recovery. Both means and goals. Several persons also mention the importance of successively obtaining more secure sources of income within the social insurance system: from social welfare payments, to disability benefits, from disability benefits to early retirement pension. On the other hand, these allowances are seldom very substantial. The size of pensions is based on the person's lifetime earnings but most of the persons in our interview group have little experience of paid work. Basic security makes life possible, one has the basic necessities to preserve life, but it does not give the person access to the city's social and cultural life. For many of the interview subjects, there is a constant worry about how to make ends meet over and above the basic necessities of life.

To relinquish the security of the social insurance system, to reject early retirement and take the step of entering the labour market is a hard challenge. People who have recovered have experienced problems that are usually regarded as chronic. They have been told that symptom-free periods do not indicate a cure, but rather are merely intervals of respite between relapses.

The social insurance system, which plays such a crucial role in a person's life situation, is made invisible in the medical world which prevents us from seeing what contradictions it creates in the lives of those concerned. The contradictions are therefore rarely open to discussion, despite the emphasis policy makers give today to patients' rights.

On the general level

On a comprehensive level a main outcome of this study is that it has problematised psychiatry's goal to establish itself as a natural science.

• *Evidence-based treatment – one road among many*

The attempt to define certain behaviours as symptoms and to group these symptoms into diagnostic categories corresponding to precisely delineated pathologies is a dominant preoccupation of psychiatry. With the etiology of the illness as a basis, the goal is to develop specific treatments that attack and eliminate or neutralise the causes of the illness.

However, it has proved very difficult to clearly define symptoms and diagnostic categories and to link specific recovery factors to specific diagnoses. This could depend, of course, on the uncertainty of the diagnosis. But it could also indicate that the kinds of factors that have a positive effect are not specific for different forms of treatment or diagnoses. It could very well be that at different times in life a person is susceptible in different degrees to what transpires in different interpersonal relationships.

The treatment interventions described in the interviews suggest a diversity of actions and words. Diversity and complexity are problematic concepts for the possibility to define evidence-based treatment:

- There is a diversity of aspects regarding which behaviours are to be regarded as symptoms and to what extent and in what combinations they should occur in order to justify a specific diagnosis.
- There is a diversity of recovery factors and whether they depend how the person understands them.

Because of this diversity, it is difficult to realise in practice the hopes that lie behind the production of narrowly defined evidence-based treatments (as a constantly refined technical model). The answers in this study indicate, rather, that there is not one road to recovery, but many.

• *Diagnosis and treatment – coincidence and random events*

Against the idea that knowledge makes it possible to predict and direct a particular course of events is juxtaposed the idea that the recovery process involves coincidences and random events. The present study points at a number of necessary but insufficient factors. It is possible to create the conditions that will allow efficacious factors to come into play, but neither the factors themselves nor the situations in which they occur can be created. For example, it is not possible to develop a technique for establishing a good and helpful relationship, not least because people have different ideas about what characterises a good relationship. Consequently, it is not possible to force a recovery process into being.

Here we are touching upon the schism that exists between the object of study in natural science and the object of study in the human and social sciences. It also concerns, therefore, psychiatry's position as a area of endeavour that has always been characterised by its borderline position – both; but whose leading representatives have traditionally proceeded in a single direction – either/or.

- *Treatment – support, service and common humanity*

The term "non-specific" factors is usually defined as successful factors that are common to the interventions of professional groups, although the groups themselves regard their interventions as fundamentally at variance in that they build on different theories on the causes of mental disorders and on different techniques for treating them.

In recent years there has been an attempt to separate treatment from support and service in the care of persons with severe mental disorders. This goal is based on certain assumptions:

- Treatment impacts on the symptomology by attacking the processes that cause the illness.
- The purpose of providing support and service is to prevent from becoming handicaps the disabilities that are thought to be a consequence of the illness.
- Support and service have no impact on the symptoms and causes of mental disorders. If they do have an impact, then they are not support and service, but treatment.

Treatment is the responsibility of psychiatry, support and services are the responsibility of the social welfare authorities. Thus, non-specific factors remain within the professional groups' sphere of responsibility, just as the placebo effect in medicine lies within the sphere of responsibility of a few treatment professions.

In this view, the contributions of family and friends lack any real meaning for the disorder but are probably comparable to the contributions of the social services. Nevertheless, the efforts of both groups represent different expressions of common humanity, and can, if family members are trained by suitable treatment staff, result in extending the intervals between relapses.

The efficacy of this attempt to establish lines of demarcation between medical and psychotherapeutic interventions, support and service and common humanity is questioned in the interviews in this study. The same non-specific factors, the same "placebo effect", that contribute to recovery, that have a "treatment effect", can emerge in patients' interactions with staff whether the staff work in psychiatry or the social services and whether they have advanced training or are untrained; and they can emerge in the patients' interactions with friends, peers, family members, and so on. The conditions under which these various groups meet the patient differ and besides the non-specific factors that their work brings into play, they provide different forms of intervention depending on their specific fields of knowledge and their positions of authority.

• *Meaning – truth*

A guiding principle behind much of the research in psychiatry is that by finding the underlying causes of specific diagnoses, specific forms of treatment can be devised for each of them. Each diagnosis, each illness, has its objective truth.

The life stories about recovery indicate that a crucial component of the process is that the persons who have recovered have found a truth – their own truth. They have found a meaning to what has happened in their lives, a meaning that can be accepted either by their earlier social network or their current one. It is a subjective truth, one that can build on different and contradictory explanatory models.

Problematising the truth concept in this way is linked to a discussion within psychoanalysis where several authors (Schafer 1976, Spence

1982, Viderman 1982,) asserted that psychoanalytic therapy did not reveal an actual historical truth about what had happened in the analysand's growing years, rather it supplied the analysand with a coherent and acceptable story about his/her life that gave it substance and meaning. The crucial aspect was the "narrative truth", regardless of whether it had anything to do with what actually transpired in the person's earlier life. To manage the contradiction between the idea of one objective truth and the idea of several subjective truths remains a central task for psychiatric research and practice.

Therefore...

In presenting Burke's pentad, Asplund (1980) describes Burke the scientist as an "antireductionist" (p. 128). Contrary to many theoreticians, Burke did not base his explanations on simple cause and effect relationships: "Burke's speciality is rather ambiguity and uncertainty." (Asplund 1980, p. 132)

Asplund (1987a) questions whether Burke's pentad, or indeed any theoretical tool, can help us explain the variance of social processes where:

> Relationships and patterns can be determined, but they are changeable or "unreliable"; the patterns can be broken. (p. 14)

But:

> What characterises an ordinary conversation about sports [or mental problems, my comment] is, I think, that it encompasses the whole cycle of Burke's five key terms or aspects, and that it does so repeatedly. In this respect we have not, in a strict sense, explained anything, we have not deduced success (or failure) in sports [or recovery from severe mental problems, or chronicity, my comment] from any set of necessary and sufficient conditions. Nevertheless, we reach a more profound insight. We sharpen and broaden our understanding. (p. 21)

To reach a more profound level of understanding can be said to be the primary aim of this study.

Appendix 1 – Interview guide

This is not an interview guide in the strict sense of the word, but rather a collection of areas of interest that have emerged during the course of the interviews and the parallel work of analysing the respondents' statements.

We used the same question to start each interview: How did it all begin? We purposely remained ambiguous about what we meant by "it" in order that the interviews would be as open-ended as possible.

During the course of the work to collect the interview data, five themes of special interest emerged; these we have termed the Self, Others, Meaning, Events and Structural factors. In connection with these five themes, the following areas were investigated in depth:

- What has contributed to your recovery?
- What kinds of treatment did you receive and what effect, if any, did they have on your recovery?
- Were you ever medicated; did the medicine(s) help and, if so, how?
- Did hospital stays help, and if so, how?
- What contacts have you had with psychiatry and the social services in community-based programmes; have these forms of support helped at all, and if so, how?
- Have contacts with other organisations or associations, or with anyone in private practice (such as psychotherapists) helped at all? How?
- Have contacts with personnel in psychiatry and the social services helped at all? How?
- Have your family, friends of other people been of any help? How?
- Is there anything in your overall social situation that has been especially important for your recovery?

The purpose of the interviews was to explore more fully concrete situations mentioned by the respondents as being important for their recovery. Each situation was examined in as much detail as possible by means of such questions as: What? Who? When? Where? How? and What happened next?

Appendix 2 – The respondents

Person	Richard	Sven	Susanne
Gender	Man	Man	Woman
Age	47	30	32
Civil status	Partner	Divorced	Married
Children	None	None	1
Diagnosis	Schizophrenia	Schizophrenia	Personality disorder
Age at onset	30	20	17
At first hospital stay	30	20	20
At latest hospital stay	43	23	22
Assistance at time of interview	Medication Support therapy	Medication Work training	None
Vocational activities	Paid work	Unpaid work	Paid work
Housing	Own	Own	Own
Social network	Neighbours Family, Friends Colleagues	Family, Friends	Family, Friends
Own assessment of condition	Feel good, feel safe	Feel hopeful, believe it's going to be all right	Feel great
Factors contributing to recovery	Own efforts Psychotherapy Work, Own home, Female friend	Own efforts Right medicine	Own efforts Psychotherapy
Other factors			

Irene	Ruth	Ester	Sören	Nils
Woman	Woman	Woman	Man	Man
40	42	63	47	63
Married	Single	Single	Partner	Married
3	None	None	None	3
Schizophrenia	Borderline psychotic personality	Affective psychosis	"Schizoid"	"Schizoid"
Early adolescence	20	33	25	Early childhood
	24-25	34	26	45
More than 8 years ago	34	56	30	56
None	Work training, Medicine when needed	Physician Day care centre Medication	Day care centre (sporadically)	Therapeutic contact (sporadically)
Paid work Continuing education	Paints, Exhibitions of own artwork, Work as course leader	Voluntary organisation	Art, Courses, Exhibitions of own artwork	Art, Exhibitions of own artwork Public performances
Own	Own	Own	Own	Own
Family, Friends Colleagues	Family, Work training programme	Patient organisation, Family Friends	Friends	Family Friends
Feel great	Some anxiety	No symptoms	Feel great	Much better
Own efforts Endurance, Psychotheapy	Own efforts Psychotherapy	Own efforts Strong family ties, Support from staff	Own efforts Support from network	Own efforts Good therapist
Pet dog				

Person	Elin	Tina	Lars
Gender	Woman	Woman	Man
Age	55	37	34
Civil status	Married	Single	Single
Children	None	None	None
Diagnosis	Schizophrenia	Paranoid psychosis	Schizophrenia
Age at onset	16	21	13
At first hospital stay	21	24	13
At latest hospital stay	46	32	31
Assistance at time of interview	None	Social services Medication	Psychotherapy Medication
Vocational activities	Unpaid work	Paid work	Artistic activity
Housing	Own	Own	Own
Social network	Husband User organisation	Friends Colleagues, Family Neighbours, Contact person	Contact person Maternal grand-mother
Own assessment of condition	Feel good	Don't know if I'll ever be completely well; can manage own problems	Much better, have good resources – can be completely well
Factors contributing to recovery	Own efforts Psychotherapy User organisation	Own efforts Right medicine Home nurse	Own efforts A good therapist/ psychotherapy
Other factors			

Maria	David	Anne	Erik	Jan
Woman	Man	Woman	Man	Man
54	29	36	47	50
Single	Single	Single	Divorced	Divorced
None	None	None	2	1
Schizophrenia	Schizophrenia	Schizophrenia	Schizophrenia	Affective psychosis
22	22	22	27	28
23	0	24	37	28
32	0	33	44	48
Social services Medication	Psychotherapy Medication	Work training centre Outpatient care Medication Support	Work training centre Outpatient care Medication	Medication
Unpaid work	Studies	Unpaid work	Paid work	Unpaid work
Own	Lives with parents	Own	Own	Own
Family Friends in user organisation	Family Friends in user organisation Contact person	Family, Contact person	Family, A few friends Contact person	Friends Patient organisation Mother
Found a level where I can function	No symptoms	No symptoms	No symptoms	Feel great
Own efforts Right to make mistakes Support from psychiatrist and nurse	Own efforts Right medicine Different therapists for different purposes	Own efforts Several good helpers for different purposes	Own efforts Own decision to stay out of hospital Contact persons	Own efforts Faith in God Right medicine
	Pet dog		Pet dog	Pet dog

References

Alanen, Y (1997). Schizophrenia – its origins and need-adapted treatment. London: Karnac Books.

Alvesson, M & Sköldberg, K (1994). Tolkning och reflektion – Vetenskapsfilosofi och kvalitativ metod. Lund: Studentlitteratur. [Interpretation and reflection – scientific philosophy and qualitative method].

American Psychiatric Association (1980). *Diagnostic and statistical manual of mental disorders* (Third Edition). Washington: APA.

American Psychiatric Association (1994). *Diagnostic and statistical manual of mental disorders* (Fourth Edition). Washington: APA.

Andersson, W (2001). *Berättelser – Verkligheter och möjligheter och sociala entreprenörer.* Malmö: Égalité. [*Stories – Realities and possibilities and social entrepreneurs*].

Andreoli, A (1986). Crise et intervention de crise en psychiatrie. In: Andreoli, A & Lalive, J & Garrone, G (eds). *Crise et intervention de crise en psychiatrie.* Paris: SIMEP.

Anthony, WA & Liberman, R (1986). The practice of psychiatric rehabilitation: Historical, conceptual and research base. *Schizophrenia Bulletin,* Vol 12, No 4, p 542–559.

Anthony, WA (1993). Recovery from mental illness: The guiding vision of the mental health service system in the 1990s. *Psychosocial Rehabilitation Journal,* Vol 16, No 4, p 11–21.

Anthony, WA & Buell, G & Sharratt, S & Althoff, M (1972). Efficacy of psychiatric rehabilitation. *Psychological Bulletin,* Vol 78, p 447–456.

Antonovsky, A (1987). *Unraveling the Mystery of Health.* San Francisco : Jossey-Bass Inc Publishers.

Asplund, J (1970). *Om undran inför samhället.* Lund: Argos. [*On wondering about society*].

Asplund, J (1980). Noter till Kenneth Burkes motivationsgrammatik. In: Asplund, J. *Socialpsykologiska studier.* Stockholm: Almqvist & Wiksell Förlag. [Notes to Kenneth Burke's motivational grammar. In: Asplund, J. *Social psychological studies*].

Asplund, J (1987a). Idrott och samhällsordning. In: Bergryd, U (ed). *Den sociologiska fantasin – teorier om samhället.* Stockholm: Rabén & Sjögren. [Sports and social order. In: Bergryd, U (ed). *The sociological imagination – theories on society*].

Asplund, J (1987b). *Det sociala livets elementära former.* Göteborg: Korpen. [*The social life's elementary forms*].

Bachrach, L (1976). *Deinstitutionalization: An analytical review and sociological perspective.* Rockville, US departement of health, education and welfare, National Institute of Mental Health.

Bachrach, L (1988). Defining chronic mental illness: a concept paper. *Hospital and Community Psychiatry*, Vol 39, No 4, p 383–388.

Barham, P (1984). *Schizophrenia and human value – Chronic schizophrenia, science and society*. Oxford: Basil Blackwell.

Barnes, M & Berke, J (1971). *Two accounts of a journey through madness*. New York: Harcourt, Brace & Jovanovitch.

Barrett, R (1996). *The psychiatric team and the social definition of schizophrenia*. Cambridge: Cambridge University Press.

Barton, R (1959). *Institutional neurosis*. Bristol: Wright.

Basaglia, F (1968). *L'istituzione negata*. Torino: Einaudi.

Basaglia, F (1982). *Salute/malatia – Le parole della medicina*. Milano: Einaudi.

Basaglia, F (1983). Psykiatrin utan mentalsjukhus. In: Costa, F & Topor A (eds). *Alternativ till psykiatrin*. Stockholm: Prisma. [Psychiatry without mental hospitals. In: Costa, F & Topor A (eds). *Alternatives to psychiatry*].

Basaglia, F (1987). *Psychiatry inside out – Selected writings of Franco Basaglia*. New York: Columbia University Press.

Bateson, G (red) (1961). *Perceval's narrative – A patient's account of his psychosis 1830-1832*. Stanford: Stanford University Press.

Beels, C (1978). Social networks, the family, and the schizophrenic patient. Introduction to the issue. *Schizophrenia Bulletin*, Vol 4, No 4, p 512–521.

Beels, C (1979). Social networks and schizophrenia. *Psychiatric Quarterly*, Vol 51, No 3, p 209–215.

Beels, C (1981). Social support and schizophrenia. *Schizophrenia Bulletin*, Vol 7, No 1, p 58–72.

Beiser, M (1995). Transcending scientific and parochialism in the service of the mentally ill. *International Journal of Mental Health*, Vol 24, No 1, p 20–38.

Beiser, M & Iacono, W (1990). An update on the epidemiology of schizophrenia. *Canadian Journal of Psychiatry*, Vol 35, No 8, p 657–668.

Belfrage, H (1994). Criminality and mortality among a cohort of former mental patients in Sweden. *Nordic Journal of Psychiatry*, Vol 48, p 343–347.

Belfrage, H (1995). *"Sundby-rapporten" - En undersökning av kriminalitet och dödlighet hos före detta mentalpatienter*. Karolinska Institutet, Sektionen för social- och rättspsykiatri, Rapport 1995:1. [*"The Sundby report" – A study of criminality and mortality in former mental patients*].

Belfrage, H (1996). *Kriminalitet, sjuklighet och dödlighet hos mentalsjukhus-patienter*. Socialstyrelsen (National Board of Health and Welfare): Psykiatri-uppföljningen 1996:1. [*Criminality, morbidity, and mortality in mental hospital patients*].

Belin, S (1994). *Schizofrenibehandling. Psykiatri på liv och död*. Stockholm: Natur & Kultur. [*Schizophrenia treatment. Psychiatry: a matter of life and death*].

Belliveau Krauss, J & Tomaino Slavinsky, A (1982). *The chronically ill psychiatric patient and the community*. Boston: Blackwell Scientific Publications.

345

Bental, R (1990). The syndromes and symptoms of psychosis. In: Bental, R (ed). *Reconstructing schizophrenia*. London: Routledge.

Bergh, A (1998). En text om arbete för psykiskt funktionshindrade. In: Topor, A (ed). *Perspektiv på psykiatrireformen*. Stockholm: FoU-enheten/psykiatri, Västra Stockholms Sjukvårdsområde. [A text on work for the mentally disabled. In: Topor, A (ed). *Perspectives on psychiatric reforms*].

Bergin, A & Lambert, M J (1978). The evaluation of therapeutic outcome. In: Garfield, S L & Bergin, A (eds). *Handbook of psychotherapy and behavior change*. 2nd ed. New York: John Wiley.

Berner, P (1992). L'approche clinique dans la recherche des causes: spécificité ou bon sens. In: Pichot, P & Rein, W (eds). *L'approche clinique en psychiatrie – Histoire, role, applications*. Vol I. Paris: Les empêcheurs de penser en rond.

Bertaux, D (red) (1981). *Biography and society. The lifehistory approach in the social sciences*. Beverly Hills: Sage Publications.

Bertaux, D (1986). Fonctions diverses des récits de vie dans le processus de recherche. In: Desmarais, D & Grell, P (eds). *Les récits de vie – Théorie, methodes et trajectoires types*. Montréal: Editions St Martin.

Bertaux, D (1997). *Les récits de vie*. Paris: Nathan.

Bettelheim, B (1943). Individual and mass behavior in extreme situations. In: Bettelheim, B (1980). *Surviving and other essays*. New York: Vintage Books.

Bettelheim, B (1986). *Surviving the Holocaust*. Glasgow: Flamingo.

Blanch, A & Fisher, D & Tucker, W & Walsh, D & Chassman, J (1993). Consumer-practitioners and psychiatrist share insights about recovery and coping. *Disability Studies Quaterly*, Vol 13, No 2, p 17–20.

Bleuler, E (1950). *Dementia praecox or the group of schizophrenia*. 1:a uppl. New York: International Universities Press.

Bleuler, M (1963). Conception of schizophrenia within the last fifty years and today. *Proceedings of the Royal Society of Medicine*, Vol 56, p 25–32.

Bleuler, M (1978). *The schizophrenic disorders – Long-term patient and family studies*. New Haven and London: Yale University Press.

Bleuler, M (1991). The concept of schizophrenia in Europe during the past one hundred years. In: Flack, W & Miller, D & Wiener, M (eds). *What is schizophrenia?* New York: Springer-Verlag.

Blomqvist, J (1996). Paths to recovery from substance missuse: change of lifestyle and the role of treatment. *Substance Use and Misuse*, Vol 31, No 13, p 1807-52.

Blumer, H (1954). What is wrong with social theory? *American Sociological review,* 19, p 3–10.

Boker, W (1987). On self-help among schizophrenics: Problem analysis and empiri-cal studies. In: Strauss, J S & Boker, W & Brenner, H (eds). *Psychosocial treatment of schizophrenia*, p 160–166. New York: Hans Huber.

Borell, P (1995). Beteendeterapeutisk behandling vid schizofreni. *Scandinavian Journal of Behaviour Therapy*, Vol 24, No 2-3, p 45–61. [Behavioral therapy treatment of schizophrenia].

Borg, M (1999). *Virksomme relasjoner – Hva inneboerer dette sett fra psykiatriske pasienters ståsted?* Oslo: Universitetet i Oslo, Det medicinske fakultet, Sekjon for helsefag. [*Active relations – What does this mean from the position of the psychiatric patient?*]

Borg, M & Topor, A (2001) (red). *Perspektiv på bedringsprosesser ved alvorlige psykiske lidelser*, Dialog, Vol 11, No 2. [*Perspectives on recovery processes in severe mental disorders*].

Borg, M & Bjerke, C & Kufås, E & Topor, A & Svensson, J (1998). Veier ut av alvorlig psykisk lidelse – en pilotstudie. *Dialog*, nr 2, s 7–21. [Paths out of severe mental disorders – a pilot study].

Borgå, P (1993). *Studies of long-term functional psychosis in three different areas of Stockholm county*. Umeå: Umeå University Medical Dissertations nr 358.

Boström, H (2000). Placebo och placeboeffekter. In: Boström, H & Dahlgren, H (eds). *Placebo*. Stockholm: Liber/SBU.

Bott, E (1976). Hospital and society. *British Journal of Medical Psychology*, Vol 49, No 2, p 97–140.

Bourdieu, P (1994). L'illusion biographique. In: Bourdieu, P. *Raisons pratiques – Sur la théorie de l'action*. Paris: Editions du Seuil.

Bourdieu, P et al. (1999). *The Weight of the World: Social suffering in contemporary society*. Oxford: Polity Press (First published 1993 as *La misère du monde*. Paris: Editions du Seuil.

Boyle, M (1990). The non-discovery of schizophrenia. In: Bentall, P (ed). *Reconstructing schizophrenia*. London: Routledge.

Boyle, M (1993). *Schizophrenia – A scientific delusion?* London: Routledge.

Breier, A (1988). Small sample studies: unique contributions for large sample outcome studies. *Schizophrenia Bulletin*, Vol 14, No 4, p 589–593.

Breier, A & Strauss, JS (1983). Self-control in psychotic disorders. *Archives of General Psychiatry*, Vol 40, No 10, p 1141-1145.

Breier, A & Strauss, JS (1984). The role of social relationships in the recovery from psychotic disorders. *American Journal of Psychiatry*, Vol 141, No 8, p 949–955.

Brenner, H & Boker, W & Muller, J & Spichtig, L & Wurgler, S (1987). On auto-protective efforts of schizophrenics, neurotics and controls. *Acta Psychiatrica Scandinavica*, Vol 75, No 4, p 405–414.

Brockington, IF & Nalpas, A (1993). L'approche clinique et le concept de schizophrénie. In: Pichot, P & Rein, W (es.d). *L'approche clinique en psychiatrie*. Vol II. Paris: Les empecheurs de penser en rond.

Bruner, J (1987). Life as narrative. *Social Research*, Vol 54, No. 1, p 11–32.

Burish, T & Bradley, L (1983). Coping with chronic disease: definitions and issues. In: Burish, T & Bradley, L (eds). *Coping with chronic disease – Research and applications*. New York: Academic Press.

Burke, K (1945). *A grammar of motives*. New York: Prentice-Hall.

Burkitt, I (1991). *Social selves – Theories of the social formation of personality*. London: Sage Publications.

Bury, M (1982). Chronic illness as biographical disruptions. *Sociology of health and illness*, Vol 4, No 2, p 167–182.

Butler, S & Strupp, H (1986). Specific and non-specific factors in psychotherapy: a problematic paradigm for psychotherapy research. *Psychotherapy*, Vol 23, No 1, p 30–40.

Carpenter, W & Kirkpatrick, B (1988). The heterogeneity of the long-term course of schizophrenia. *Schizophrenia Bulletin*, Vol 14, No 4, p 645–652.

Carr, V (1988). Patients' techniques for coping with schizophrenia: An exploratory study. *British Journal of Medical Psychology*, Vol 61, Pt 4, p 339–352.

Carr, V & Katsikitis, M (1987). Illness behaviour and schizophrenia. *Psychiatric Medicine*, Vol 5, No 2, p 163–170.

Castel, R (1973). *Le psychanalysme*. Paris: Francois Maspero.

Castel, R (1976). *L'ordre psychiatrique. L'age d'or de l'aliénisme*. Paris: Les éditions de minuit.

Castel, R (1981). *La gestion des risques. De l'anti-psychiatrie à l'après psychiatrie*. Paris: Les éditions de minuit.

Castel, R (1987). Avinstitutionaliseringen. *Kritisk Psykologi*, nr 4.

Castel, R (1992). (sous la direction de). *Les sorties de la toxicomanie. Types, trajectoires, tonalités*. Paris: MIRE.

Chadwick, P (1997). Recovery from psychosis: Learning more from patients. *Journal of Mental Health*, Vol 6, No 6, p 577-588.

Chamberlin, J (1978). *On our own - Patient-controlled alternatives to the mental health system*. New York: Hawthorn Books, Inc.

Charmaz, K (1983). Loss of self: a fundamental form of suffering in the chronically ill. *Sociology of Health and Illness*, Vol 5, No 2, p 168–195.

Chase, S E (1995). Taking narrative seriously: Consequences for method and theory in interview studies. In: Josselson, R & Lieblich, A (eds). *Interpreting experiences, The narrative study of lives*. Vol 3. New York: Sage Publications.

Ciompi, L (1980). The natural history of schizophrenia in the long term, *British Journal of Psychiatry*, Vol 136, May, p 413–420. [Sv övers. (1993) Schizofrenins naturhistoria på lång sikt. *Kritisk Psykologi* nr 1:1993].

Ciompi, L (1984). Is there really a schizophrenia? The long-term course of psychotic phenomena. *British Journal of Psychiatry*, Vol 145, December, p 636–640.

Cohen, P & Cohen, J (1984). The clinician's illusion. *Archives of General Psychiatry*, Vol 41, No 12, p 1178-1182.

Cohen, CI & Berk, LA (1985). Personal coping styles of schizophrenic outpatients. *Hospital and Community Psychiatry*, Vol 36, No 4, p 407-10.

Cole, J & Goldberg, S & Klerman, GL (1964). Phenothiazine treatment in acute schizophrenia. *Archives of General Psychiatry*, Vol 10, p 246–261.

Coleman, R (1999). *Recovery – an alien concept*. Gloucester: Handsell Publishing.

Collé, M & Quétel, C (1987). *Histoire des maladies mentales*. Paris: PUF.

Conrad, P & Schneider, J (1992). *Deviance and medicalization - From badness to sickness*. Philadelphia: Temple University Press.

Corin, E (1990). Facts and meaning in psychiatry. An anthropological approach to the lifeworld of schizophrenics. *Culture, Medicine and Psychiatry*, Vol 14, No 2, p 153–188.

Corin, E & Lauzon, G (1992). Positive withdrawal and the quest for meaning: The reconstruction of experience among schizophrenics. *Psychiatry*, Vol 55, No 3, p 266–278.

Coyne Plum, K (1987). How patients view recovery: what helps, what hinders. *Archives of Psychiatric Nursing*, Vol 1, No 4, p 285–293.

Crafoord, C (1987). *Den möjliga och omöjliga psykiatrin – Utveckling och erfarenheter av sektoriserad psykiatri*. Stockholm: Natur & Kultur. [*The possible and the impossible psychiatry – Developments in and experiences of comparte-mentalized psychiatry*].

Cullberg, J (1975). *Kris och utveckling*. Stockholm: Natur & Kultur. [*Crisis and development*].

Cullberg, J (1991). Recovered versus nonrecovered schizophrenic patients among those who had intensive psychotherapy. *Acta Psychiatrica Scandinavica*, Vol 84, No 3, p 242–245.

Cullberg, J (1993). Kliniska konsekvenser av en flerdimensionell syn på schizo-freniernas etiologier. *Kritisk Psykologi*, No 1, p 16–21. [Clinical consequences of a multi-dimensional view of schizophrenia's etiologies].

Cullberg, J (1999). *Dynamisk psykiatri i teori och praktik*. 5:e rev. utg. Stockholm: Natur och Kultur. [*Dynamic psychiatry in theory and practice*].

Cullberg, J (2000a). *Psykoser. Ett humanistiskt och biologiskt perspektiv*. Stockholm: Natur och Kultur. [*Psychoses. A humanistic and biological perspective*].

Cullberg, J (2000b). *Tal vid Nordkalottkonferensen*. Stencil. Falun. [*Speech at Nordkalott conference*].

Cullberg, J & Grunewald, K (1988). Schizofreni och den nya synen på handikapp – ställ krav på kommunerna! *Läkartidningen,* Vol 86, No 51, p 4501-4504. [Schizophrenia and the new view of disabilities – make demands on the munici-palities!].

Cullberg, J & Levander, S (1991). Fully recovered schizophrenic patients who received intensive psychotherapy – A Swedish case-finding study. *Nordisk Psykiatrisk Tidskrift*, Vol 45, p 253–262.

Cutting, J & Dunne, F (1989). Subjective experience of schizophrenia. *Schizophrenia Bulletin*, Vol 15, No 2, p 217–231.

Danziger, K (1990*). Constructing the subject: historical origins of psychological research*. New York: Cambridge University Press.

Danziger, K (1997). The historical formation of selves. In: Ashmore, R & Jussim, L (eds). *Self and identity. Fundamental issues*. Oxford: Oxford University Press.

Davidson, L & Stayner, D (1997). Loss, loneliness, and the desire for love: Perspectives on the social lives of people with schizophrenia. *Psychiatric Rehabilitation Journal*, Vol 20, No 3, p 3–12.

Davidson, L & Strauss, JS (1992). Sense of self in recovery from severe mental illness. *British Journal of Medical Psychology*, Vol 65, June (pt 2), p 131–145.

Davidson, L & Strauss, JS (1995). Beyond the biopsychosocial model: Integrating disorder, health and recovery. *Psychiatry*, Vol 58, No 1, p 44–55.

Deegan, P (1988). Recovery: The lived experience of rehabilitation. *Psychosocial Rehabilitation Journal*, Vol 11, No 4, p 11–19.

Deegan, P (1997a). Recovery as a journey of the heart. In: Spaniol, L & Gagne, C & Koehler, M (eds). *Psychological and social aspects of psychiatric disability.* Boston: Center for Psychiatric Rehabilitation, Boston University.

Deegan, P (1997b). Recovering our sense of value after being labelled. In: Spaniol, L & Gagne, C & Koehler, M (eds). *Psychological and social aspects of psychiatric disability.* Boston: Center for Psychiatric Rehabilitation, Boston University.

Dell'Acqua, G & Mezzina, R (1988). Responding to crisis – Strategies and intentionality in community psychiatric intervention. *Per la salute mentale/For mental health*, No 1, p 139–158.

Denhov, A (2000). *Personalens bidrag till återhämtning – Ett brukarperspektiv.* Stockholm: FoU-enheten/psykiatri. Västra Stockholm. Rapport 11/2000.

di Paola, F (2000a). *L'istituzione del male mentale – critica dei fondamenti scientifici della psichiatria biologica.* Roma: Manifesto Libri.

di Paola, F (2000b). *The flaw in the medical model of mental health; the right to dissent from treatment.* Paper addressed to the conference "Making or breaking barriers?", Centre for Mental Health Policy, University of Central England, Birmingham, 7th July 2000.

Diderichsen, F & Janlert, U (1983). Krisen i Malmfältet – är psykiatrin ett alternativ? In: Costa, F & Topor, A (eds). *Alternativ till psykiatrin.* Stockholm: Prisma. [Crisis in the Minefield– is psychiatry an alternative? In: Costa, F & Topor, A (eds). *Alternatives to psychiatry*].

Distefano, MK Jr & Pryer, MW & Garrison, JL (1991). Validity of psychiatric patients self-report of rehospitalization. *Hospital and Community Psychiatry*, Vol 42, No 8, p 849–850.

Eisenberg, L (1988). The social construction of mental illness. *Psychological Medicine*, Vol 18, No 1, p 1–9.

Ekströmer, CJ (1847). *Underdånig berättelse om Länslasaretterne, kurhusen och hospitalen i riket.* Stockholm: Norstedt & söner. [*Humble tale of county hospitals, health spas, and hospitals in the country*].

Estroff, S (1985). *Making it crazy.* Berkeley: University of California Press.

Estroff, S (1989). Self, identity and subjective experiences of schizophrenia: In search of the subject. *Schizophrenia Bulletin*, Vol 15, No 2, p 189–196.

Ewertzon, M & Forssell, H (1999). *Patienter och anhörigas nätverk – Kartläggning och uppföljning av det sociala nätverket hos första gångsinsjuknade patienter med psykotiska symtom och för deras anhöriga.* Stockholm: FoU-enheten/VSPS, Rapport nr 7/1999. [*Patients and relatives' network – Survey and follow-up of the social network in first-time patients with psychotic symptoms, and their relatives*].

Ey, H (1977). *La notion de schizophrénie.* Séminaire de Thuir, Alencon: Desclée de Brouer.

Falloon, IR & Talbot, RE (1981). Persistent auditory hallucinations: Coping mechanisms and implications for management. *Psychological Medicine,* Vol 11, No 2, 329–339.

Fenichel, O (1971). *The psychoanalytic theory of neurosis.* London: Routledge & Keegan.

Forsberg, E & Starrin, B (1996). The Millhill. A study of discharged patients' experiences of care at a therapeutic community in Sweden, *Scandinavian Journal of Social Welfare,* Vol 5, No 1, p 2–11.

Foucault, M (1972). *Histoire de la folie à l'age classique,* Paris: Gallimard.

Frank, A & Gunderson, J (1987). The psychotherapy of schizophrenia: patient and therapist factors related to continuance. *Psychotherapy,* Vol 24, No 3, p 392–403.

Frank, A (1995). *The wounded storyteller. Body, illness and ethics.* Chicago: The University of Chicago Press.

Frank, JD (1963). *Persuasion and healing. A comparative study of psychotherapy.* New York: Schocken Books.

Frank JD (1968). The role of hope in psychotherapy. *International Journal of Psychiatry,* Vol 5, No 5, p 383 – 395.

Frank, JD (1971). Eleventh Emil A. Gutheil memorial conference. Therapeutic factors in psychotherapy. *American Journal of Psychotherapy,* Vol 25, No 3, p 350–361.

Frank, JD (1974). Psychotherapy: The restoration of morale. *American Journal of Psychiatry,* Vol 131, No 3, p 271–274.

Fredén, L (1991). Schizofreni enligt DSM-III-R i kritisk belysning. In: Fredén, L & Svensson, T (eds). *Perspektiv på psykisk sjukdom.* Linköping, Tema Hälso- och sjukvården i samhället, SHS 13. [Schizophrenia according to DSM-III-R in a critical light. In: Fredén, L & Svensson, T (eds). *Perspectives on mental illness*].

Freud, S (1905). *Bruchstück einer Hysterie-Analyse. Gesemmelte Werke V.* V.S. Fischer Verlag, Frankfurt am Main.

Freud, S (1959). Psycho-analytic notes upon an autobiographical account of a case of paranoia (dementia paranoides). In: *Collected papers.* Vol 3. New York: Basic Books.

Freud, S (1980). *Orientering i psykoanalys.* Stockholm: Natur och Kultur. [*Orientation in psychoanalysis*].

Fuchs Ebaugh, HR (1988). *Becoming an ex. The process of role exit.* Chicago: The University of Chicago Press.

Gallio, G (red) (1991). *Nell'impresa sociale – cooperazione, lavoro, ri-habilitazione, culture di confine nell politiche di salute mentale.* Trieste: Edizioni E.

Gardell, B (1983). Effektivitetskrav och hälsorisker i ett teknifierat samhälle. In: Costa, F & Topor, A (eds). *Alternativ till psykiatrin.* Stockholm: Prisma. [Efficiency demands and health risks in a technology society. In: Costa, F & Topor, A (eds). *Alternatives to psychiatry*].

351

Garrabé, J & Winkelmuller, P (1994). Les neuroleptiques ont-ils réellement modifié le pronostic à long terme des psychoses schizophréniques? In: Fédération francaise de psychiatrie/Union nationale des amis et familles de malades mentaux. *Conférence de consencus. Stratégies thérapeutiques à long terme dans les psychoses schizophréniques – Textes des experts.* Paris: Editions Frison-Roche.

Garrabé, J (1992). *Histoire de la schizophrénie.* Paris: Seghers.

Gauchet, M & Swain, G (1980). *La pratique de l'esprit humain. L'institution asilaire et la révolution démocratique.* Paris: Gallimard.

Gentis, R (1969). *Les schizophrènes.* Paris: Editions du scarabée.

Gergen, KJ (1989). Warranting voices and the elaboration of the self. In: Shotter, J & Gergen K J (eds). *Texts of identity,* London: Sage Publications.

Gergen, KJ (1991). *The saturated self – Dilemmas of identity in contemporary life.* New York: Basic Books.

Gergen, KJ & Gergen, M (1988). Narrative and the self as relationship. *Advances in Experimental Social Psychology,* Vol 21, p 17–56.

Gerhardt, U (1989). *Ideas about illness – an intellectual and political history of medical sociology.* London: Macmillan.

Glaser, B (1978). *Theoretical sensitivity.* San Francisco: The Sociology Press.

Glaser, B & Strauss, A (1967). *The discovery of grounded theory: strategies for qualitative research.* New York: Aldine de Gruyter.

Goffman, E (1961). *Asylums – Essays on the social situation of mental patients and other inmates.* New York: Doubleday & Co.

Goffman, E (1968). *Stigma – Notes on the management of spoiled identity.* Harmondsworth: Pelican Books.

Goffman, E (1972). Role distance. In: Goffman, E. *Encounters – Two studies in the sociology of interaction.* Harmondworth: Penguin University Books.

Green, H (1967). *I never promised you a rose garden.* London: Pan Books.

Greenberg, G (1994). *The self on the shelf – Recovery books and the good life.* New York: State University of New York Press.

Greenfeld, D & Strauss, JS & Bowers, M & Mandelkern, M (1989). Insight and interpretation of illness in recovery from psychosis. *Schizophrenia Bulletin,* Vol 15, No 2, p 245–252.

Gronfein, W (1985). Psychotropic drugs and the origins of deinstitutionalisation. *Social Problems,* Vol 32, No 5, p 437–454.

Grunewald, K (1997). *Psykiska handikapp: möjligheter och rättigheter.* Stockholm: Liber. [*Mental disability: opportunities and rights*].

Grunewald, K (1999). Psykiskt sjuk eller psykiskt handikappad? *Revansch!* No 3. [*Mentally ill or mentally disabled?*].

Guelfi, J-D (1994). Critères cliniques d'évaluation des stratégies thérapeutiques à long terme dans les psychoses schizophréniques. In: Federation francaise de psychiatrie/Union nationale des amis et familles de malades mentaux. *Conférence de consencus. Stratégies thérapeutiques à long terme dans les psychoses schizophréniques – Textes des experts.* Paris: Editions Frison-Roche.

352

Gunderson, JG & Frank, AF & Katz, HM & Vannicelli, ML & Frosch, M & Knapp, PH (1984). Effects of psychotherapy in schizophrenia: II. Comparative outcome of two forms of treatment. *Schizophrenia Bulletin*, Vol 10, No 4, p 564–598.

Gylling, M (1996). *Det första mötet med psykiatrin – en studie av bemötanderutiner på en akut- och korttidsavdelning, Beckomberga sjukhus.* Stockholm: FoU-enheten/psykiatrin, VSSO, Rapport 9/96. [*The first encounter with psychiatry – a study of encounter procedures at an emergency and acute care ward, Beckomberga hospital*].

Hagnell, O (1966). *A prospective study of the incidence of mental disorder. A study based on 24.000 person – years of the incidence of mental disorders in a Swedish population together with an evaluation of the aetiological significance of medical, social and personality factors.* Lund: Scandinavian University Books.

Haley, J (1982). *Leaving Home: The Therapy of Disturbed Young People.* 2nd edition. New York: Taylor & Francis.

Halldin, J (2000). Avinstitutionaliseringens betydelse för hemlösheten – myter och fakta. In: Runquist, W & Swärd, H (eds). *Hemlöshet – En antologi om olika perspektiv och förklaringsmodeller.* Stockholm: Carlssons. [The importance of deinstitutionalisation for the homeless – myths and facts. In: Runquist, W & Swärd, H (eds). *Homelessness – An anthology of different perspectives and explanatory models.* Stockholm: Carlssons].

Hansson, JH (1993). *Organizing normality – essays on organizing day activities for people with severe mental disorders.* Linköpings Universitet: Tema Hälsa och Samhälle.

Harding, CM (1986). Speculations on the measurement of recovery from severe psychiatric disorder and the human condition. *The Psychiatric Journal of the University of Ottawa*, Vol 11, No 4, p 199–204.

Harding, CM (1988). Course types in schizophrenia: an analysis of European and American studies. *Schizophrenia Bulletin*, Vol 14, No 4, p 633–643.

Harding, CM (1997). Personal communication.

Harding, CM & Brooks, GW & Ashikaga, T & Strauss, JS & Breier, A (1987a). The Vermont longitudinal study of persons with severe mental illness. In: Methodology, study sample, and overall status 32 years later. *American Journal of Psychiatry*, Vol 144, No 6, p 718–726.

Harding, CM & Brooks, GW & Ashikaga, T & Strauss, JS & Breier, A (1987b). The Vermont longitudinal study of persons with severe mental illness. II: Long-term outcome of subjects who retrospectively met DSM III criteria for schizophrenia. *American Journal of Psychiatry*, Vol 144, No 6, p 727–735.

Harding, CM & Strauss, JS (1984). How serious is schizophrenia? Comments on prognosis. *Biological Psychiatry*, Vol 19, No 12, p 1597-1600.

Harding, CM & Zubin, J & Strauss, JS (1987). Chronicity in schizophrenia: fact, partial fact or artefact. *Hospital and Community Psychiatry*, Vol 38, No 5, p 477–486.

Harding, CM & Zubin, J & Strauss, JS (1992). Chronicity in schizophrenia: Revisited. *British Journal of Psychiatry*, Vol 161 (Suppl 18), October, p 27–37.

Hastings, D (1958). Follow-up results in psychiatric illness. *American Journal of Psychiatry*, June, p 1057-1066.

Hatfield, A & Lefley, H (1993). *Surviving mental illness – Stress, coping and adaptation*. New York: The Guildford press.

Hegarty, JD & Baldessarini, RJ & Tohen, M & Waternaux, C & Oepen, G (1994). One hundred years of schizophrenia: a meta-analysis of the outcome literature. *American Journal of Psychiatry*, Vol 151, No 10, p 1409-1416.

Heilig, M (1999a). Återskapa den medicinska kulturen inom psykiatrin! *Läkartidningen*, Vol 96, No 41, p 4427-4433. [Recreate the medical culture in psychiatry!].

Heilig, M (1999b). Förenklade sanningar har skadat psykiatrin! *Läkartidningen*, Vol 96, No 47, p 5184-5186. [Simplified truths have damaged psychiatry!]

Heinritz, C & Rammstedt, A (1991). L'approche biographique en France. *Cahiers Internationaux de Sociologie*, Vol XCI, p 331–370.

Hogarty, GE (1984). Depot neuroleptics: The relevance of the psychosocial factors. *Journal of Clinical Psychiatry*, Vol 45, May (pt 2), p 36–42.

Hogarty, GE & Anderson, CM & Reis, DJ & Kornblith, SJ & Greenwald, DP & Javna, CD & Madonia, MJ (1986). Family psychoeducation, social skills training and maintenance chemotherapy in the aftercare treatment of schizophrenia – I. One-year effects of a controlled study on relapse and expressed emotions. *Archives of General Psychiatry*, Vol 43, p 633–642.

Hogarty, GE & Anderson, CM & Reis, DJ & Kornblith, SJ & Greenwald, DP & Ulrich, RF & Carter, M (1991). Family psychoeducation, social skills training and maintenance chemotherapy in the aftercare treatment of schizophrenia – II. Two-years effects of a controlled study on relapse and adjustment. *Archives of General Psychiatry*, Vol 48, p 340–347.

Huber, G (1997). The heterogeneous course of schizophrenia. *Schizophrenia Research*, Vol 28, No 2-3, p 177–185.

Huber, G & Gross, G & Schuttler, R & Linz, M (1980). Longitudinal studies of schizophrenic patients. *Schizophrenia Bulletin*, Vol 6, No 4, p 592–605.

Hydén, LC (1995a). *Psykiatri samhälle patient – Psykisk sjukdom i socialt och kulturellt perspektiv*. Stockholm: Natur & Kultur. [*Psychiatry society patient – Mental illness in social and cultural perspective*].

Hydén, LC (1995b). The rhetoric of recovery and change. *Culture, Medicine and Psychiatry*, Vol 19, No 1, p 73–90.

Hydén, L-C (1997). Illness and narratives. *Sociology of Health & Illness*, Vol. 19, No. 1, p 48-69.

Hydén, LC & Karlsson, I (1994). *Arbetsverksamheter i tre psykiatriska sektorer. En uppföljning*. Nacka: Psykosociala forskningsenheten, Rapport nr 1994:4. [*Working operations in three mental sectors. A follow-up*].

354

Hydén, M (1992). *Woman battering as marital act. The construction of a violent marriage*. Stockholm: Studies in Social Work, No 7. Stockholm University.

Jones, M (1968). *Social psychiatry in practice. The idea of the therapeutic community*. Harmondsworth: Penguin.

Jonsson, D (1993). Hälsoekonomiska aspekter på schizofreni. *Socialmedicinsk Tidskrift*, Vol 70, No 6, s 280–283. [Health-economics aspects of schizophrenia].

Jonsson, E (1986). *Tokfursten*. Stockholm: Rabén & Sjögren. [*The crazy prince*].

Kanfer, FH (1971). The maintenance of behaviour by self-generated stimuli and reinforcement. In: Jacobs, A & Sachs, LB (eds). *The psychology of private events: Perspectives on covert response systems*. New York: Academic Press Inc.

Karebo Larsén, I (1996). *Istället för slutenvården? Sveaborg. Äldre deprimerade kvinnliga patienters väg från den slutna psykiatriska vården. En slutenvårdskonsumtionsstudie*. FoU-enheten/psykiatri, VSSO, Arbetspapper 3/96. [*Instead of institutional care? Sveaborg. The route taken by older depressed female patients from institutionalized psychiatric care. A study of consumption of institutionalized care*].

Kaufmann, J-C (1996). *L'entretien compréhensif*. Paris: Nathan Université.

Kirk, S & Kutchins, H (1992). *The selling of the DSM. The rhetoric of science in psychiatry*. New York: Walter de Gruyter.

Kleinman, A (1988). *The illness narratives – suffering, healing and the human condition*. New York: Basic Books.

Kopelowicz, A & Liberman, R (1996). Biobehavioral treatment and rehabilitation of schizophrenia. *Harvard Review of Psychiatry*, July/August, p 55–64.

Kraepelin, E (1971). *Dementia praecox and paraphrenia*. (From the 8th German edition 1919). New York: Robert E. Krieger Publishing Co Inc.

Kramer, M (1969). Cross-national study of diagnosis of the mental disorders: origin of the problem. *American Journal of Psychiatry,* 10 Suppl, April, p 1–11.

Kramer, PJ & Gagne, C (1997). Barriers to recovery and empowerment for people with psychiatric disabilities. In: Spaniol, L & Gagne, C & Koehler, M (eds). *Psychological and social aspects of psychiatric disability*. Boston: Center for Psychiatric Rehabilitation, Boston University.

Kvale, S (1996). *Interviews. An Introduction to Qualitative Research Interviewing*. London: Sage Publications

Lally, SJ (1989). "Does being in here mean there is something wrong with me?" *Schizophrenia Bulletin*, Vol 15, No 2, p 253–265.

Lamb, R (1976). Individual psychotherapy: Helping the long-term patient achieve mastery. In: Lamb, R et al (eds). *Community survival for long-term patients*. San Francisco: Jossey-Bass Publishers.

Langfeldt, G (1937). The prognosis in schizophrenia and the factors influencing the course of the disease – A katamnestic study, including individual re-examinations in 1936 with some considerations regarding diagnosis, pathogenesis and therapy. *Acta Psychiatrica et Neurologica*, suppl XIII.

Lantéri-Laura, G (1997). La chronicité dans la psychiatrie francaise moderne – note d'histoire théorique et sociale. In: Lantéri-Laura, G. *La chronicité en psychiatrie*. Paris: Les Empécheurs de Penser en Rond.

Lee, PW & Lieh-Mak, F & Yu, KK & Spinks, JA (1993). Coping strategies of schizophrenic patients and their relationship to outcome. *British Journal of Psychiatry*, Vol 163, August, p 177–182.

Leete, E (1989). How I perceive and manage my illness. *Schizophrenia Bulletin*, Vol 15, No 2, p 197–200.

Leff, JP (1977). International variations in the diagnosis of psychiatric illness. *British Journal of Psychiatry*, Vol 131, October, p 329–338.

Leff, J & Sartorius, N & Jablensky, A & Korten, A & Ernberg, G (1992). The international pilot study of schizophrenia: five-year follow-up findings. *Psychological medicine*, Vol 22, No 1, p 131–145.

Leff, JP & Wing, JK (1971). Trial maintenance therapy in schizophrenia. *British Medicine Journal*, Vol 3, No 775, p 559–604.

Leff, J &Wig, NN & Bedi, H & Menon, DK & Kuipers, L & Korten, A & Ernberg, G & Day, R & Satorius, N & Jablensky, A (1990). Relatives' Expressed Emotions and the course of schizophrenia in Chandigarh. A two-year follow-up of a first-contact sample. *British Journal of Psychiatry*, Vol 156, March, p 351–356.

Leff, J & Wig, NN & Ghosh, A & Bedi, H & Menon, DK & Kuipers, L & Korten, A & Ernberg, G & Day, R & Satorius, N & Jablensky, A (1987). Influence of relatives' Expressed Emotions on the course of schizophrenia in Chandigarh. *British Journal of Psychiatry*, Vol 151, August, p 166–173.

Lemoine, P (1996). *Le mystère du placebo*. Paris: Editions Odile Jacob.

Lerman, P (1984). *Deinstitutionalization and the welfare state*. New Brunswick: Rutgers.

Lévi-Strauss, C (1962). *La pensée sauvage*. Paris: Plon. [Sv övers. (1971) *Det vilda tänkandet*. Stockholm: Bonniers].

Liberman, RP & Mueser, KT & Wallace, CJ & Jacobs, HE & Eckman, T & Massel, HK (1986). Training skills in the psychiatrically disabled: Learning coping and competence. *Schizophrenia Bulletin*, Vol 12, No 4, p 631–647.

Ljungberg, L (1975). *Schizofreni*. Stockholm: Essex Läkemedel AB. [*Schizophrenia*].

Ludwig, A (1971). *Treating the treatment failures – The challenge of chronic schizophrenia*. New York: Grune & Stratton.

Läromedelförlagen Språkförlaget (1969). *Engelsk-svensk ordbok*. Stockholm: Norstedt & söner. [*English-Swedish dictionary*].

Machiavelli, N (1532/2000). *Fursten*. Stockholm: Natur och Kultur. [*Il Principe*].

Marin, I (2000). *La riabilitazione psicosociale nella prospetiva dell'utente. Cinque percorsi di recovery in salute mentale*. Universita degli studi di Trieste.

Mattingly, C (1994). The concept of therapeutic "emplotment", *Social Science and Medicine*, Vol 38, No 6, p 811–822.

Mauss, M. (1950/1923-1924). Essai sur le don – Forme et raison de l'échange dans les sociètés archaiques. In Mauss, M. *Sociologie et anthropologie*, Paris: Presses Universitaires de France.

Mayer, JE & Rosenblatt, A (1974). Clash in perspective between mental patients and staff. *American Journal of Orthopsychiatry*, Vol 44, No 3, p 432–441.

McGlashan, TH (1984). The Chestnut Lodge follow-up study. II. Long-term outcome of schizophrenia and the affective disorders. *Archives of General Psychiatry*, Vol 41, No 6, p 586–601.

McGlashan, TH (1987). Recovery style from mental illness and long-term outcome. *The Journal of Nervous and Mental Disease*, Vol 175, No 11, p 681–685.

McGlashan, TH (1988). A selective review of recent north American long-term follow-up studies of schizophrenia. *Schizophrenia Bulletin*, Vol 14, No 4, p 515–542.

McGorry, P (1992). The concept of recovery and secondary prevention in psychotic disorders. *Australian and New Zealand Journal of Psychiatry*, Vol 26, No 1, p 3–17.Minkoff, K (1978). A map of chronic mental patients. In: Talbott, J (red). *The chronic mental patient – Problems, solutions and recommendations for a public policy*. Washington: The American Psychiatric Association.

Mosher, LR & Burti, L (1988). *Community mental health – Principles and practice*. New York: W. W Norton & company.

Nathan, T (1994). *L'influence qui guérit*. Paris: Editions Odile Jacob.

Nathan, T (1998). Elements de psychothérapie. I : Nathan, T (red). *Psychothérapies*. Paris: Editions Odile Jacob.

National Board of Health and Welfare (1989). *Psykoterapins effekter vid psykos – En forskningsöversikt*. SoS-rapport 1989:4. [*The effects of psychotherapy in psychoses – A research overview*].

National Board of Health and Welfare (1996). *Psykiatrireformen – Årsrapport 1996*. Socialstyrelsen följer upp och utvärderar 1996:4. [*Psychiatric reform – Annual report 1996*].

National Board of Health and Welfare (1997). *God psykiatrisk vård på lika villkor? - En nationell översyn av innehåll och kvalitet i den psykiatriska vården*. Socialstyrelsen följer upp och utvärderar 1997:8. [*Good psychiatric care on equal terms? – A national overview of content and quality in psychiatric care*].

Nilson, G (1997). Hur är livskonsten möjlig? In: Oddner, F & Isenberg, B (eds). *Seendets pendel*. Stockholm: Brutus Östlings Bokförlag Symposion. [How is the art of life possible? In: Oddner, F & Isenberg, B (eds). *The pendulum of vision*].

Official Reports of the Swedish Government 1992:37. *Psykiatrin och dess patienter – levnadsförhållanden, vårdens innehåll och utveckling*. Delbetänkande av Psykiatriutredningen. [SOU (Swedish Government Official Reports). *Psychiatry and its patients – living conditions, content and development of care*].

Official Reports of the Swedish Government 1992:73. *Välfärd och valfrihet – service, stöd och vård för psykiskt störda*. Slutbetänkande av Psykiatriutredningen. [SOU (Swedish Government Official Reports). *Welfare and freedom of choice – service, support and care for the mentally disturbed*]. Official Reports of the Swedish Government 2000:14. *Adressat okänd. Om hemlöshetens bakgrund, orsaker och dynamik*. Delbetänkande av Kommittén för hemlösa. [SOU (Swedish Government Official Reports). *Address unknown. On the background, causes, and dynamics of homelessness*].

Olofsson, B (2000). *Use of coercion in psychiatric care as narrated by patients, nurses and physicians*. Umeå University Medical Dissertation, No 655.

Parsons, T (1951). Illness and role of the physician: A sociological perspective. *American Journal of Orthopsychiatry*, Vol 21, p 452–460.

Pattison, EM & Defrancisco, D & Wood, P & Frazier, H & Crowder, J (1975). A psychosocial kinship model for family therapy. *American Journal of Psychiatry*, Vol 132, No 12, p 1246-1251.

Penn, DL & Mueser, KT (1996). Research update on the psychosocial treatment of schizophrenia. *American Journal of Psychiatry*, Vol 153, No 5, p 607–617.

Pilgrim D & Rogers, A (1993). *A sociology of mental health & illness*. Buckingham: Open University Press.

Plummer, K (1995). *Telling sexual stories*. London: Routledge.

Podvoll, E (1990). *The seduction of madness*. New York: Harper & Row Publishers Inc.

Polanyi, L (1985). *Telling the American story: A structural and cultural analysis of conversational storytelling*. Norwood, NJ: Ablex.

Punell, G (1970). Det psykiatriska artefactsyndromet och dess behandling. *Läkartidningen*, Vol 67, No 32, s 3560-3567. [The psychiatric artefact syndrome and its treatment].

Qvarsell, R (1982). *Ordning och behandling. Psykiatri och sinnessjukvård i Sverige under 1800-talets första hälft*. Stockholm: Almqvist & Wiksell International. [*Order and treatment. Psychiatry and mental care in Sweden during the first half of the nineteenth century*].

Racamier, PC (red) (1973). *Le psychanalyste sans divan*. Paris: Payot.

Radley, A (1994). *Making sense of illness – The social psychology of health and disease*. London: Sage Publications.

Rakfeldt, J & Strauss, JS (1989). The low turning point. A control mechanism in the course of mental disorder. *The Journal of Nervous and Mental Disease*, Vol 177, No 1, p 32–37.

Regeringens proposition 1979/80:1. *Om socialtjänsten*. [Government Bill. *On social services*].

Roazen, P (1995). *How Freud worked. First-hand accounts of patients*. New Jersey: Jason Aronson Inc.

Romme, M & Escher, S (1989). Hearing Voices. *Schizophrenia Bulletin*, Vol 15, No 2, p 209–216.

Romme, M & Escher, S (1996). Empowering people who hear voices. In: Haddock, G & Slade, P (eds). *Cognitive behavioural interventions with psychotic disorders.* London: Routledge.

Roos, JP (1992). Livet – berättelsen – samhället: En bermudatriangel? In: Tigerstedt, C & Roos, J P & Vilkko, A (eds). *Självbiografi, kultur, liv – Levnadshistoriska studier inom human- och samhällsvetenskap.* Stockholm: Brutus Östlings Bokförlag Symposion. [Life – the story – society: A Bermuda triangle? In: Tigerstedt, C & Roos, J P & Vilkko, A (eds). *Autobiography, culture, life – History of life studies in the humanities and social sciences*].

Rose, N (1996). *Inventing our selves. Psychology, power, and personhood.* Cambridge: Cambridge University Press.

Rosen, B & Engelhardt, DM & Freedman, N & Margolis, R (1968). The hospitalization proneness scale as a predictor of response to phenothiazine treatment. *Journal of Nervous and Mental Disease,* Vol 146, No 6, p 476–480.

Rosen, B & Engelhardt, DM & Freedman, N et al (1971). The hospitalization proneness scale as a predictor of response to phenothiazine treatment. II. Delay of psychiatric hospitalization. *Journal of Nervous and Mental Disease,* Vol 152, No 6, p 405–411.

Rotelli, F & de Leonardis, O & Mauri, D (1987). Avinstitutionaliseringen – en annorlunda väg – Den italienska mentalvårdsreformen. *Kritisk Psykologi,* nr 4. [Deinstitutionalization – a different path – The Italian mental health care reform].

Rotelli, F (1994). Per un'impresa sociale. In: Rotelli, F. *Per la normalita – Taccuino di uno psychiatria.* Trieste: Edizione E.

Rund, B R (1990). Fully recovered schizophrenics: a retrospective study of some premorbid and treatment factors. *Psychiatry,* Vol 53, No 2, p 127–139.

Sacks, MH & Carpenter, WT & Strauss, JS (1974). Recovery from delusions. Three phases documented by patient's interpretation of research procedures. *Archives of General Psychiatry,* Vol 30, No 1, p 117–120.

Salokangas, R (1996). Living situation and social network in schizophrenia. A prospective 5-year follow-up study. *Nordisk Psykiatrisk Tidskrift,* 50/1, p 35–42.

Sampson, EE (1989). The deconstruction of the self. In: Shotter, J & Gergen, KJ (eds). *Texts of identity.* London: Sage Publications.

Sander, R & Smith, R & Weinman, B (1967). *Chronic psychoses and recovery.* San Francisco: Jossey-Bass Inc. Publishers.

Sandin, B (1986). *Den zebrarandiga pudelkärnan.* Stockholm: Rabén & Sjögren. [*The zebra-striped poodle core*].

Sartre, J-P (1971). *L'idiot de la famille.* Vol I-III. Paris: Gallimard.

Schafer, R (1976). *A new language for psychoanalysis.* New Haven: Yale University Press.

Scheff, T J (1984). *Being mentally ill – A sociological theory.* 2nd ed. New York: Aldine Publishing Company.

Schreiber, R (1996). (Re)defining my self: Women's process of recovery from depression. *Qualitative Health Research,* Vol 6, No 4, p 469–491.

Scull, AT (1979). *Museums of madness. The social organization of insanity in nineteenth-century England.* Harmondsworth: Penguin books.

Scull, AT (1984). *Decarceration. Community treatment and the deviant – a radical view.* Worcester: Polity press.

Sedgwick, P (1982). *Psychopolitics.* New York: Harper and Row.

Sève, L (1972). *Marxisme et théorie de la personalité.* 2eme edition. Paris: Editions sociales.

Shepherd, M & Watt, D & Falloon, I & Smeeton, N (1989). The natural history of schizophrenia: a five-year follow-up study of outcome and prediction in a representative sample of schizophrenics. *Psychological medicine,* Monograph Supplement 15.

Sjöström, R (1985). Effects of psychotherapy in schizophrenia – a retrospective study. *Acta Psychiatrica Scandinavica,* Vol 71, No 5, p 513–522.

Slavney, P & McHugh, P (1984). Life stories and meaningful connections: Reflections on a clinical method in psychiatry and medicine. *Perspectives in Biology and Medicine,* Vol 27, No 2, p 279–288.

Spence, D (1982). *Narrative truth and historical truth: Meaning and interpretation in psychoanalysis.* New York: W. W. Norton.

Stanton, AH & Gunderson, JG & Knapp, PH & Frank, AF & Vannicelli, ML & Schnitzer, R & Rosenthal, R (1984). Effects of psychotherapy in schizophrenia: I. Design and implementation of a controlled study. *Schizophrenia Bulletin,* Vol 10, No 4, p 520–563.

Starrin, B & Larsson, G & Willebrand, K (1984). Upptäckande metodologi. *Sociologisk forskning,* No 3–4, p 15–28. [Discovering methodology].

Starrin, B & Larsson, G & Dahlgren, L & Styrborn, S (1991). *Från upptäckt till presentation – Om kvalitativ metod och teorigenerering på empirisk grund.* Lund: Studentlitteratur. [*From discovery to presentation – On qualitative method and theory generation on empiric grounds*].

Starrin, B (1996) Grounded Theory – En modell för kvalitativ analys. In: Svensson, P-G & Starrin, B (eds) *Kvalitativa studier i teori och praktik.* Lund: Studentlitteratur. [Grounded Theory – A model for qualitative analysis. In: Svensson, P-G & Starrin, B (eds). *Qualitative research in theory and practice*].

Stefansson, CG (1991). Lång väg kvar innan psykiatriplanens intentioner om nya vårdformer för schizofrena förverkligas. *Läkartidningen,* Vol 88, No 25, p 2304-2306. [Long road left before the psychiatric plan's intentions on new forms of care for schizophrenic patients become reality].

Stein, L & Test, MA (ed) (1978). *Alternatives to mental hospital treatment.* New York, Plenum Press.

Stein, L & Test, MA (1980). Alternative to mental hospital treatment. In: Conceptual model, treatment program and clinical evaluation. *Archives of General Psychiatry,* Vol 37, No 4, p 392–397.

Steinholtz Ekecrantz, L (1995). *Patienternas psykiatri – En studie av institutionella erfarenheter.* Stockholm: Carlssons. *[The patients' psychiatry – A study of institutional experiences].*

Stephens, J & Astrup, C (1963). Prognosis in process and non-process schizophrenia. *American Journal of Psychiatry*, Vol 119, p 945–953.

Strauss, A & Corbin, J (1990). *Basics of qualitative research – Grounded theory Procedures and Techniques.* Newbury Park: Sage Publications.

Strauss, A & Corbin, J & Fagerhaugh, S & Glaser, B & Maines, D & Suczek, B & Wiener, C (1984). *Chronic Illness and the quality of life.* St Louis: Mosby.

Strauss, JS (1980). Chronicity: causes, prevention and treatment. *Psychiatric Annuals*, Vol 10, No 9, p 23–29.

Strauss, JS (1989a). Mediating processes in schizophrenia – Towards a new dynamic psychiatry. *British Journal of Psychiatry*, July (Suppl), p 22–28.

Strauss, JS (1989b). Subjective experiences of schizophrenia: Toward a new dynamic psychiatry. II. *Schizophrenia Bulletin*, Vol 15, No 2, p 179-187.

Strauss, JS (1992a). The person – Key to undersanding mental illness: Towards a new dynamic psychiatry. III. *British Journal of Psychiatry*, October (Suppl), p 19–26.

Strauss, JS (1992b). The person with schizophrenia as a person. In: Werbart, A & Cullberg, J (eds). *Psychotherapy of schizophrenia: Facilitating and obstructive factors.* Oslo: Scandinavian University Press.

Strauss, JS (1994). The person with schizophrenia as a person II: Approaches to the subjective and complex. *British Journal of Psychiatry*, April (Suppl), p 103–107.

Strauss, JS & Carpenter, WT (1978). The prognosis of schizophrenia: rationale for a multidimensional concept. *Schizophrenia Bulletin*, Vol 4, No 1, p 56 - 67.

Strauss, JS & Carpenter, WT (1981). *Schizophrenia.* New York: Plenum Medical Book Company.

Strauss, JS & Carpenter, WT & Bartko, JJ (1974). The diagnosis and understanding of schizophrenia. Part III. Speculations on the process that underlie schizophrenic symptoms and signs. *Schizophrenia Bulletin*, Winter, No 11, p 61–69.

Strauss, JS & Estroff, S (1989). Foreword. *Schizophrenia Bulletin,* Vol 15, No 2, p 177–178.

Strauss, JS & Gabriel, R & Kokes, R & Ritzler, B & Vanord, A & Tamara, E (1979). Do psychiatric patients fit their diagnoses? Patterns of symptomatology as described with the biplot. *The Journal of Nervous and Mental Disease*, Vol 167, No 2, p 105 – 113.

Strauss, JS & Hafez, H (1981). Clinical questions and "real" research. *American Journal of Psychiatry,* Vol 138, No 12, p 1592-1597.

Strauss, JS & Hafez, H & Lieberman, P & Harding, CM (1985). The course of psychiatric disorder, III: Longitudinal principles. *American Journal of Psychiatry*, Vol 142, No 3, p 289-296.

Strauss, JS & Harding, CM & Hafez, H & Lieberman P (1987). The role of the patient in recovery from psychosis. In: Strauss, J S & Boker, W & Brenner, H (eds). *Psychosocial treatment of schizophrenia*, p 160–166, New York: Hans Huber.

Strauss, JS & Rakfeldt, J & Harding, C & Lieberman, P (1989). Psychological and social aspects of negative symptoms. *British Journal of Psychiatry*, Vol 155, suppl. 7, p 128–132.

Strupp, H & Hadley, S (1979). Specific vs nonspecific factors in psychotherapy. A controlled study of outcome, *Archives of General Psychiatry*, Vol 36, No 10, p 1125-1136.

Suczek, B & Wiener, C (1984). *Chronic Illness and the quality of life*. St Louis: Mosby.

Sullivan, WP (1994). A long and winding road: The process of recovery from severe mental illness. *Innovations and Research*, Vol 3, No 3, p 19–27.

Swain, G (1977). *Le sujet de la folie. Naissance de la psychiatrie*. Toulouse: Privat.

Swain, G (1994). *Dialogue avec l'insensé*. Paris: Editions Gallimard.

Svenska Akademien (1985). *Svenska Akademiens ordlista över svenska språket*. Stockholm: P. A. Norstedt & söners förlag. [*Swedish Academy's list of words in the Swedish language*].

Svenska Psykiatriska Föreningen & Spri (1996). *Kliniska riktlinjer för utredning och behandling av schizofreni och schizofreniliknande tillstånd*. Stockholm: Spri förlag. [*Clinical guidelines for work-up and treatment of schizophrenia and schizophrenia-like conditions*].

Szecsödy, I (1989). Att förvärva och överbringa psykoanalytisk kunskap. In: Crafoord, C (ed). *Psykoanalytiker utan soffa*. Stockholm: Natur och Kultur. [*Acquiring and conveying psychoanalytical knowledge. In: Crafoord, C (ed). Psychoanalyst without a couch*].

Talbott, J (1981). *Chronic mental patients: Treatment, programs, systems*. New York: Human Sciences Press.

Tatossian, A (1994). La notion de qualité de vie subjective: evidences et illusions. In : Terra, J-L (ed). *Qualité de vie subjective et santé mentale*. Paris: Ellipses.

Terra, J-L (ed) (1994). *Qualité de vie subjective et santé mentale*. Paris: Ellipses.

Test, MA & Stein, L (1978). Community treatment of the chronic patient: research overview.*Schizophrenia Bulletin*, Vol 4, No 3, p 350–364.

The New National Dictionary (1959). *Dictionary of the English language*. London: William Collins Sons & co.

Thomas, W. I. & Znaniecki, F. (1927) The polish peasant in Europe and America, New York: Octacon Press.

Tidemalm, D (1996). *Från psykiatrisk avdelning till gruppbostad – Flyttning i samband med psykiatrireformen*. Stockholm: FoU-enheten/psykiatri, VSSO, Rapport 5/1996. [*From mental ward to group housing – Moving in connection with the psychiatry reform*].

Tooth, B & Kalyanansundaram, V & Glover, H (1997). *Recovery from schizophrenia – a consumer perspective*. Queensland University of Technology, Center for Mental Health Nursing Research.

362

Topor, A (1985), *Mentalvård i frihet.* Stockholm: Liber. [*Mental care in freedom*].

Topor, A (1987). *EMMA – en studie i brott med den psykiatriska vårdens och socialtjänstens traditionella metoder.* Stockholm: Stockholms socialförvaltning, FoU-byrån, Rapport 73. [*EMMA – a study in crime with the traditional methods of mental care and social services*].

Topor, A (1993). *Socialpsykiatri i utveckling. Kontinuitet, tillgänglighet och helhetssyn. Fallet Enskede-Skarpnäcks Psykiatriska Sektor.* Stockholm: Bonnier Utbildning. [*Social psychiatry in development. Continuity, accessibility, and a holistic approach. The case of Enskede-Skarpnäck Psychiatric Sector*].

Topor, A (1995). *Hemtjänsten, kunskap och erfarenheter – lirkandets svåra konst.* Stockholm: Bonnier Utbildning. [*Home services, knowledge, and experiences – the difficult art of coaxing*].

Topor, A (1996a). *Krisverksamheten för nyinsjuknade patienter med psykosproblematik inom Hässelby-Vällingby psykiatriska sektor – Nya arbetssätt för en ny psykiatri.* Stockholm: FoU-enheten/psykiatri, VSSO, Rapport 10/1996. [*Crisis operations for patients recently ill with psychosis problem complex within Hässelby-Vällingby psychiatric sector – New methods for a new psychiatry*].

Topor, A (1996b). *På patientens planhalva – socialt psykiatriskt behandlingsarbete med långtidsvårdade patienter i deras hem.* Stockholm: FoU-enheten/psykiatri, VSSO, Rapport 1/1996. [*In the patient's court – social psychiatric treatment with chronically ill patients receiving care at home*].

Topor, A (1997). *Att återhämta sig från svåra psykiska störningar – en litteraturstudie.* Stockholm: FoU-enheten/psykiatri, VSSO, Rapport 9/1997. [*Recovering from severe mental disorders – a literature study*].

Topor, A (1998). Om det obetydligas betydelse – återhämtning från svåra psykiska störningar. *Psykisk Hälsa,* Vol 39, No 4. [On the significance of the insignificant – recovery from severe mental disorders].

Topor, A (2000). Den psykiatriska slutenvården – nedlagd eller förflyttad? *Läkartidningen,* Vol 97, No 51/52, p 6095-6099. [Institutionalized psychiatric care – closed or moved?]

Topor, A & Karebo Larsén, I (2000). *Vart har den slutna psykiatriska vården tagit vägen?* Stockholm: FoU-enheten/psykiatri, VSPS, Rapport No 10/2000. [*Where has institutionalized psychiatric care gone?*]

Topor, A & Schön, UK (1998). *Den sociala vardagen. En studie av 115 verksamheter för personer med psykiska funktionshinder.* Socialstyrelsen: Psykiatri uppföljningen 1998:4. [*Everyday social life. A study of 115 operations for people with mental disabilities*].

Topor, A & Svensson, J & Bjerke, C & Borg, M & Kufås, E (1998). *Vägen tillbaka – Att återhämta sig från svår psykisk störning, rapport från en pilotundersökning.* Stockholm: FoU-enheten/psykiatri, VSSO, Rapport 4/1998. [*The road back – Recovering from severe mental disorders, report from a pilot study*].

Vail, DJ (1966). *Dehumanization and the institutional career.* Springfield: Charles Thomas Publisher.

363

Vaillant, GE (1964). Prospective prediction of schizophrenic remission, *Archives of General Psychiatry*, Vol 11, p 509–518.

Vaillant, GE (1978). A 10-year followup of remitting schizophrenics. *Schizophrenia Bulletin*, Vol 4, No 1, s78-85.

Warner, R (1985). *Recovery from schizophrenia – Psychiatry and political economy*. New York: Routledge & Kegan Paul.

Watzlawick, P & Weakland, J & Fish, R (1978). *Change – Principles of Problem Formation and Problem Resolution*. New York: Norton & Company Inc.

Waxler, N (1979). Is outcome for schizophrenia better in nonindustrial societies? The case of Sri Lanka. *The Journal of Nervous and Mental Illness*, Vol 167, No 3, p 144–158.

Weiss, KM (1989). Advantages of abandoning symptom-based diagnostic systems of research in schizophrenia. *American Journal of Orthopsychiatry*, Vol 59, No 3, p 324–330.

Werner, E (1995). *Mot alla odds*. Svenska föreningen för psykisk hälsa. [*Overcoming the odds*].

WHO (1979). *Schizophrenia – an international follow-up study*. Chichester: John Wiley & sons.

Viderman, S (1982). *La construction de l'espace analytique*. Paris: Gallimard.

Wing, JK & Brown, GW (1970). *Institutionalism and schizophrenia. A comparative study of three mental hospitals 1960-1968*. Cambridge: Cambridge University Press.

Winokur, G & Tsuang, M (1996). *The natural history of mania, depression and schizophrenia*. Washington: American Psychiatric Press.

Wynne, L., Cromwell, R. & Matthysse, S. (red) (1978). *The nature of schizophrenia - New approaches to research and treatment*. New York: John Wiley & sons.

Young, SL & Ensing, DS (1999). Exploring recovery from the perspective of people with psychiatric disabilities. *Psychiatric Rehabilitation Journal*, Vol. 22, No. 3, p 219-231.

Zarifan, E (1988). *Les jardiniers de la folie*. Paris: Editions Odile Jacob.

Zubin, J (1985). General discussion. In: Alpert, M (ed). *Controversies in schizophrenia: Changes and constancies*. New York: Guilford Press.

Zubin, J & Spring, B (1977). Vulnerability – a new view of schizophrenia. *Journal of Abnormal Psychology*, Vol 86, No 2, p 103–126.

Zubin, J & Steinhauer, SR & Condray, R (1992). Vulnerability to relapse in schizophrenia. *British Journal of Psychiatry Supplement,* Vol 18, October, p 13-18.

Ågren, G & Beijer, U & Finne, E (2000). Hemlösa i Stockholm. In: Runquist, W & Swärd, H (eds). *Hemlöshet – En antologi om olika perspektiv och förklaringsmodeller*. Stockholm: Carlssons. [Homeless in Stockholm. In: Runquist, W & Swärd, H (eds). *Homelessness – An anthology on different perspectives and explanatory models]* .

Ågren, G & Berglund, E & Franér, P (1984).*Hemlösa i Stockholm – Hemlösa med psykisk störning. Undersökningar av hemlösa i Stockholm 1993 och 1994*.

Stockholm: FoU-byrån, Socialtjänsten i Stockholm, Rapport 1994:18. [*Homeless in Stockholm – Homeless people with mental disturbances. Studies of the homeless in Stockholm 1993 and 1994*].

Åsberg, M (2000). Placebo inom psykiatrin. In: Boström, H & Dahlgren, H (eds). *Placebo*. Stockholm: Liber/SBU. [Placebos in psychiatry. In: Boström, H & Dahlgren, H (eds). *Placebo*].

Öberg, P (1997). *Livet som berättelse – om biografi och åldrande*. Uppsala: Acta Universitatis Upsaliensis. [*Life as a story – on biography and aging*].

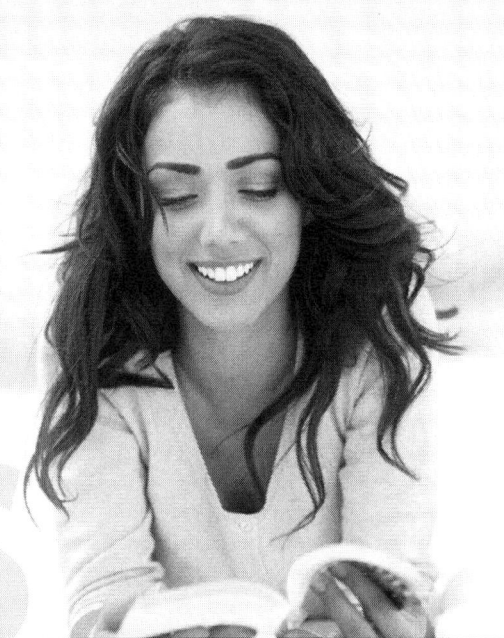
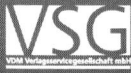

Printed in Great Britain
by Amazon.co.uk, Ltd.,
Marston Gate.